THE COMPLETE

Prebiotic

&

Probiotic

Health Guide

A Vegetarian Plan for Balancing Your Gut Flora

+**175** RECIPES

Dr. Maitreyi Raman, MD, MSc, FRCPC
Angela Sirounis, BSc, RD
Jennifer Shrubsole, BSc, RD

Robert
ROSE

For complete cataloguing information, see page 336.

Disclaimer
This book is a general guide only and should never be a substitute for the skill, knowledge and experience of
a qualified medical professional dealing with the facts, circumstances and symptoms of a particular case.

The nutritional, medical and health information presented in this book is based on the research,
training and professional experience of the authors, and is true and complete to the best of their knowledge.
However, this book is intended only as an informative guide for those wishing to know more about health,
nutrition and medicine; it is not intended to replace or countermand the advice given by the reader's
personal physician. Because each person and situation is unique, the authors and the publisher urge the
reader to check with a qualified health-care professional before using any procedure where there is a
question as to its appropriateness. A physician should be consulted before beginning any exercise program.
The authors and the publisher are not responsible for any adverse effects or consequences resulting from
the use of the information in this book. It is the responsibility of the reader to consult a physician or other
qualified health-care professional regarding his or her personal care.

This book contains references to products that may not be available everywhere. The intent of
the information provided is to be helpful; however, there is no guarantee of results associated with
the information provided. Use of brand names is for educational purposes only and does not imply
endorsement.

The recipes in this book have been carefully tested by our kitchen and our tasters. To the best of our
knowledge, they are safe and nutritious for ordinary use and users. For those people with food or other
allergies, or who have special food requirements or health issues, please read the suggested contents of each
recipe carefully and determine whether or not they may create a problem for you. All recipes are used at the
risk of the consumer. We cannot be responsible for any hazards, loss or damage that may occur as a result of
any recipe use. For those with special needs, allergies, requirements or health problems, in the event of any
doubt, please contact your medical adviser prior to the use of any recipe.

Design and Production: Joseph Gisini/PageWave Graphics Inc.
Editors: Sue Sumeraj and Fina Scroppo
Copy editor: Kelly Jones
Proofreader: Gillian Watts
Indexer: Gillian Watts
Nutrient analysis: Magda Fahmy
Illustrations: Kveta/threeinabox.com

The publisher gratefully acknowledges the financial support of our publishing program by the Government
of Canada through the Canada Book Fund.

Published by Robert Rose Inc.
120 Eglinton Avenue East, Suite 800, Toronto, Ontario, Canada M4P 1E2
Tel: (416) 322-6552 Fax: (416) 322-6936
www.robertrose.ca

Printed and bound in Canada

1 2 3 4 5 6 7 8 9 MI 23 22 21 20 19 18 17 16 15

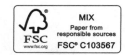

Contents

Introduction 5

PART I: Understanding the Gut Microbiome

Chapter 1: The Gut Microbiome 8
Chronic Disease and the Gut 9
History of the Microbiome 10
The Influence of Diet 11
Defining Microbiota 13
Gastrointestinal Tract Anatomy 13
The Forgotten Organ 16
Bacterial Colonization 18
Lifestyle Changes Contributing to Changes in Gut Microbiota 20
Groups of Bacteria 21
The Impact of Diet on the Microbiome 22

Chapter 2: Antibiotics and the Gut Microbiome 30
Antibiotics: History and Future 31
Susceptibility to Harmful Bacteria 35

Chapter 3: Beneficial Bacteria 40
Functional Foods and Probiotics 40
What Are Probiotics? 41
How Do Probiotics Work? 41
Probiotics in the Treatment of GI Conditions 43
Probiotics in the Treatment of Non-GI Conditions 51
The Safety of Probiotics 55

Chapter 4: The Impact of Fiber on Gut Microbiota 57
What Is Fiber? 58
How Much Fiber Should I Eat? 59
Forms of Fiber 60
Benefits of a High-Fiber Diet 63
What Are Prebiotic Fibers? 64
Effects of Prebiotic Fibers 68
Treating Disease with Prebiotics 69
Prebiotic Fiber Safety 72
Prebiotic Health Claims 73

PART II: How to Achieve a Healthy Microbiome

Chapter 5: The Vegetarian Diet 76
History of Vegetarianism 77
What Exactly Is a Vegetarian Diet? 78
Health Benefits of the Vegetarian Diet 79
Vegetarian Diets and the Microbiome 82

Chapter 6: The Vegetarian Diet in Detail 85

Vitamin B$_{12}$ 86

Iron 89

Protein 95

Calcium and Vitamin D 102

Zinc 104

Chapter 7: Optimizing Dietary Fiber and Prebiotics 107

Dietary Fiber Through the Ages 108

Adding Prebiotic-Rich Foods to Your Diet 109

Tips to Increase Your Fiber Intake 113

Prebiotic Supplements 114

Prebiotic Claims 114

Chapter 8: How to Optimize Dietary Probiotics 116

Top 8 Probiotic-Rich Foods 117

Tips for Probiotic Living 121

PART III: The 8-Step Biotic-Balanced Program

Chapter 9: Nutrition Prescription for Healthy Living 124

Overview of the 8-Step Biotic-Balanced Program 125

The 8 Steps Expanded 126

Chapter 10: Changing Your Eating Habits 133

Setting a SMART Goal 134

Introduction to the 14-Day Meal Plan 135

PART IV: Recipes for a Healthy Microbiome

Introduction to the Recipes 142

Breakfast and Brunch 145

Smoothies, Juices and Other Beverages 161

Baked Goods 173

Snacks, Appetizers, Dips and Spreads 187

Soups 211

Salads and Dressings 227

Pasta and Grains 245

Legumes, Tofu and Tempeh 269

Vegetables 285

Desserts 309

References 324

Contributing Authors 326

Index 327

Introduction

With the prevalence of chronic diseases at an all-time high, there has never been so much urgency among researchers, doctors, patients and the motivated individual to find useful, sustainable solutions to address chronic diseases. Although medications are often used to treat them, medical literature is showing us that most patients would benefit instead from nutritional interventions. In fact, many chronic diseases may even be treated and cured with diet alone.

Although this concept is not new to doctors and patients, it begs us to examine the compliance or lack of compliance associated with dietary reform. Why are so many motivated individuals not successful in changing their dietary habits? Why don't doctors emphasize the importance of diet in more granular and compelling terms? Why is there a perceived lack of emphasis on disease prevention? I have been struggling to answer these questions for years, and have come to a few conclusions.

First, patients may not appreciate the value of dietary and lifestyle modifications, perhaps as a consequence of inadequate research funding dedicated to better understanding the science guiding nutritional and dietary optimization. Although many accept motherhood statements like "You are what you eat" at face value, there isn't a compelling need for change. Second, doctors are not adequately trained to make in-depth nutrition and dietary recommendations. I hope this paradigm is changing, as nutrition education is increasing in medical schools. Third, even doctors who are keenly interested in this area are stretched with patients who have more acute problems, so dietary and nutritional therapies take a backseat. Finally, patients must become more engaged in managing their own diseases and take ownership of their own health by seeking out resources to maintain good health and prevent disease. It can be particularly challenging to distinguish credible from less credible sources of information in the era of information technology. These complex factors may inhibit people from realizing the full health potential they can achieve through dietary and nutritional interventions.

> Many chronic diseases may be treated and cured with diet alone.

Nutrition is critical in maintaining the health of the gut microbiome (the bacteria living in the intestines and the metabolic consequences of the residing bacteria). The emerging research on the gut microbiome is reframing our knowledge of acute and chronic diseases, showcasing the critical role of diet and nutrition therapies in shaping a favorable microbiome to improve health and prevent disease.

In this book, we explore the impact of the microbiome on health and disease, as well as the factors — in particular, diet and the environment — that interact and shape the microbiome. Specific strategies to create a more healthful microbiome are detailed, with a focus on diet, such as increasing your intake of probiotic-rich foods and your intake of dietary fiber, found in prebiotic-rich foods. In the latter part of the book, exercises are recommended, including steps for maintaining a food diary for 7 days, as well as strategies to follow a vegetarian diet. By critically assessing your food intake and meal patterns, you will be able to bring your microbiome into tip-top shape to fight disease.

PART I

Understanding the Gut Microbiome

CHAPTER 1

The Gut Microbiome

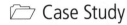 Case Study

Modifying Diet

Jacques is a 49-year-old male patient who came to see me to discuss his interest in natural foods and holistic therapies for health and wellness, following some symptoms of abdominal bloating and a change in his bowel habit. A year ago, I saw him to discuss colon cancer screening. His recent symptoms started to appear soon after he used antibiotics that his family physician had prescribed for a sore throat and phlegm. When his symptoms had cleared up after 4 days, he stopped taking his antibiotics — even though they were prescribed for 7 days.

His father was diagnosed with ulcerative colitis, an inflammatory disorder of the large bowel, in his 60s, and his aunt developed colon cancer in her mid-50s. Jacques is presently healthy, without any medical conditions, and determined to make every effort to maintain his health and minimize his risks for disease. He has read a variety of literature about diet and health, and recently came across a recurring theme involving the relationship between the "bugs" in the gut and their influence on health and disease. In his reading, Jacques noted that the gut bugs may be protective against illness and that certain diet components might help to improve and maintain gut health.

Given Jacques' family history of colon cancer, I recommended a colonoscopy, the results of which were completely normal. There was no evidence of polyps, which are precancerous growths. In addition, I asked Jacques to have a complete set of blood work done to rule out other conditions, such as celiac disease. I told him that his symptoms were most likely related to the recent antibiotic use, which can disrupt the gut microbiome and result in a change in bowel movements. We discussed how to make modifications to his diet, such as increasing his intake of yogurt and kefir to boost his probiotic exposure, and to focus on fiber-rich foods such as fruits, vegetables and grain products and minimize exposure to processed foods in order to restitute his gut flora.

During Jacques' follow-up visit 6 months later, he reported that his bowels were back to normal and his overall quality of life had improved substantially because of more healthful choices.

Scientists and researchers used to believe that gut bacteria live harmoniously with our human cells without any significant interaction. However, a recent explosion of research has emerged exploring the interaction between the gut microbiome and disease prevention and treatment. Perhaps it may come as no surprise that diet and environment are contributors to the composition and function of the gut microbiome. Altering the microbiome to reflect a healthy ecosystem may, in fact, prevent and curb disease. The gut ecosystem is readily impacted by dietary choices, and with more and more evidence appearing, it is difficult to ignore the fact that changes in the gut microbiome may stem from poor dietary choices and may be a driver of disease.

Did You Know?

Flourishing Bacteria

The bacterial cells in our intestines outnumber our own human cells. In fact, we have 10 times as many bacteria in our gut than we have total number of human cells.

Chronic Disease and the Gut

The most common chronic diseases in North America are obesity, diabetes, heart disease and cancer. Two-thirds of adults are either overweight or obese, and the estimated number of deaths in the United States associated with being overweight is approximately 300,000 a year. More than 64 million Americans have heart disease, which represents the leading cause of mortality (40%) in all deaths in the U.S. Fifty million Americans have high blood pressure, the leading cause of stroke and heart disease, and 11 million adults have type 2 diabetes. More than 1.5 million Canadians have heart disease, claiming 34,000 lives a year. Fifty percent of Canadians are either overweight or obese, with 7% of Canadians suffering from diabetes. Cancer is the second leading cause of death: 25% in the U.S. and 30% in Canada. Wouldn't it be remarkable if these major chronic diseases could be addressed through nutritional and dietary therapies?

Through advancing research regarding the microbiome, it is conceivable, indeed, that dietary therapies that adjust the microbiome may be instrumental in modifying the course of chronic diseases. The science in this field is novel and rapidly growing, creating a very compelling argument for researchers and doctors to cast a second glance at preventive nutritional treatments that address the health of the microbiome.

Two-thirds of adults are either overweight or obese, and the estimated number of deaths in the United States associated with being overweight is approximately 300,000 a year.

History of the Microbiome

> Beneficial microbes are required for metabolism and the production of essential vitamins, and as a first line of defense against potentially harmful bacteria that could cause diseases.

Throughout most of human history, we have been fearful of microbes. Historically, the plague, smallpox and typhoid, for example, posed serious threats to human life, and in modern times, infectious diseases such as HIV and malaria, to name just a couple, are associated with poor outcomes. The scientific study of microbiology grew out of the need to conquer the organisms responsible and eradicate infectious diseases. However, a new paradigm is emerging that addresses the need for humans and microbes to coexist for mutual benefit.

If microbes cause illness, how can we possibly benefit from them? We are now learning that beneficial microbes are required for metabolism and the production of essential vitamins, and as a first line of defense against potentially harmful bacteria that could cause diseases. We know that the human body is made up of about 10 times more microbial cells than human cells. Furthermore, there may be millions more microbial genes than human genes, and therein lies the secret of health and disease. Scientists now believe that the way in which these microbial genes interact with the human body may ultimately determine our overall health.

FAQ

 I've been hearing that some factors over time have affected the health of gut bacteria. Is this true?

Yes. As we are beginning to appreciate the gut microbiome, researchers are also growing concerned about factors that may disturb its delicate balance. Exposure to antibiotics, for example, could have undesirable effects on the microbiome while treating an underlying infectious problem. A detailed discussion follows later regarding antibiotics and their impact on the microbiome (see Chapter 2). Beyond antibiotic use, other modern societal practices that have impacted the human microbiome are clean water, sanitation, delivery by caesarean section and antibacterial soaps, to name a few. Over many generations, these practices may alter the human microbiome and, ultimately, the human genome. An impoverished microbiome may lead to decreasing numbers and types of microbiota, compromising human health. This hypothesis will be subject to scrutiny over the next decade of research.

The Influence of Diet

Similarly, diet is critically important to the microbiome. Before the development of agriculture, dietary choices would have been limited to wild, minimally processed plant and animal foods. With the domestication of plants and animals, the original nutrient characteristics of these once-wild foods changed, especially with the start of the Industrial Revolution. In the 21st century, there is an abundance of prepared convenience foods. The typical North American diet is 50% carbohydrate, 15% protein and 35% fat, which differs from the health guidelines proposed by many experts, which recommend limiting fat to less than 30% of total energy consumed. However, the quality of carbohydrate, protein and fat consumed is at least as important as the quantity of food consumed.

Until very recent years, the concept of food quality was missing from many food guides. As a result, many consumers have focused on food quantity, calorie counting and big nutrient categories, and are missing the finer details when it comes to the nutritional composition of food on their plates.

In terms of carbohydrates, complex carbohydrates such as starch are healthier than simple carbohydrates like refined sugars. In industrialized nations, diets are high in saturated fat compared to other fats in the diet. Similarly, an increase in omega-3 fatty acids in the diet may be associated with a decrease in cancer and heart disease. Shifts in dietary composition that reflect a low-fiber, high-saturated-fat, high-sugar diet over the decades may contribute to changes in the microbiome that predispose individuals to disease.

It is entirely conceivable and plausible that dietary changes reflecting a more favorable composition are beneficial to health largely because of diet's impact on the microbiome. For example, Asian and Mediterranean diets have long been seen as healthful diets. Recent research shows that people who live in areas of the Mediterranean with the lowest recorded rates of chronic diseases and the highest adult life expectancy follow a diet that is abundant in food from plant sources, including fruits, vegetables, breads, grains, legumes, nuts and seeds. In addition, there is an emphasis on a variety of minimally processed foods and, where possible, seasonally fresh and locally grown foods. Also, olive oil is the principal fat, displacing other fats and oils. Meat consumption, in particular red meat consumption, is low in these diets, and when meat is

---

Did You Know?

Replacing Bad Fats with Good

Research tells us that for every 1% of saturated fat energy replaced with polyunsaturated fat in the diet, there could be a reduction of more than 3% in heart disease.

An increase in omega-3 fatty acids in the diet may be associated with a decrease in cancer and heart disease.

---

consumed, the emphasis has been placed on fish and poultry, albeit in small quantities and with moderate frequency.

Although this is an area of much-needed research, there is scientific speculation that the microbiome in people who follow these diets will be different and more favorable than for those who follow a typical North American diet.

A Shift in Diet

Throughout much of history, humans have been hunter-gatherers, collecting a diverse variety of fruits, vegetables, seeds and root vegetables rich in starch and complex carbohydrates. The ancient diet is very different from our current North American diet, which is higher in fat, sugars and salt, often based on animal protein, and low in fiber, polyphenols, healthy fats, minerals and vitamins. The dietary shift that has happened over the past several centuries, which has accelerated in the last three to four decades, has undoubtedly affected the largest ecosystem in our body, the gut microbiome.

High dietary sugar intake can lead to dysbiosis, a disorganized microbiome structure favoring the proliferation of some organisms over others. For example, harmful bacteria tend to predominate over beneficial bacteria in a sugar-rich environment. The story with higher fat intake is perhaps less direct. High fat intake appears to increase inflammation and affect the immune system's interaction with the gut's bacterial environment. What is perhaps of larger concern is that the harmful effects of diet can actually stretch across generations. Children inherit their microbiome from their mother at the time of delivery and through breastfeeding. When the mother's diet provokes an unbalanced microbiome, she passes this imbalance on to her child, who will have less than ideal bacteria for proper immune functioning.

Other Influences

Although the numbers of bacteria in our gut are not new, the impact of diet and environment is shaping the microbiome in a way that is perhaps more harmful than ever before — due to an increased emphasis on hygiene, easy access to fast food and availability of antibiotics, to name just a few of the big players. An altered microbiome may predispose individuals to many chronic diseases, such as obesity, diabetes and cardiovascular diseases, in addition to an increase in inflammatory diseases.

Did You Know?

Inheriting Taste

A mother's diet may shape her child's flavor preferences even before birth, predisposing the child's future food intake in the direction of the mother's.

The harmful effects of diet can actually stretch across generations. Children inherit their microbiome from their mother at the time of delivery and through breastfeeding.

Defining Microbiota

"Gut microbiota" refers to all the bacteria living in the gut. The gut microbiota have a number of functions in human health, including:

- Protecting the gut from the "bad bacteria," otherwise known as pathogens.
- Extracting nutrients and energy from our food.
- Assisting with the digestion of certain foods that the small intestine has not been able to digest.
- Maintaining a normal immune system.

Given the multitude of functions of the gut microbiota, some experts consider the gut bacteria a separate organ. "Gut microbiome" refers to gut microbiota and all their associated functions.

> **Major Functions of the Gut Microbiota**
> - Digestion
> - Regulation of immunity
> - Maintenance of bacterial balance in the gut
> - Nutrient and energy regulation

Gastrointestinal Tract Anatomy

Before we can have a meaningful discussion regarding the gut microbiota, we need to define the anatomy of the gastrointestinal (GI) tract. The GI tract is the system that is primarily responsible for the digestion and absorption of food. The digestion process begins in the mouth immediately after food is eaten. Food then travels down the esophagus, or food pipe, and enters the stomach.

> The stomach produces a number of hormones and chemicals, such as acid, required for optimal digestion.

Stomach

The stomach is a highly acidic environment. It is very sterile and has very few to no organisms. It is responsible for the digestion or initial breakdown of the three major macronutrients — protein, fat and carbohydrates. The stomach does this through mechanical and chemical processes. Mechanical functions include churning food into smaller particles until they can pass into the small intestine for further processing. The stomach produces a number of hormones and chemicals, such as acid, required for optimal digestion.

The Gastrointestinal Tract

The gastrointestinal system can be seen as a long pipe, or tract, that begins at the mouth and ends at the anus, with separate sections throughout that each have a particular function.

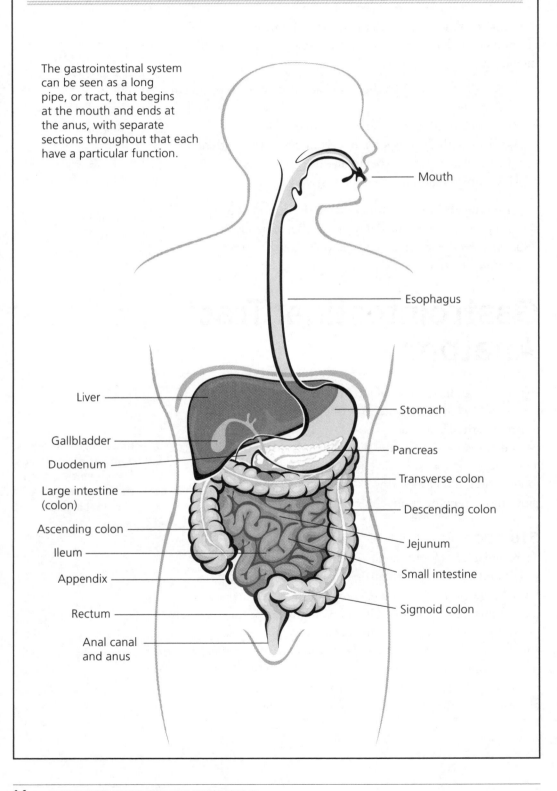

Mouth

Esophagus

Liver

Stomach

Gallbladder

Pancreas

Duodenum

Transverse colon

Large intestine (colon)

Descending colon

Ascending colon

Jejunum

Ileum

Small intestine

Appendix

Sigmoid colon

Rectum

Anal canal and anus

Small Intestine

The small intestine, also called the small bowel, is the most important site for nutrient absorption. It is approximately 235 to 275 inches (600 to 700 cm) in length and is divided into three sections — the duodenum, jejunum and ileum. Each section of the small intestine has specialized functions in terms of vitamin and mineral absorption. For example, the duodenum is primarily responsible for the absorption of iron. The absorption of folate tends to occur exclusively in the jejunum, while vitamin B_{12} absorption only occurs in the last part of the ileum. This is particularly important in the context of disease. Inflammation or abnormalities involving any of these specific segments of bowel may cause nutrient deficiencies.

The main function of the small bowel is to absorb major nutrients — carbohydrates, protein, fat and water — as well as vitamins, minerals and trace elements. Once partially digested food enters the small bowel from the stomach, the digestion process is then completed in the first part of the small intestine. Nutrients are absorbed into the bloodstream and distributed throughout the body.

> Each section of the small intestine has specialized functions in terms of vitamin and mineral absorption.

Colon

The colon, also known as the large intestine, is approximately 40 to 60 inches (100 to 150 cm) in length and its major function is to absorb residual water. The colon is divided into three segments — the ascending colon, transverse colon and descending colon. Each segment of the colon is approximately 16 inches (40 cm) in length.

Some digested products are not absorbed in the small intestine and pass into the colon. The remaining unabsorbed material is stored in the large intestine until it is ready to be eliminated through a bowel movement. The large intestine is home to close to 1,000 species of bacteria. The majority of human waste is made up of undigested fiber and bacteria. Bacteria in the colon act on the undigested colonic fibers and break them down into fatty acids, which are a source of energy and fuel for the colon cells. These fatty acids are then absorbed back into circulation.

Did You Know?

Big Reserves

Although other human organs, such as the skin, also have bacteria, the large intestine has the largest reservoir of microbes.

The Brain-Gut Axis

Researchers are very aware of the tight relationship between the brain and gut. How our state of mind influences the gut is evident in many gut disorders, such as irritable bowel syndrome. However, the opposite is not so well known. While the brain communicates with the gastrointestinal tract to sense pain and gut motility, gut microbes make hormones that influence the nervous system, in particular the brain, as well as make neurotransmitters that directly communicate with the brain to influence mood and thinking.

Research using an animal study showed that when mice were bred in sterile conditions, thus lacking intestinal microbes, they did not recognize other mice with which they had had previous interactions. Other animal studies suggested that disruptions of the microbiome induce behavior that mimics anxiety, depression and even autism. The majority of research exploring the gut–brain axis as it relates to the microbiota has been conducted in mice to study how selective exposure to various microbes may alter behavior and function. Human studies are still in their very early stages.

The Forgotten Organ

The gut contains more than 100 trillion bacteria, which come from about 500 different bacterial species, the majority of which live in the large intestine. The metabolic activities of these bacteria resemble those of an organ. It is estimated that these gut microbes have 100 times as many genes as there are in the entire human genome.

Functions of the Gut Microbiome

The primary function of the gut microbiome is to optimize digestive function and absorb nutrients that are critical in maintaining good health. Ultimately, the gut excretes undigested food particles as waste. The colon serves as the primary repository for waste storage. Consequently, the bacterial load in the colon is exceptionally high — higher than in any other location in the GI tract. The microbiome in the gut is responsible for fermenting unused energy sources from food eaten. The end products of digestion that are not absorbed accumulate in the colon — it's here where residing colonic bacteria produce either additional energy for bodily functions or essential nutrients, such as biotin and vitamin K. Biotin is required for cell growth and the production of fatty acids and amino acids. It also helps to maintain stable blood sugar. Vitamin K is essential for clotting and preventing bleeding.

It is estimated that gut microbes have 100 times as many genes as there are in the entire human genome.

In addition, the gut microbes produce short-chain fatty acids from the fermentation of carbohydrates. The most important of these fatty acids are butyrates, which are protective for heart disease and cancer cells, among other benefits to health.

Since the GI tract is the biggest immunological organ in the body, it also plays a large role in maintaining immunity and fighting infection. Even many scientists appear to forget this fact. Most of the gut microbes are either harmless or have substantial benefit to humans. Given the enormous number of bacteria that reside in the colon, it is easy to see why the intestinal tract has developed multiple layers of protection to limit the ability of the gut bacteria or microbes to escape the colon. If bacteria in the colon gained access to other parts of the body, it could be very dangerous. Even good gut bacteria are not harmless and are capable of causing life-threatening infections. Equipping the gut, and in particular the colon, with a favorable microbiome will strengthen the immune system by reducing its predisposition to infectious or inflammatory diseases.

Another important role of the gut microbiome is to prevent harmful bacterial species from colonizing the gut. This happens through competitive exclusion, an activity that creates a barrier in the gut to keep harmful organisms out, thereby reducing the risk of GI infections.

FAQ

 What types of bacteria are typically found in the gut?

 The four dominant phyla (groups) in the human gut are Firmicutes, Bacteroidetes, Actinobacteria and Proteobacteria. From a clinical perspective, the two most common bacterial phyla in adults are Bacteroidetes and Firmicutes. Within each of these two groups are many classes and subclasses of microbes that are shaped early in life and are subject to change through diet and environment. Some of the microbes in each of these two groups are protective of health, while others may predispose the body to disease. The balance and ratios of these microbes likely play a role in determining overall health. In recent years, with the advent of high-resolution techniques and novel scientific tools, we know much more about gut bacteria than ever before.

> Research Spotlight

A Link to Crohn's Disease

Background: There is a link between the gut microbiome and the development of Crohn's disease, which is an autoimmune disease affecting the entire gastrointestinal tract. A change in the microbiome in patients affected by Crohn's disease has been previously reported.

Objective: To review all the published works investigating this topic, using a systematic review.

Methods: Seventy-two research studies assessing the microbiome in Crohn's disease were reviewed.

Results: The largest class of bacteria, Bacteroidetes, was increased while the second largest class of bacteria, Firmicutes, was decreased. Specifically, the bacteria *Escherichia coli* (otherwise known as *E. coli*) are enriched and *Faecalibacterium prausnitzii* are decreased in patients with Crohn's disease. The findings also showed lower levels of butyrate and other short-chain fatty acids.

Conclusions: Changes in microbial composition have been noted in Crohn's disease. Therapeutic strategies to address these changes may be of value in the treatment of this disease.

Bacterial Colonization

Major Contributing Factors Shaping Gut Microbiota

- Diet
- Genetics
- Sanitation/ environmental cleanliness
- Environmental exposures (for example, to pollution)

The only time the human body is germ-free or devoid of microbes is during pregnancy, in the mother's uterus. At birth, the newborn becomes colonized with bacteria from the mother's vagina, skin, feces and breast milk. The initial bacteria the newborn is exposed to lay the foundation for future growth and colonization of the complex bacteria that will change throughout the years. Over time, a relatively stable, diverse bacterial community is formed.

Diet may be the most critical factor shaping the gut bacteria, and we will explore it throughout the book. However, there are other significant indicators that mark a person's gut microbiota.

Bacterial samples obtained from the same person over time are very similar, indicating bacterial stability. One individual's microbiome, however, may differ significantly from the microbiome of another individual. Twins and mother–daughter pairs have more similar microbial compositions compared to unrelated individuals, suggesting there may be a genetic component in regulating the bacterial population. However, identical twins compared to fraternal twins have fairly similar bacterial patterns, suggesting that perhaps environment is a strong factor in shaping an individual's bacterial populations.

Populations of individuals can also be separated by the differences in their gut microbiota. For example, people born in Rome, Italy, have a different and unique gut microbial composition compared to those born in Cape Town, South Africa. Similarly, people who live in rural towns may have a different microbial composition from urban dwellers, although further research is required to substantiate this statement.

Although these groups of people are genetically different, their exposure to various environments, levels of sanitation and cleanliness, and exposure to antibiotics may all play a significant role in shaping the gut bacteria.

Did You Know?

Similar Species

Studies show that healthy adults share most of the same bacterial species, or a common core of microbiota.

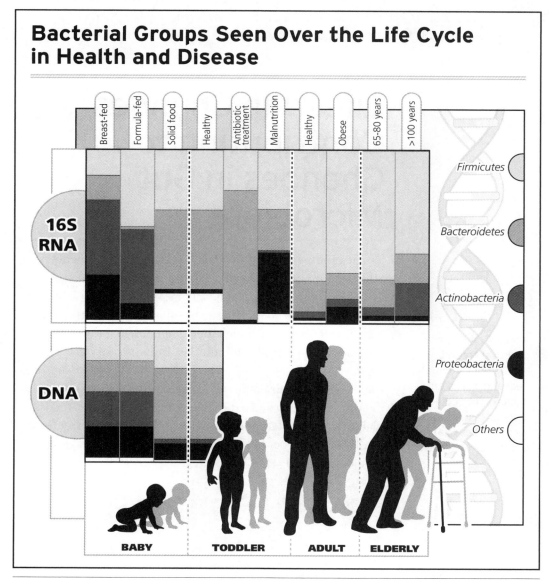

Bacterial Groups Seen Over the Life Cycle in Health and Disease

Q
A

Is it true that modern sanitation may be adversely affecting our gut microbiome?

North Americans generally feel fortunate to have clean drinking water and good sanitation. However, these are two factors that could be causing a barrier to developing beneficial microbiomes. A recent study showed that American adults lacked approximately 50 bacterial types that were key members of the gut microbiome found in adults of two rural, non-industrialized regions of Papua New Guinea. Jens Walter, the senior scientist of this study, hypothesized that the ability of bacteria to be transmitted from person to person may be linked to water. The results confirm that hygiene practices could be limiting the ability of beneficial bacteria to be transmitted among humans, and while hygiene practices also contribute to fewer infectious diseases, they may be making North Americans susceptible to other ill effects not yet well known.

Lifestyle Changes Contributing to Changes in Gut Microbiota

Understanding how cultural traditions and environments have affected gut microbiota could give us insight into diseases associated with these microbes.

Understanding how cultural traditions and environments have affected gut microbiota could give us insight into diseases associated with these microbes. For example, Crohn's disease, a chronic disease characterized by inflammation of the small and large intestines, is much more common in industrialized societies than in rural communities. Inflammatory diseases like Crohn's disease may be exacerbated by Western exposures, such as rampant air pollution, lower microbial presence due to rigorous sanitation and a diet that is rich in processed foods, high in saturated fats and low in fiber. Similarly, the frequency of allergies is higher in the developed world compared to the developing world.

Historical Lifestyle vs. Modern Lifestyle

Historical Lifestyle	Modern Lifestyle
Vaginal delivery at home	Increasing rate of caesarean delivery
Large family size and overcrowding	Small family size
Rural lifestyle, in contact with soil microorganisms	Urban setting, surrounded by concrete
Lack of antibiotics in infant life	Antibiotic usage early in life
Limited access to hot water and soap	Daily body wash with hot water and soap
Parasitic worm infections	Decline in parasites
Food conserved by microbial fermentation	Food conserved by refrigeration
Consumption of natural foods	Consumption of natural and processed foods

FAQ

Q **Is there a link between air pollution and the gut?**

A An estimated 5 million people worldwide suffer from Crohn's disease or ulcerative colitis, the terms used collectively to describe inflammatory bowel disease. Researchers have hypothesized that the environment is instrumental in the onset of disease. A small but growing number of studies now suggest that air pollutants may play a role in disease of the gut. Dr. Karen Madsen, a senior researcher from the University of Alberta in Canada, claims that fine pollution particles are cleared from the respiratory tract by mucus and ultimately find their way to the gut. Some evidence affirms that inhaling fine particles or soot may disrupt the immune system and trigger gut inflammation by altering its normal bacteria, predisposing a person to disease.

Groups of Bacteria

Recent research suggests that a healthy gut microbiota is made up of a well-balanced community of three highly evolved groups of bacteria. These three groups are symbionts, commensals and pathobionts.

Symbionts are the bacteria, primarily found in the colon, that offer beneficial health effects.

Commensals are bacteria that thrive within the gut but really have no positive or negative effects on humans.

The primary purpose of commensal bacteria is to ensure an optimum balance of bacteria, essentially acting as a checkpoint to prevent overgrowth of pathobiont bacteria while limiting the entry of pathogens.

Pathobionts are part of the normal gut microbiota but they have the potential to cause disease under certain situations. In certain circumstances, these native bacteria can predispose the body to illness and disease. If the composition or number of bacteria is altered from a normal baseline, it may promote the overgrowth of pathobionts and, ultimately, immune-mediated diseases.

Collectively, the gut microbiome protects against the colonization of "bad" bacteria, also known as pathogens, and reduces the overgrowth of pathobionts.

There is also some evidence that genetic changes, a failing immune system, or a less desirable living environment may encourage the growth of pathobionts, which may cause inflammation or even allow these bacteria to enter the bloodstream. Entry of these bacteria into the blood circulation could cause diseases of variable severity. Keep in mind that pathobionts are different than pathogens. Pathogens are not part of the normal gut microbiota. They gain access to the intestine from outside the human body, potentially causing infections or inflammation in an otherwise healthy person.

The Impact of Diet on the Microbiome

Diet shapes the composition of the intestinal bacterial community. Many studies have highlighted the links between diet and distinct gut microbiota. Understanding how diet influences microbiota is critical in understanding why diet affects the onset of disease.

Macronutrients

The amount, type and balance of the three main dietary nutrients — carbohydrates, fats and proteins — have a profound impact on the gut microbiota.

Carbohydrates range from simple sugars to complex starchy substances. Examples are whole grains such as wheat, oats, barley, rye, rice and potatoes. Carbohydrates are the main energy source for daily activities. Glucose, one of the main building blocks of carbohydrates, is needed for our brains and central nervous system to function.

Proteins are the nutrients needed for building new muscles and are critical to the successful repair and regeneration of muscles and other tissues in the body. Proteins may be derived from either plant-based or animal sources. Plant sources of proteins are legumes such as beans, peas and lentils. Examples of animal-based sources of protein are poultry, fish, milk, eggs and red meats.

Fats are the most energy-dense macronutrient. Fat provides 9 calories per gram, which is more than double the ratio for a protein or carbohydrate, which each provides 4 calories per gram. This means that when equal amounts of protein, fat and carbohydrates are consumed, fats will provide the most energy, otherwise known as calories. But not all fat sources are created equal.

There are four major types of dietary fats in the foods we eat. These include the naturally occurring saturated, monounsaturated and polyunsaturated fats. The fourth fat is trans fat, which is used in processing and manufacturing certain foods. The undesirable fats are the saturated fats and trans fats, which are solid at room temperature. The more desirable fats are the monounsaturated and polyunsaturated fats, which are liquid at room temperature.

There is growing concern that the average North American diet, which is high in both fat and sugar, has altered our gut bacteria. In particular, there is concern that a high-fat, high-sugar diet can alter the genes in the bacteria and, subsequently, bacterial actions within the gut, leading to chronic illness. Until recently, it was unclear how quickly and predictably gut bacteria respond to dietary change. Research in animal subjects has shown that shifting the macronutrient composition of a diet can broadly and consistently alter the gut microbiome within a single day.

Did You Know?

Rapid Fix
Gut bacteria adapt to a change in diet within 24 hours.

Did You Know?

Fat Facts
The four types of fats — saturated, monounsaturated, polyunsaturated and trans fat — each have different chemical structures and properties.

Meat vs. Plant Diets

Background: The composite gut microbiomes of Western populations have changed over the past century, brought on by new environmental triggers that may have a negative impact on health. Those who eat diets low in fiber and high in both saturated fats and refined sugars are at risk for developing inflammatory diseases.

Objective: To evaluate the impact of diets based entirely on animal or plant products on the microbial community.

Methods: Researchers recently completed an interesting study in which healthy volunteers followed two distinct diets that varied according to their primary food source. Study subjects received either a plant-rich diet, consisting of whole grains, legumes, fruits and vegetables, or an animal-rich diet, composed of meats, eggs and cheese.

Results: Not surprisingly, subjects that followed the animal-based diet had a higher concentration of end products of protein digestion compared to subjects who followed the plant-based diet, who had more end products of carbohydrate digestion. Bacteria that are able to tolerate high levels of bile acids in the gut, particularly *Bilophila wadsworthia*, were seen far more frequently in the animal-based diet group compared to the plant-rich group. Higher levels of bile acid have been linked to a variety of cancers. The microbiota in subjects who followed the plant-based diet showed an increase in the numbers of bacteria that produce a very beneficial fatty acid called butyrate. Butyrate, a short-chain fatty acid, is important for the health of the colon and is known to reduce inflammation in the colon.

Conclusions: The bacteria identified in the animal diet group have been associated with greater rates of inflammation and, in particular, may be linked to inflammatory bowel diseases like Crohn's disease. In contrast, the end products of plant digestion are of great health benefit.

Dietary Carbohydrates

The bacterial action of carbohydrates occurs largely in the right side of the colon and the bacterial action of undigested proteins occurs in the left colon. Approximately 40 grams of unabsorbed dietary carbohydrates reach the colon each day. The main types of carbohydrates that are not absorbed include resistant starches (dietary fibers) and certain sugars. There is some evidence to show that changing the amount and/or type of carbohydrate consumed over a period of up to 4 weeks can have an intense and rapid influence on the gut microbiota.

Carbohydrates are divided into four groups based on their chain length:

- Monosaccharides (one sugar)
- Disaccharides (two sugars)
- Oligosaccharides (few sugars)
- Polysaccharides (many sugars)

Consuming complex carbohydrates that are rich in fiber is invaluable to health and will be discussed in detail later in the book (see "Fiber in the Gut," page 58). Dietary fiber is fermented by gut microbes to become short-chain fatty acids, primarily butyrate, propionate and acetate.

Agrarian diets high in fruits and legumes are associated with a greater diversity in the microbiome, which is associated with good health. In contrast, Western diets that are rich in fat and sugar and low in fiber result in gut microbes that are less diverse, which increases the risk for diseases. In addition, two human clinical trials have suggested that consumption of whole-grain cereals increases the number of health-promoting bifidobacteria in the gut.

Whole grains have been shown to decrease protein fermentation by the gut microbes. Protein fermentation may be associated with undesirable fermentation end products, and whole grains can reduce the impact of this effect. The beneficial effects of whole grains on health are likely to be a combined result of multiple components within the grain, rather than one specific component.

FAQ

  What is butyrate and how does it benefit the gut?

Butyrate is a short-chain fatty acid produced when the body ferments dietary fiber. It is the preferred energy source for the cells in the colon and is known to lower the risk of colon cancer and reduce inflammation. Butyrate helps keep the gut wall healthy and sealed, thereby suppressing the development of gut inflammation and improving the intestinal barrier. This may be related to enhancement of the gut immune system. In addition, butyrate is known to inhibit the toxic effect of certain compounds in colonic cells. Through these mechanisms, butyrate lessens inflammation in the colon, which is important for people with colitis.

Factors that reduce butyrate formation can negatively affect inflammation, predisposing an individual to disease. Because there are very few sources of butyrate in the diet, humans rely on gut bacteria to synthesize it. Consequently, diets that are rich in plant sources, which are known to improve butyrate formation by altering the gut microbiome, are highly recommended.

Dietary Protein

In a typical North American diet, approximately 12 to 18 grams of protein reach the colon daily. The proportion of undigested protein, otherwise known as residual protein, is approximately 10% of total protein consumed, depending on the amount and kind of protein. The colon is an active site of protein metabolism, which provides nitrogen for bacterial growth. Some of the end products resulting from protein fermentation by bacteria have harmful health-related consequences.

- **Ammonia:** Ammonia is an end product of protein fermentation. Ammonia is known to alter the structure of intestinal tissue, and it may promote cancer in the gut and increase tumor formation.

- **Nitrosamines:** Other end products of protein are nitrosamines, which are known carcinogens. It is believed the gut microbiota plays a role in generating these protein metabolites, so altering gut microbiota may promote bacteria that are less capable of achieving these harmful metabolic processes, which may be important in reducing tumor risk.

There have been only a few studies assessing the impact of dietary protein on the microbial composition in the gut. The current published works confirm that diets high in red meat consumption increase nitrosamine levels, which are associated with tumor promotion.

Diets high in red meat consumption increase nitrosamine levels, which are associated with tumor promotion.

- **Lower SCFAs:** In addition, higher meat intake has been associated with lower short-chain fatty acid (SCFA) production, which has been shown to be critical to good health. Fatty acids are the end products of fat digestion and are classified by their chain length — short chain, medium chain or long chain. SCFAs have fewer than six carbon atoms in their chemical structure, while medium chains have between six and 12 carbons, and long chains have 13 or more carbons. Each of these types of fatty acids has unique characteristics.

- **Hydrogen Sulfide:** Protein can also become hydrogen sulfide through fermentation. A diet rich in meat is linked to higher stool concentrations of sulfide. Hydrogen sulfide has been shown to decrease the positive effects of butyrate in the colon. However, increasing dietary fiber in high-protein diets has been shown to increase SCFAs and decrease ammonia concentrations, both of which favorably impact health.

Diet Intervention

Background: We coexist with our gut microbes, but this relationship sometimes becomes unfriendly in conditions such as obesity and inflammatory bowel disease. Dietary factors are known to influence the microbiome, and diet presents the simplest route for therapeutic intervention.

Objective: To assess the impact of a short-term controlled feeding experiment to test the stability of the gut microbiome and interactions between nutrients and the microbiome.

Methods: For 98 healthy volunteers, information about their diet was collected using two types of questionnaire to ensure validity of content. A subset of these individuals was sequestered in a hospital and given a very specific diet. The diets tested included a diet that was high in fat and protein but low in fiber, compared to a diet that was low in fat, low in protein and high in fiber.

Results: Distinct microbial associations were observed with nutrients from proteins versus diets rich in carbohydrates. Particularly, diets rich in protein had a microbiome high in species from the *Bacteroides* family and low in species from *Prevotella*. In contrast, diets rich in carbohydrates and fibers were rich in *Prevotella* compared to *Bacteroides*. Self-reported vegetarians showed a high representation of the *Prevotella* group. One self-reported vegan also had an enriched *Prevotella* microbiome.

Conclusions: Dietary factors offer potential clues to differences in the microbiome. Future research would involve assessing the impact of a *Bacteroides*-based microbiome on the incidence of health and disease.

Dietary Fats

Dietary fats are mostly absorbed in the small intestine. In a healthy person, the majority of fat eaten is absorbed. However, up to 7% of fat may not be absorbed into the cells for use. Fat that is not absorbed moves into the colon and is eventually excreted in a bowel movement. As with protein, there have been only a handful of studies investigating the effect of dietary fat on the gut microbiota. What we do know is that consuming a high-fat diet compared to a low-fat diet lowers the SCFA levels substantially. Remember that short-chain fatty acids are important to overall gut health.

An interesting animal study using mice fed a high-fat diet for 12 weeks, followed by a standard laboratory chow diet for another 10 weeks, showed that the microbiota composition during the high-fat diet was different for the first phase but returned to normal following exposure to their usual diet.

> In a healthy person, the majority of fat eaten is absorbed. However, up to 7% of fat may not be absorbed into the cells for use.

This study provides preliminary evidence that microbial response to a high-fat diet is reversible. This area certainly needs further scientific investigation. Other researchers have shown that the negative effects of a higher-fat diet may be improved or lessened by adding prebiotic fibers to the diet.

Future Dietary Studies

Some unanswered questions at the present time relate to the impact of the quality of each of the macronutrients. For example, are there differences between plant and animal proteins regarding their effect on the microbiome? Similarly, are there differences between the effects of low- and high-glycemic-index carbohydrates on the microbiome? These types of questions are imperative for researchers to understand, and scientifically rigorous work is still needed to make definitive statements.

However, there is some pioneer work underway exploring these themes. A recent research group tested the hypothesis that the type and quantity of dietary fat and carbohydrate significantly affected the gut microbes and the end products of fermentation by these microbes. In this European study, 88 participants completed the 24-week experiment. The participants were required to have at least two metabolic risk factors, such as diabetes, high cholesterol, obesity or high blood pressure. These participants were assigned different diets:

- A diet high in saturated fat and with a high glycemic index
- A diet high in monounsaturated fat and with a high glycemic index
- A diet high in monounsaturated fat and with a low glycemic index
- A diet high in carbohydrates and with a high glycemic index
- A diet high in carbohydrates and with a low glycemic index

The researchers observed significant changes in total numbers of bacteria in the experimental groups. In particular, diets rich in fat (either monounsaturated or saturated fat) experienced a decrease in total bacterial content compared to the other groups. The two high-carbohydrate groups showed the largest increase in *Bifidobacterium* species (highly beneficial to health). Participants in the high-carbohydrate and high-glycemic-index group had a greater abundance of *Bacteroides* species compared to the baseline. The significance of this is unknown at the present time.

> The negative effects of a higher-fat diet may be improved or lessened by adding prebiotic fibers to the diet.

In addition, diets rich in monounsaturated fats and high in carbohydrates yielded lower blood cholesterol results, which is not surprising. The impact of a total decrease in bacteria observed in the high-fat groups is unknown, but the potential for increased disease due to inflammation may be higher because of the loss of protective bacteria such as *Bifidobacterium*. These studies are still in their infancy and further work is required to tease out the effects of the quality of macronutrients.

Diet and Mental Health

A growing number of observational studies have been documenting the associations between diet quality and the risk of depression. These associations have been consistently observed in adults and children and in myriad countries and cultures. For example, studies investigating the protective effects of a Mediterranean diet on brain diseases have shown a reduced risk of depression and a reduced risk of decline in cognition. Moreover, children who consume more unhealthy sugar-laden and fat-rich foods seem to have more psychological disorders than children who follow a healthier diet.

The evidence that gut microbes influence brain and behavior is gaining traction. We are seeing how gut microbes can affect behaviors such as anxiety in animal models and, when specific probiotics are introduced, can improve depression-like behaviors. In small studies, the consumption of *Bifidobacterium* or *Lactobacillus* species of probiotics has been associated with a significant improvement in anxiety symptoms and depression.

Depression is strongly associated with a number of diseases, including irritable bowel syndrome (IBS), fibromyalgia and migraines, so it's exciting to think that exploring the health of the gut microbiome may offer effective preventive and treatment strategies in the future. In fact, probiotics and dietary manipulation to produce a healthy microbiome may be a treatment option in the coming years for many psychiatric disorders, including depression, anxiety, autism, schizophrenia and bipolar disorders.

CHAPTER 2

Antibiotics and the Gut Microbiome

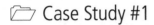 Case Study #1

Treating Fever without Antibiotics

Annie brought her 3-year-old daughter, Kate, to her family doctor's office following 24 hours of fever. She was visibly perturbed because her daughter had been treated with antibiotics 3 months earlier for another episode of fever without a clear underlying cause being identified.

Kate was otherwise healthy, born at 38 weeks' gestation and average in size. She started daycare at 2 years of age, and it seems that she has since had a perennial battle with coughs and a runny nose. Three months ago, she had 2 days of fever documented at 101.3°F (38.5°C). At that time, she had a cough but no other symptoms. She was playing and interacting normally with her siblings. Annie was quite concerned at the time but could not see her family doctor for another 24 hours, so she treated Kate with antibiotics that were left over from 3 months ago.

Since then, Annie had been reading about the association of antibiotic exposure with the development of asthma in young children, and was quite concerned that self-treating Kate could result in her developing asthma and/or other allergic diseases in the future. She was also unsure how to deal with the fever and was seeking advice in this regard.

Kate's family physician took a detailed history and conducted a thorough physical examination. There was no evidence of an ear infection and her throat was normal. The respiratory exam was normal and pneumonia was ruled out. In addition, a urine sample was negative, with no sign of a urinary tract infection. The child was well hydrated and interacted normally. The family physician assured Annie that young children are at increased risk of viral infections and are predisposed toward fevers, which are a symptom of the body mounting a response against the virus.

Annie was reassured that no further treatment was indicated at the present time, and that antibiotics in this setting might be of greater harm than benefit. Annie was advised to manage the symptoms with fluids and pain medication. Specifically, she was advised not to administer any antibiotics, including leftover antibiotics from the previous encounter with illness.

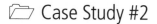 Case Study #2

Antibiotic Complications

Roberto is a 43-year-old diabetic male who had developed a leg infection 5 days before visiting his doctor. He had a fever and a swollen, hot and red shin. He was diagnosed with cellulitis and it was recommended that he be admitted to hospital for administration of intravenous antibiotics.

Four days after starting antibiotics, he started having diarrhea. In fact, he noted seven episodes of loose, watery bowel movements. The diarrhea was associated with abdominal pain and cramping. This happened for 2 days. Roberto was convinced he had *Clostridium difficile* colitis, otherwise known as the superbug infection associated with antibiotics.

His family doctor requested that I see him for a consultation, while Roberto was admitted to hospital. During the assessment, we established that his diarrhea was acute, and apart from his diabetes (for which he required insulin), Roberto was otherwise reasonably well. Typically he reported one to two bowel movements daily without blood or mucus. Therefore, his current presentation was clearly a departure from his baseline bowel habits.

I shared Roberto's concern about an antibiotic-associated diarrhea or *Clostridium difficile* colitis. After all, the timing after antibiotic exposure was a significant risk for this. In addition, I mentioned to Roberto that sometimes antibiotic exposure itself may disrupt bowel frequency and routine, resulting in altered bowel habits. I recommended that he have his stool specimens assessed for *Clostridium difficile* toxin, along with a full stool assessment for parasites and bacteria. They tested positive for *Clostridium difficile* toxin, and Roberto started antibiotics to manage this illness, along with a discussion surrounding the use of probiotics.

Antibiotics: History and Future

There is absolutely no question that the discovery and rise of antibiotics changed medicine in a positive way.

Antibiotics can be defined as medicines that inhibit the growth of or destroy bacteria. The history of antibiotics can be divided into two segments: early and modern history. During ancient times, Greeks and South Asians used molds and other plants to treat infections. Interestingly, in Greece and Serbia, moldy bread was traditionally used to treat wounds and infections. In Russia, warm soil was used by peasants to cure infected wounds, and it has been reported that Babylonian doctors healed eyes plagued with infection with a sour milk concoction.

One of the most significant medical advances of the 20th century was the newfound ability to treat infectious diseases. Since then, deaths from these diseases have declined markedly in North America. This decline contributed to a sharp drop in infant and child mortality, and to the 30-year increase in life expectancy. Antibiotics have arguably been solely responsible for the reduction in childhood mortality and increase in longevity. There is no doubt that antibiotics historically have saved millions of lives.

However, a new era has arrived. Antibiotics have been misused and overused for the past few decades, and as a result, many antibiotics are now no longer effective against certain bacteria. Antibiotic resistance happens when bacteria evolve to protect themselves from an antibiotic and are then no longer sensitive to the effects of that antibiotic. When this happens, antibiotics that previously would have been effective in either controlling the multiplication of bacteria or killing the bacteria no longer work. We have become familiar with the term "superbug," which refers to these bacteria that are resistant to antibiotics.

A common example of a superbug is methicillin-resistant *Staphylococcus aureus* (MRSA), which was once confined to hospitalized patients and, more recently, is now seen in community settings. Other superbugs are *Clostridium difficile* (*C. diff*) as well as *Mycobacterium tuberculosis*, the bacteria that causes tuberculosis, which is now becoming difficult to treat as there are mounting concerns about antibiotic resistance.

Changes in Microbiota

The ability of antibiotics to dramatically alter the microbiota in the GI tract was observed as early as 1950, when high doses of a particular antibiotic were shown to eliminate the intestinal bacteria in patients who were preparing for intestinal surgery. In just a few years of regular antibiotic use, there was already mounting evidence that altering the host microbiota with antibiotics could lead to a gut microbiome that predisposes to opportunistic pathogens or bacteria that can cause illness, rather than to friendly bacteria. We know that antibiotics change the microbiota composition in the gut. What is less known is whether the microbial community regains its original composition after treatment. A few research studies have

<h2>Did You Know?</h2>

Saving Lives

In 1900, 30% of all deaths in North America occurred in children younger than 5 years old. In 1997, only 1% of children younger than 5 years of age died. In 1900, the three leading causes of death were pneumonia, tuberculosis and uncontrolled diarrhea — and they accounted for one-third of all deaths. In 1997, heart disease and cancer accounted for more than 50% of all deaths, with only 4% attributed to pneumonia or influenza.

attempted to answer this question, but with mixed results; we need to explore it further.

For example, one study assessed six patients treated with a short course of various antibiotics. Only one individual did not regain his original gut microbial profile within 60 days of treatment. However, in another study, which used a more advanced technology to better profile gut bacteria, the vast majority of individuals treated with antibiotics had permanent changes in the microbial species in the gut. Although the findings are unclear, their impact is noteworthy, since functions associated with regaining a normal gut microbiota, along with overall health, may be compromised.

> Our normal microbiome is critical for a variety of functions, and environmental bacteria are the foundation on which all life on earth exists.

Antibiotic Resistance

What is the impact of antibiotic resistance and should we be concerned about this? Microbes will never stop adapting to whatever selective pressure we throw at them. It is reasonable to surmise that antibiotic resistance ranks close to death and taxes as a third inevitable truth in life. Some experts have claimed that we will never win a war against microbes. Nor should we want to. We have previously described the commensal relationship we have with our microbes and the benefits gained by coexisting harmoniously with microbes. Our normal microbiome is critical for a variety of functions, and environmental bacteria are the foundation on which all life on earth exists, literally speaking.

The antibiotic crisis is the predictable outcome of how we have developed and used antibiotics since their discovery. If we continue to develop and use antibiotics for the next 80 years in the same way that we have done in the past 80 years, future resistance will continue to explode, and our treatment options will decline. We will reenter a paradigm previously seen in the pre-antibiotic era, when there was a resurgence of life-threatening infections without effective weapons to abate the impact of resistant organisms. Infectious-disease experts have claimed that if we want to change that prediction and have long-term availability of effective antimicrobial therapy for infections, we need to challenge long-standing and sometimes cherished assumptions.

Preventing antibiotic abuse is critical to modernizing antibiotic use. This can be accomplished largely through behavioral change, such as education and restricting prescribing practices.

> **Did You Know?**
>
> **Resistance Increases**
>
> Data suggest that more than 60% of specialists have seen a bacterial infection resistant to innumerable antibiotics within the previous year.

➤ Research Spotlight

Antibiotic Use

Background: Using antimicrobial agents can cause several adverse effects on gut microbes. The emergence of resistance among bacteria in the normal microbiome can contribute to an increased load of microbes that may be harmful.

Objective: To assess the effect of two commonly used antibiotics, ciprofloxacin and clindamycin, on the microbiome.

Methods: Thirty healthy volunteers were recruited for the study. They were randomly assigned to receive ciprofloxacin, clindamycin or a placebo. Stool samples were collected at various times.

Results: There was a decrease in one large group of bacteria, known as gram-negative bacteria, 11 days after initiating ciprofloxacin antibiotics, but this normalized at the end of 30 days. Interestingly, in the same group of volunteers, the numbers of another large group of bacteria, known as gram-positive bacteria, were stable until day 11, then remained persistently elevated until 12 months later. In the clindamycin group, no changes regarding gram-negative bacteria were observed. A decrease in gram-positive bacteria was observed 11 days after initiating clindamycin antibiotics, and this did not normalize until 12 months. The numbers and distribution of bacteria did not change in the placebo group.

Conclusions: The time required for the normal microbes to normalize after antibiotics is different for various bacterial species. It may take between 1 and 12 months to normalize the gut microbiome, which could pose a risk to health until that time. The study demonstrates that an increased exposure to antibiotics may prevent the microbiome from regaining normalcy.

Susceptibility to Harmful Bacteria

Antibiotic use increases the susceptibility to harmful bacteria. Unfortunately, even when using antibiotics for appropriate medical conditions, it may result in serious side effects related to imbalances in the microbiome. *Clostridium difficile* is the prototype example of this relationship.

Clostridium Difficile

Many of you might be familiar with the superbug *Clostridium difficile*, otherwise known as *C. diff*. It is fast emerging as a health threat, especially in hospitalized patients and patients living in long-term care facilities. The majority of patients with *C. diff* have had recent exposure to antibiotics. In other words, antibiotics, in fact, may lead to other infections. How is this even possible if antibiotics are designed to kill or reduce the amount of bacteria present? Under normal circumstances, the good bacteria in the gut keep *C. diff* — a naturally occurring organism — under control, not allowing this bacterium to proliferate. However, when antibiotics are administered, both the good and bad bacteria are suppressed, allowing *C. diff* to grow out of control and cause symptoms.

Identifying and Treating C. *Diff*
- **How do you know if you have C. *diff*?** Symptoms of *C. diff* are typically multiple large-volume stools per day, abdominal pain, bloating and cramping. In serious situations, the body's white blood cell count rises and there is evidence of inflammation on abdominal X-rays. Usually *C. diff* is diagnosed using a stool test for the *C. diff* toxin. Sometimes a limited colonoscopy, otherwise known as a flexible sigmoidoscopy, is needed to confirm the diagnosis of *C. diff* and rule out additional contributing diagnoses. Most cases of *C. diff* respond to standard treatment, which is a beneficial antibiotic. However, some people with *C. diff* do not respond to standard antibiotics and may require a more potent antibiotic. In very serious cases of *C. diff*, surgery may be required to remove the affected bowel, although this is extremely rare. In rare cases, *C. diff* can be life-threatening.

Did You Know?

New Strain

In more recent years, a new strain of *C. diff* has developed, producing an even more severe colon infection. Although first identified in Canada, it has spread to all the U.S. states.

- **How do you prevent and treat C. *diff*?** Unfortunately, once you get C. *diff*, it is tough to get rid of it permanently. The first-line antibiotic to try is metronidazole, otherwise known as Flagyl. Treatment is usually given for 10 to 14 days. If metronidazole does not work, the second-line antibiotic, vancomycin, is used. In special circumstances, a medical practitioner might combine treatments to include both Flagyl and vancomycin. Vancomycin is generally more effective than metronidazole, especially if the disease is more severe. The recurrence rate of C. *diff*, once it has been treated, can be as high as 20%. Regrettably, this means that even if C. *diff* was treated successfully, one in five people will have it rear its ugly head again.

- **What can you do to avoid C. *diff*?** It is critical that you avoid casual antibiotic use. This means limiting antibiotics for only those conditions that have a clear reason for treatment. Keep in mind that a sore throat and runny nose may happen for a number of reasons and do not necessarily mean that you have a bacterial infection. Remember that antibiotics can only treat bacteria, not viruses. Practice good hand hygiene at all times.

How to Prevent Antibiotic Resistance

1. Ask if tests will be done to make sure the right antibiotic is prescribed when needed.
2. Take antibiotics exactly as your doctor prescribes. Do not skip doses.
3. Complete the prescribed course even when you start feeling better.
4. Do not save antibiotics to treat a future illness.
5. Do not ask for antibiotics when your doctor thinks you do not need them.
6. Prevent infections by practicing good hand hygiene and getting your recommended vaccines.

Antibiotic-Associated Diarrhea

We have established that antibiotics can be disruptive to gut bacteria. Depending on the proportion of bacteria residing in the colon, this disruption can also damage the bowel wall lining and trigger diarrhea. Typically, diarrhea that is a direct result of taking antibiotics is self-limited and resolves without any specific treatment. However, the symptoms and severity of diarrhea may impact quality of life.

Antibiotics in Children

During the past two decades, allergic diseases have rapidly grown to afflict more than 20% of the population in industrial countries. However, explanations for the dramatic increase and prevalence are still less than satisfying.

Although regional antibiotic prescription rates vary, the use of antibiotics in early childhood markedly increased in the late 1980s and early 1990s. This phenomenon coincides with the increase in the prevalence of allergic diseases during the past decades. Early research studies suggested a positive association between antibiotic exposure early in life and the development of allergic diseases. Allergic diseases, such as asthma, dermatitis and rhinitis, are chronic inflammatory disorders resulting from the complex interaction between the genetics of individuals and the environment in which they reside.

Although subsequent studies have shown conflicting results, the largest recent study, which involved more than 250,000 subjects, confirmed a link. Information about the types of antibiotics used, doses and duration of antibiotics prescribed are not noted. It is believed that broad-spectrum antibiotics, or antibiotics targeted at a broad number and types of bacteria, are more potent in reducing bacteria in the gut than more focused antibiotics. What is interesting is that the association of early-life exposure to antibiotics and allergies and asthma seems more prominent in children without any family history of asthma or other allergic diseases.

Did You Know?

Hygiene Effect

The hygiene hypothesis, first proposed by a group of researchers in 1989, suggests that the lack of microbial exposures as a result of very hygienic conditions early in life may have an impact on the balance of the immune system.

Modern Environments

Many researchers have observed that the onset of allergic diseases is associated with a modern lifestyle and that their increase is parallel to the decrease in infectious diseases, which may be in part attributed to vaccination policies and greater use of antibiotics, among other factors. Since human genetics has not really changed in the past few decades, it is reasonable to surmise that the environment has changed, and it is likely the greater driver in the development of allergic diseases.

Treating Symptoms in Children without Antibiotics

Children are particularly predisposed to developing symptoms like cough, runny nose and fevers, especially early in life while the immune system is growing and maturing. Daycares and preschools are prime breeding grounds for children to contract infectious diseases. Most fevers in young, healthy, immunized children are due to viral illnesses, which will not respond to antibiotics. In such cases, seek medical advice and follow your doctor's suggestions. Refrain from asking to treat symptoms with antibiotics when not medically appropriate. If your child's symptoms do not improve within the expected time or if your child's health deteriorates, schedule another appointment with the primary-care physician — further testing may be warranted before exposing your child to antibiotics.

Sore Throat

Sore throat is a very common symptom of upper respiratory tract infections. A sore throat may be caused by either a bacteria or a virus, but is more commonly viral than bacterial. The majority of sore throats are *not* caused by streptococcal bacteria. However, it is important to accurately diagnose and treat strep throat (officially known as Group A streptococcal pharyngitis) to prevent any complications. Strep throat is very rare in children under the age of 3. In fact, most children with upper respiratory tract infections do not have a sore throat. The American Academy of Pediatrics, the American Heart Association and the Infectious Diseases Society of America recommend testing with a throat culture in suspected cases of strep throat, and avoiding treatment with antibiotics until test results are available. It is safe to await results before treatment, since it is aimed at preventing complications.

Earaches

Painful earaches occur commonly in young children. In 2009, the Canadian Paediatric Society published comprehensive guidelines on the management of acute otitis media (acute ear infections). In children over the age of 6 months, careful observation is recommended, as most symptoms resolve on their own. However, if symptoms persist beyond 48 to 72 hours, then antibiotics should be prescribed. Most parents are generally satisfied with this strategy, which decreases the complications associated with antibiotic therapy.

Cough and Cold

There is a minimal role for antibiotics in the treatment of pediatric upper respiratory tract infections. In young children, bacterial pneumonia is relatively rare — the more common causes of pneumonia are viruses such as respiratory syncytial virus (RSV) or influenza. Many parents have fever phobia. They seek medical care because they believe fever is dangerous and indicates a serious infection that needs to be treated with antibiotics.

FAQ

If my child has a fever, how can I be reassured that he doesn't need antibiotics?

Remember, fever is a normal immune system response and is not dangerous in itself. However, use these guidelines to assess the situation:

- Remember that most fevers in healthy immunized children are caused by viruses.
- A medical history and physical examination are the best approach to identify the source of the fever and determine the need for any further testing.
- Children should be interacting normally and playing well once their fever has been treated and temperature has decreased.

Doc Talk

Antibiotics have forever altered the field of modern medicine, notably improving the quality of life in countless individuals. However, with advances in scientific methods, researchers are just beginning to understand the damage caused to the gut microbiota, which protects individuals from bacteria that may cause serious damage and disease. In the future, more work needs to be done to detail the composition of the gut microbiome so that clear connections can be understood between the microbiota and health and disease. This will allow scientists to better understand how antibiotic-altered bacteria may affect the development of diseases.

CHAPTER 3

Beneficial Bacteria

 Case Study

Probiotic Therapy

Mira, a 30-year-old woman, came to see me after experiencing abdominal bloating, alternating diarrhea and constipation, and abdominal cramping for the past 3 years. Her symptoms had increased in frequency and severity in the past year, following a trip to Mexico, at which time she experienced 3 days of severe diarrhea. Mira did not have any unexpected weight loss, blood in bowel movements or a family history of colon cancer or inflammatory bowel disease. She had been uncomfortable and felt a sense of urgency about being close to a bathroom in case of stool incontinence.

Her family physician referred Mira to me, her gastroenterologist, for further assessment and management. I sent her for some blood tests, including a test for celiac disease. All the tests were negative. Her stool samples were clear of infection. I diagnosed Mira with irritable bowel syndrome (IBS) and suspected her symptoms had accelerated after her presumed viral infection when traveling in Mexico. I felt that her symptoms were predominantly post-infectious in nature.

Her treatment plan consisted of dietary modifications, including reducing simple sugar intake from sources like fruits, fruit juice and soda pop, while increasing her intake of probiotic-rich foods such as yogurt and kefir. I recommended she start taking a specific probiotic consisting of *Bifidobacterium infantis*.

Mira tried out these therapies and I saw her in a follow-up visit after 3 months, at which time her symptoms had markedly improved and her quality of life was restored.

Functional Foods and Probiotics

Recent advances in the field of gut microbiota have set the stage for a focus on functional foods. Optimal gut bacteria are achieved by eating a well-balanced diet with an increased intake of functional foods, specifically prebiotics and probiotics.

Prebiotics are dietary fibers that are non-digestible in the GI tract. Once consumed, prebiotic fibers selectively alter the bacterial composition in the intestine.

Probiotics, in contrast, are live bacteria that are ingested and have a beneficial effect by changing the gut microbiome in a favorable way.

Prebiotics and probiotics are two of the most powerful strategies to alter the microbiome in a health-promoting manner.

What Are Probiotics?

More than 100 years ago, Russian scientist Élie Metchnikoff suggested that milk fermented with lactic acid bacteria improves health. And so the term "probiotics" was born. Around the same time, bifidobacteria — bacteria known for optimizing digestive health that are native to the intestine of all human beings — were isolated from breast-fed infant stool and associated with decreased infections in breast-fed babies. However, the term "probiotic" has been more clearly defined only in the past few years to properly categorize commercialized functional foods.

Probiotics are defined as "living organisms that when administered in sufficient numbers confer a beneficial effect to the host." We know that they may have beneficial effects in an array of areas involving the gut, and beyond, to impact other organs. While probiotics are typically consumed in fermented foods with active live cultures, such as yogurt, they are also available in supplement forms such as capsules.

The idea of consuming live bacteria may seem strange at first. After all, don't we take antibiotics to fight bacteria? Aren't bacteria associated with infections? Hopefully, the background information so far has convinced you that our genetic makeup of good and bad bacteria works in a delicate yet complex balance to promote health and wellness.

How Do Probiotics Work?

It is not completely understood how probiotics work, but some basic principles are accepted by most scientists and doctors. These include the following:

- **Limit bad bacteria:** Probiotics limit the ability of bad bacteria (also called pathogens) to live in the gut. They help produce substances that make the gut more acidic, which reduces bacterial growth. Probiotics may also have an antimicrobial effect, which limits bacterial growth as well. Finally, probiotics themselves may bind to the gut wall, preventing other bacteria from binding to it — meaning that bad bacteria cannot move to other sites in the body.

- **Improve the barrier function of the gut:** Barrier function is related to the quality, or integrity, of the intestinal cell. Increased tightness between intestinal cells, achieved by increasing their mucus production, prevents bad bacteria from escaping as freely into other areas within the body. Probiotics contribute to maintenance of the thick mucous layer, thereby providing a greater defense within the gut.

- **Modulate the immune system:** The gut is the largest immune organ in the body, with more than 70% of the immune cells residing there. Probiotic bacteria activate immune system responses that have beneficial effects. In particular, certain bacteria in the gut influence immune system responses such as correcting immune deficiencies and increasing certain types of white blood cells, in particular T cells, which are critical in maintaining a strong immune system.

Diseases That Probiotics May Beneficially Impact

GI Conditions

- Infectious diarrhea
- Antibiotic-associated diarrhea
- *Clostridium difficile* colitis (*C. diff*)
- Inflammatory bowel disease (Crohn's disease and ulcerative colitis)
- Irritable bowel syndrome
- Stomach ulcers

Non-GI Conditions

- Urinary tract infections
- Bacterial vaginosis
- Nonalcoholic fatty liver disease
- Allergies, especially dermatitis
- Diabetes
- Obesity
- Respiratory infections (pneumonia)
- Hepatic encephalopathy

Probiotics in the Treatment of GI Conditions

GI illnesses are among the most frequently encountered illnesses and often result in poor quality of life and poor functioning. Probiotics have been shown to significantly treat many medical problems and prevent the onset of such diseases. Consequently, there is a robust rationale for increasing the intake of probiotic-rich foods in preventive medicine and health maintenance. In this section, we will review the most common gastrointestinal diseases that have benefited from the use of probiotics.

Infectious Diarrhea

At least a dozen research studies, many conducted with infants or children, involve the use of probiotics to either treat or prevent acute diarrhea from infections. The majority of studies show a very positive benefit from probiotics in reducing the severity and duration of infectious diarrhea symptoms. The benefits of probiotics did extend to multiple strains, including *Lactobacillus rhamnosus* GG and *Saccharomyces boulardii*.

People traveling to warmer climates and less developed countries experience a high incidence of diarrhea. In fact, up to 50% of travelers may experience problematic diarrhea, resulting in significant dehydration, weakness and lethargy. With traveler's diarrhea, the only recourse is to sit, wait and let nature run its course. If the diarrhea is serious enough, an emergency room visit may be in order for rehydration. Probiotics have been shown to add significant protection and reduce both the onset and severity of diarrhea in this situation. Based on studies, the best probiotic for treating traveler's diarrhea is the strain *Lactobacillus* GG. Eat more probiotic-rich foods, such as yogurt and kefir, while on vacation and consider a probiotic supplement if you are suffering from an infectious diarrhea.

Eat more probiotic-rich foods, such as yogurt and kefir, while on vacation and consider a probiotic supplement if you are suffering from an infectious diarrhea.

Probiotics for Acute Diarrhea

Background: Probiotics may offer a safe intervention in acute diarrhea related to infections, reducing the duration and severity of illness.

Objective: To assess the impact of probiotics on the treatment of acute diarrhea.

Methods: All randomized controlled studies comparing a specific probiotic agent with a placebo in people with acute diarrhea were included. Sixty-three studies met the inclusion criteria, for a total of more than 8,000 patients. The majority of trials were in children, although seven studies were in adults.

Results: Probiotics reduced the duration of diarrhea by 24 hours and reduced stool frequency significantly.

Conclusions: There was clear benefit from probiotics in improving the course of infectious diarrhea; however, no conclusions could be reached regarding the probiotic strain or dosage of organisms in reaching these outcomes.

Did You Know?

Common Symptom

Diarrhea is a common symptom that arises from antibiotic use.

Antibiotic-Associated Diarrhea

Your digestive system is a complex ecosystem that is home to trillions of organisms. Antibiotics can be especially disruptive to the gut bacteria because they destroy both the helpful bacteria and the harmful ones. Sometimes, without the good bacteria, the dangerous ones can grow with abandon, producing toxins that damage the bowel lining and trigger inflammation. This may cause diarrhea. Probiotics have been shown to reduce the severity of diarrhea by 70% in people who have taken antibiotics. Although scientific evidence exists that shows benefits from a few different probiotic strains, the best evidence is for the probiotic yeast *Saccharomyces boulardii* (*S. boulardii*). This strain has been shown to cause improvements in the symptoms of antibiotic-associated diarrhea in at least three high-quality research trials.

Here is a list of probiotic regimens that may provide benefit in preventing and treating antibiotic-associated diarrhea:

- *Saccharomyces boulardii*: 10×10^9 colony-forming units (CFU)/day for the duration of the antibiotic course
- *Lactobacillus acidophilus* CL1285 and *Lactobacillus casei*: 25×10^9 CFU/day for 2 days, then 50×10^9 CFU/day for the duration of the antibiotic course

- *Lactobacillus plantarum* 299v: 10 x 10^9 CFU/day within 48 hours of starting antibiotic therapy until 7 days after the antibiotic course
- *Lactobacillus rhamnosus* GG: 40 x 10^9 CFU/day within 72 hours of starting antibiotic therapy, then for 14 days
- VSL#3: 900 x 10^9 CFU/day for the duration of the antibiotic course until 7 days after the antibiotic course

---

➢ Research Spotlight

Probiotic Prevention of Antibiotic-Associated Diarrhea

Background: Antibiotic-associated diarrhea is a common complication when taking antibiotics and when diagnosed with *Clostridium difficile* (*C. diff*). The use of probiotics for these two related diseases remains controversial.

Objective: To compare the efficacy of probiotics for the prevention of antibiotic-associated diarrhea and the treatment of *C. diff*.

Methods: A large meta-analysis included 31 randomized controlled trials. More than 3,000 patients were included for analysis.

Results: In 25 randomized controlled trials, probiotics significantly reduced the risk of developing antibiotic-associated diarrhea by 57%. In six randomized controlled trials, probiotics had significant benefit, reducing the risk of developing *C. diff* by 40%.

Conclusions: A variety of different types of probiotics show promise as effective therapies for these two diseases. These include *Saccharomyces boulardii* and *Lactobacillus rhamnosus* GG. Only *S. boulardii* was effective for *C. diff*.

Clostridium Difficile Colitis

Probiotics may be effective in the prevention and treatment of *C. diff*–associated diarrhea. That's because probiotics colonize the gut and encourage antibacterial activity while at the same time promoting competition among microbes for nutrients and a favorable position on the gut lining. These effects appear to reduce the friendliness of the gut to *C. diff*. Probiotics such as *Lactobacillus* and *S. boulardii* curb the growth of *C. diff*. Probiotics, in particular *Bifidobacterium* and *Saccharomyces*, also improve the immune system.

Probiotics for Prevention of *Clostridium Difficile* Colitis

The role of probiotics in the prevention of C. *diff* diarrhea is a growing area of study. To date, it has been difficult to make general conclusions from one probiotic species to another, or combinations of strains. However, here is what has been investigated. A large meta-analysis, which provides the best and most accurate summary of medical results, has found that people who consume probiotics develop C. *diff* infections up to 66% less often than people who don't. Some aspects of this meta-analysis are still being evaluated and confirmed. A subsequent well-designed study involving almost 3,000 adults with antibiotic exposure failed to show a significant reduction in the development of C. *diff*. Therefore, there is uncertainty in the field of C. *diff* prevention about probiotics at the present time.

Doc Talk

The strain, dose and duration of probiotics used in the noted C. *diff* studies varied widely, as is often the case in a probiotic discussion. In designing future studies to assess the impact of probiotics in the prevention of C. *diff* diarrhea, researchers must standardize the probiotic strains used, along with the dosing and duration of therapy. In the meantime, I recommend considering probiotic supplements when using antibiotics, as the risks for adverse complications are fairly low for someone with a healthy immune system, and potential benefits from this strategy may exist. If nothing else, the risk of antibiotic-induced diarrhea (which is different than C. *diff* diarrhea) is reduced. It is important, however, that if probiotics are used for the prevention of antibiotic-associated diarrhea or C. *diff*, treatment should consist of only those regimens that have demonstrated benefit.

Probiotics for Treatment of *Clostridium Difficile* Colitis

Probiotics may be useful for the treatment of non-severe C. *diff*, particularly during a recurrence of the disease. There have been two large meta-analyses evaluating the effectiveness of probiotics for the treatment of C. *diff*, suggesting a benefit from probiotics in addition to standard antibiotic therapy. However, there have been some well-conducted clinical trials that show insufficient evidence to recommend probiotics as an addition to standard therapies. This area of research is still evolving. Most medical doctors, including specialist gastroenterologists, would conclude that probiotics may be a useful addition to antibiotic therapies in patients with a recurrent, non-severe form of the disease, as long as there are no reasons why probiotics cannot be used. Probiotic stand-alone treatment, with no antibiotics, in the case of C. *diff* is not recommended.

Did You Know?

Treatment with Recurrence

If you previously had C. *diff*, were treated with standard antibiotics and now have a recurrence of C. *diff*, adding probiotics to your regimen may have a great beneficial effect.

Antibiotics That May Induce *C. Diff* Diarrhea

Frequently Associated	Occasionally Associated	Rarely Associated
Fluoroquinolones • Ciprofloxacin • Levofloxacin • Moxifloxacin • Norfloxacin	Macrolides • Azithromycin • Clarithromycin • Erythromycin	Aminoglycosides • Gentamicin • Neomycin • Streptomycin • Tobramycin
Clindamycin	Trimethoprim	Tetracyclines • Doxycycline • Minocycline • Tetracycline
Penicillins • Amoxicillin • Ampicillin • Cloxacillin • Piperacillin/tazobactam	Sulfonamides • Sulfamethoxazole • Trimethoprim-sulfamethoxazole (TMP-SMX)	Metronidazole
Cephalosporins • Cefuroxime • Cefotaxime • Ceftazidime • Ceftriaxone • Cephalexin		Vancomycin

Inflammatory Bowel Disease

Ulcerative colitis (UC) and Crohn's disease (CD) are the major subtypes of inflammatory bowel disease (IBD). In the case of UC, inflammation is limited to the colon (large intestine); in the case of CD, inflammation can occur in any part of the GI tract, from mouth to anus.

IBD is a chronic disease; people who have IBD may experience recurring flare-ups. Remission of the disease can be controlled with medications — usually an extensive regimen that involves many combinations of drugs — some of which suppress the immune system significantly. In the case of colitis, the probiotic *Escherichia coli* strain Nissle 1917 has shown to benefit patients and maintain remission. Some gastroenterologists would consider using this probiotic strain as an alternative in patients who are intolerant or resistant to standard 5-aminosalicylic acid (5-ASA) preparations, the current first-line therapy in patients with UC. To date, no other probiotic preparation has been validated for this indication. A benefit of probiotics remains unproven for CD.

Did You Know?

IBD Factors

There are many factors that may lead to the development of IBD, including genetic factors, environmental factors (like diet) and abnormalities in the immune system.

Irritable Bowel Syndrome

There is mounting evidence to show that probiotics may benefit those with irritable bowel syndrome (IBS), although there is still debate as to which agent or group of probiotics is most beneficial. Patients with IBS may experience constipation, diarrhea or an alternating pattern between the two that brings on abdominal cramping or bloating.

There are many other conditions that can mimic IBS, and these may need to be ruled out before confirming an IBS diagnosis.

Managing IBS symptoms can often be challenging and may involve dietary modifications, stress management and easing the sensitivity of nerves that may be overactive. Medications in the treatment of IBS are often not effective. A number of research studies show that probiotics improved IBS in some patients; in particular, they reduced abdominal bloating and gas and helped with diarrhea symptoms. One particular study saw reductions in overall symptoms and improvement in quality of life.

Did You Know?

Mysterious Origins

IBS is a very common bowel disorder, but there is no identifiable disease or gut abnormality to account for its symptoms.

Doc Talk

In my practice, I see up to 25 patients a month with IBS. Inevitably, I typically recommend probiotics to most of these patients. Surprisingly, most people who suffer from IBS are already quite aware of probiotics and have either tried them or continue to use them in some capacity. However, there remains significant confusion regarding the probiotic strain to take and the duration of use. I usually recommend *Bifidobacterium infantis* (trade name Align), one capsule daily. For best results, the probiotic needs to be used every day, without missing doses. I also find the probiotic *Lactobacillus plantarum* (trade name Tuzen) effective in IBS.

Given the best evidence for these two probiotics, I typically limit my suggestions to these two strains. So when my patients report to me that they have tried other preparations purchased from a health food or grocery store, what do I generally advise? First, I inquire about their symptoms since starting the probiotic and ask about other lifestyle changes they may have made. I then assess the magnitude of symptom improvement compared to the usual burden of symptoms. If symptoms persist with significant severity, resulting in limitations and an impact on the patient's quality of life, I typically suggest discontinuing the current probiotic and replacing it with either *Bifidobacterium infantis* or *Lactobacillus plantarum* for a 6-week trial — while strongly encouraging dietary modifications and a focus on probiotic-rich foods.

Stomach Ulcers

Many of you are likely familiar with stomach ulcers. The most common types of ulcers typically seen by gastroenterologists in routine clinical practice are stomach ulcers and duodenal (small intestinal) ulcers. People with ulcers generally have symptoms of abdominal pain and it is usually localized to the upper part of the stomach. The pain may feel like a burning or hunger type of pain. Ulcers may also bleed, resulting in black, tarry, liquid stools. In addition, people may experience symptoms of nausea and vomiting, and may even vomit old blood that looks like coffee grinds. In less common situations, bright red blood is visible in the stool, and patients may feel weak, dizzy or light-headed. This is a medical emergency, likely an ulcer that is bleeding quite rapidly.

Did You Know?

Causes of Ulcers

The most common cause of ulcers is a bacterium called *Helicobacter pylori* (*H. pylori*). Contrary to popular belief, ulcers are not caused by stress or too much coffee or spicy foods.

Treating Stomach Ulcers

Stress or too much coffee or spicy foods may worsen the symptoms associated with ulcers but are not causative of ulcers in any way. The *H. pylori* bacterium was discovered in 1982 by two Australian scientists who later won the Nobel

Prize for their discovery. Many people carry this bacterium in their stomach and up to 20% of people with *H. pylori* develop ulcers as a consequence; the vast majority don't experience any symptoms. This bacterium is known to cause stomach cancer. Therefore, medical doctors usually recommend treating *H. pylori* once it is identified.

The standard treatment choices for *H. pylori* are two types of antibiotics, plus an acid-suppressive medication known as a proton-pump inhibitor (PPI). The most common prescribed first-line antibiotics are amoxicillin and clarithromycin, to be taken twice daily for 10 days. In people with a penicillin allergy, which is common, metronidazole (Flagyl) can be substituted for amoxicillin. In many areas of the world, however, resistance to standard antibiotics is a big problem. This means that the bacterium is resistant to the actions of the antibiotics, and standard treatments will not be successful in killing the bacterium. Therefore, a number of second-line regimens are also used. But these regimens are often tough for people to tolerate because of their many side effects, including nausea, vomiting and abdominal discomfort. Consequently, many patients often do not complete the second-line course of treatment, resulting in unsuccessful treatment of the *H. pylori* bacterium.

> In many areas of the world, resistance to standard antibiotics is a big problem. This means that the bacterium is resistant to the actions of the antibiotics, and standard treatments will not be successful in killing the bacterium.

Probiotics with Antibiotics for *Helicobacter Pylori* Treatment

Probiotics have been shown to be useful additions or adjuncts to improve tolerability and compliance with traditional antibiotic regimens. *Saccharomyces boulardii*, a probiotic used in the treatment of *C. diff* diarrhea, has been studied in the treatment of *H. pylori*. In a study involving more than 1,300 patients, *S. boulardii* administered along with standard therapies increased the eradication rates of *H. pylori* while decreasing therapy-related adverse effects.

Another study assessed the effect of standard antibiotics along with yogurt containing the *Lactobacillus gasseri* probiotic strain. In this study, 86% of patients who received the yogurt plus antibiotics successfully eradicated *H. pylori*, compared to 69% of people who received antibiotics alone. The study authors concluded that the major cause of treatment failure was resistance of the bacterium to one of the antibiotics, clarithromycin, and that the yogurt addition was instrumental in treating the *H. pylori*.

Probiotics in the Treatment of Non-GI Conditions

There are a number of non-GI medical conditions that benefit from probiotics. Urinary tract infections and bacterial vaginosis are two examples. The theory for the efficacy of probiotics in these conditions has to do with gut bacteria migrating or translocating to cause disease. Both have excellent responses to probiotic therapies.

Urinary Tract Infections

The urinary tract comprises the kidneys, ureter, bladder and urethra. The kidney is the workhorse of the urinary tract and is responsible for filtering toxins and providing clean blood to the rest of the body. The urine, which consists of waste products, then moves down the ureter and is stored in the bladder. Once the bladder is full, urine is excreted through the urethra.

Most urinary tract infections (UTIs) are, in fact, infections of the bladder, not the kidney. A bladder infection in adults is usually not serious if it is diagnosed and treated quickly. But if it is not addressed in a timely manner, it may travel into the

Symptoms of Urinary Tract Infections

- Burning with urination
- Frequent need to urinate
- Urgent need to urinate
- Blood in the urine
- Lower abdominal pain
- Incomplete emptying of the bladder
- Fever
- Chills

Using probiotics to manage urinary infections is a treatment supported by increasing clinical evidence and for a growing number of probiotic strains.

kidneys. A kidney infection can be quite serious and can cause permanent damage. Women are more predisposed to bladder infections than men because of a shorter urethra; bacteria have less distance to travel in a short urethra, increasing the possibility of a bladder infection.

Typical symptoms of a UTI include burning with urinating, urinating frequently, the need to urinate urgently and sometimes bleeding with urinating. Additional symptoms may include lower abdominal pain and a sense of incomplete emptying of the bladder. In serious circumstances, patients may experience a fever, along with chills or sweats. Diabetes increases the risk of urinary infections.

A urine sample is taken to confirm the diagnosis of a UTI — a positive result indicates the growth of bacteria. Antibiotics may be prescribed by your doctor as a first-line therapy. To treat the infection, doctors often prescribe antibiotics, with the type of antibiotic and the duration of treatment in part dependent on the patient's gender and other risk factors.

Since many women will experience more than one UTI, repeated exposure to antibiotics is a concern. Preventive strategies, such as using lower-dose antibiotics daily, may result in adverse antibiotic-related side effects, antibiotic resistance and even *C. diff* colitis. Therefore, women are increasingly looking for safe and effective alternatives. Using probiotics to manage urinary infections is a treatment supported by increasing clinical evidence and for a growing number of probiotic strains. Research shows a link between the loss of normal genital microbiota, particularly *Lactobacillus* species, and UTIs, and several in vitro studies have confirmed that *Lactobacillus* species inhibit the growth of *Escherichia coli* (*E. coli*), a common bug causing UTIs.

A Finnish study showed that women who consumed fermented milk products containing probiotic bacteria more than three times a week had a decrease in recurrent UTIs. More recently, in a U.S. study of 100 young women who experienced recurrent UTIs, a vaginal suppository containing *Lactobacillus* was inserted daily for 5 days, followed by a maintenance dose of once weekly for 10 weeks, and the researchers found that the regimen was superior in preventing further infections compared to women who did not receive the probiotics. When choosing a probiotic supplement, the best evidence for UTIs appears to be *Lactobacillus* species, in the magnitude of 10^9 CFUs.

UTIs and Diet

Background: Because UTIs are caused by bacteria from the stool that come in contact with a part of the urinary tract, dietary factors may affect the risk of contracting a UTI.

Objective: To study dietary factors for developing UTIs in women.

Methods: One hundred thirty-nine women with a diagnosis of UTI were compared with a similar number of women with no episodes of UTIs. Data on dietary intake were collected by questionnaire.

Results: Frequent consumption of fresh juices, especially berry juices, and fermented milk products containing probiotic bacteria was associated with a decreased risk of UTI, by 34%. Consumption of fermented milk products three times a week or more lowered the risk of UTIs significantly.

Conclusions: Dietary habits are an important risk factor in UTIs, and dietary guidance could be a first step toward prevention.

Bacterial Vaginosis

Bacterial vaginosis (BV) is an infection caused by an imbalance of bacteria in the vagina, commonly experienced by younger women of childbearing age. In BV, less desirable bacteria overgrow and crowd out the naturally occurring vaginal bacteria. Bacterial vaginosis tends to resolve on its own after a few days without any specific therapy. However, the symptoms can be cumbersome, and in certain cases, it may lead to more serious problems. The most common symptom of BV is a foul-smelling vaginal discharge, sometimes with a "fishy" smell, often worse following sexual intercourse. The diagnosis is confirmed following a sample collection of the vaginal discharge.

> **Did You Know?**
>
> **No Therapy Required**
> Up to one-third of cases of bacterial vaginosis may resolve on their own.

Antibiotics, usually first metronidazole (Flagyl), are the recommended treatment for BV. Sometimes antibiotics are ineffective and many women have high recurrence rates following treatment. In fact, one study showed that in the majority of women with BV, the most common bacteria causing the condition, *Gardnerella vaginalis*, was still present in the vaginal lining despite treatment with metronidazole.

The vaginal flora of healthy women is generally dominated by *Lactobacillus* species. Factors influencing the vaginal flora include hormonal changes (with menopause), vaginal pH and

A Possible Role for Probiotics in the Treatment of Autism

Autism is a neurodevelopmental disorder characterized by impaired social interactions and communication and restricted and repetitive behavior, and is frequently accompanied by digestive disorders. Since the original description of autism in 1943, its prevalence has exploded from 1 in 5,000 people to 1 in 68! While the cause of the prevalence is not entirely clear, there is speculation that factors involving the mother's immunity, environmental toxicity during the prenatal period or abnormalities of metabolic function may contribute toward the development of autism.

Interest in the gastrointestinal tract and dietary contributions to autism is not entirely new, as a growing medical community reports a higher incidence of gastrointestinal symptoms in children with autism. This area has been tougher to explore because recognizing gastrointestinal symptoms and other medical problems may be difficult in individuals with limited verbal capacity.

The development of the gut microbiome begins even before birth and continues during the first 3 years of life. There are differences that occur in the microbiome based on infant nutrition — the microbiome of breast-fed infants compared to formula-fed infants is different. Around the age of 3, the child's microbiome is similar to that seen in adulthood. Because children are typically diagnosed with autism between ages 1 and 3, the parallel in timing suggests that more research is worth exploring between the developing microbiome and the immune system.

Several research teams have studied the intestinal microbes in the autistic population and have found consistent differences in the composition of the microbiome compared to healthy control subjects. For example, compared to healthy children, children with autism have been found to have 10 times more *Clostridium*-class bacteria, in addition to other observed bacterial differences. Interestingly, in one study, antibiotic treatment in autistic children improved intestinal symptoms and cognitive skills.

A recent report in the prestigious journal *Cell* describes the improvement in a mouse model of autism when the animals were treated with the natural microbe *Bacteroides fragilis*, inhabiting the gut. It suggests a possible role for probiotic therapies in autism. In this study, gut leakiness was corrected and symptoms related to communication and anxiety improved.

Since microbiome interactions with the brain are a potentiating factor for autism, therapeutic interventions aimed at the microbiome may be of value. Diets that include prebiotics and probiotics and that facilitate the growth of health-promoting bacteria may all have value.

We are at the very early stages of understanding the effect of the microbiome in individuals with autism. We now have the technology to begin accurately identifying microbial species and assessing the functions of these bacterial species as they specifically relate to autism and other psychiatric disorders. Over the next decade, it is likely that researchers will capitalize on these early signals and explore the microbiome in psychiatry in more detail.

the use of antimicrobial agents. Probiotics can play a protective role. Clinical trials have studied their effects when taken in either oral form or by intravaginal application. Two excellent-quality research studies have confirmed that *Lactobacillus rhamnosus* plus *Lactobacillus reuteri* in doses of 1×10^9 CFUs a day substantially improved BV symptoms compared to patients who did not receive any therapy. A large group of women with BV who took the same probiotic combination had normal vaginal tests, indicating that BV was treated successfully, compared to women who did not take any probiotic.

Doc Talk

From my perspective, the combination of probiotics with standard antibiotics is likely to have greater value in treating BV successfully compared to antibiotics alone. Moreover, probiotics may also prevent recurrence in women with BV, improving quality of life. While promising, the data are split between different routes of administration (oral versus intravaginal) and among different strains. Although diet has not been formally evaluated when treating BV, I believe that dietary choices rich in probiotics will compound the beneficial effects of supplements.

The Safety of Probiotics

Probiotics have a long history of safety with their established use in fermented food and milk. What's more reassuring is that these bacteria are frequently encountered in nature: they naturally reside in plants, animals and humans. It is important to note, however, that probiotics are regulated as foods, not drugs. Therefore, they are not subject to the same level of scrutiny as drug monitoring and are not required to demonstrate their safety. Just the same, probiotics are considered safe for the vast majority of the population.

Risks of Probiotic Use

There are different theoretical risks related to the use of probiotics. The most important is infections due to the movement of probiotic bacteria. A probiotic bacterium may move from the digestive tract to other sites within the body where it is not usually found and, subsequently, cause

> **Future Clinical Applications of Probiotics**
> - Alcoholic liver disease
> - Cancer prevention
> - Diabetes
> - Graft versus host disease
> - Rheumatoid arthritis

infection. But this is a rare occurrence and is typically confined to cases that involve patients who have suppressed immune systems — their immune system is not functioning normally — or hospitalized patients with catheters. Catheters pose a risk for infection, which can be magnified. People with healthy immune systems and without catheters should not face any infectious complications during probiotic use. Patients with active cancer who are receiving chemotherapy or taking medications that lower the function of the immune system should discuss the risks with their doctor before taking probiotics.

> ➤ Research Spotlight

Diabetes and the Microbiome

Background: Changes in the microbiome and the interaction between the microbiome and human genes have been linked to diabetes.

Objective: To explore the possible connection between changes in the microbiome and type 1 diabetes.

Methods: Thirty-three infants who were genetically predisposed to type 1 diabetes were followed over 3 years by researchers. The research team regularly analyzed the infants' stool samples, collecting data on the composition of their gut microbiomes.

Results: In the handful of babies who developed type 1 diabetes, there was a sharp decline in the types of bacteria seen in the gut. There was also a decrease in the bacteria known to regulate health and an increase in potentially harmful bacteria known to promote inflammation.

Conclusions: By revealing patterns in the development of the microbiome in healthy individuals and in those susceptible to developing type 1 diabetes, it will become possible to guide future diagnoses and therapies.

CHAPTER 4

The Impact of Fiber on Gut Microbiota

📁 Case Study

Colon Cancer and Fiber

Jun is a 42-year-old physiotherapist who has been interested in a holistic approach to health and wellness for the majority of her adult life. She came to see me to discuss screening for colorectal cancer, since there was a family history of the disease. Her father was diagnosed with colon cancer at the age of 45. While discussing the screening strategies for colon cancer, she had many questions regarding the role of fiber in cancer protection. Jun was aware of the various forms of dietary fiber, and in particular was quite interested in learning more about the new kid on the block, prebiotic fibers, and their role in health maintenance and disease prevention. She has been committed to a lifestyle of healthy dietary choices and is interested in maximizing this strategy.

Jun does not have any specific GI symptoms. In particular, she denies abdominal pain, cramping, blood in bowel movements and any change in her bowel movements. She is at a healthy weight and does not drink alcohol. She attempts to exercise three times a week. In fact, Jun was so motivated to identify further opportunity to optimize her diet that she brought in a food diary for me to review.

I reassured Jun that she was clearly on the right track to reaching her goal of maintaining health and preventing disease. I told her that a colonoscopy was the gold standard for diagnosing colon polyps, which are the precursor to developing colon cancer, and that even people with no symptoms can have colon polyps and colon cancer. She agreed to proceed with a colonoscopy, given her family history. I was impressed with the amount of detail in her 3-day food diary — she ate three meals and one snack daily. Each meal contained fiber from grains, fruits or vegetables. I was impressed with her daily fiber intake of almost 25 grams, which is right on target — in fact, it's outstanding, given that the majority of North Americans eat only between 10 and 15 grams of fiber a day (see "How Much Fiber Should I Eat?" page 59). I encouraged her to continue with her current efforts.

What Is Fiber?

The term "dietary fiber" originated in 1953, but the health benefits of high-fiber foods have long been appreciated. In 430 BC, Hippocrates, the father of Western medicine, described the laxative effects of coarse wheat compared with refined wheat. Over the decades, other noteworthy individuals described the association between fiber and disease prevention. In particular, fiber-rich diets have been credited with protecting against chronic diseases (including diabetes), cardiovascular diseases, colon cancer and obesity. Now, in the 21st century, fiber has resurged as a potential champion for health maintenance and disease prevention, albeit through novel associations involving the shaping of the gut microbiome.

Fiber in the Gut

Dietary fiber is primarily derived from plant material and is composed of complex non-starch carbohydrates that are not digested in the small intestine. As a result, these compounds pass uninterrupted into the colon, where they are available for fermentation by the bacteria that reside there. Dietary fiber is not believed to contribute calories or energy to our diet — at least this has been the long-standing teaching imparted to doctors and health-care professionals for decades. However, what is often not taken into consideration is the impact of fermentation on fiber in the colon. When fiber ferments in the colon, metabolites are released, often resulting in fatty acids, which get reabsorbed and become a source of calories. This is a finer point that many doctors are increasingly starting to appreciate.

Fiber-rich diets have been credited with protecting against chronic diseases (including diabetes), cardiovascular diseases, colon cancer and obesity.

Fiber has long been linked to better health, but new research now shows how the gut microbes might play a role in this benefit. For example, one study showed that adding more fiber to the diet can trigger a shift from a microbiome linked to obesity to one correlated with a leaner body type. In fact, one researcher claimed that "diet is one of the most powerful tools we have for changing the microbiota." Another researcher concluded that "dietary fiber and diversity of the microbes complement each other for better health outcomes." When fiber reaches the colon, it is ready to be devoured by the resident microbes, which extract extra energy from fiber as well as nutrients, vitamins and additional compounds. In particular, a group of fatty acids called short-chain fatty acids are of particular interest — they have long been linked to improving immunity and decreasing inflammation, as discussed earlier. Therefore, the dietary potential to impact the microbiome is immense.

Research led by a group in Michigan demonstrated that mice that were fed a high-fiber diet had a healthy gut lining, while mice on a fiber-free diet had a lining layer that dramatically diminished. Because the gut's lining is critical as a layer of defense against bacteria escaping from the colon and into the bloodstream, it appears that fiber should be incorporated into the diet to decrease risk of infection.

> ### ➢ Research Spotlight

Whole Grains and Healthy Bacteria

Background: Consuming whole grains reduces the risk of major chronic diseases. It is not entirely clear how whole grains exert their beneficial impact.

Objective: To measure the impact of whole grains on the gut microbiome.

Methods: Two specific diets of either whole-grain oats or low-bran oats were administered to mice for 8 weeks.

Results: The weight gain observed was 15% less in the whole-grain oats group compared to the low-bran oats group. There was a significant increase in certain beneficial bacterial families, such as *Lactobacillus* and *Prevotella* strains. These microbial findings also showed an improved sensitivity to insulin — which may reduce the risk of developing diabetes — in the whole-grain group. *Lactobacillus* levels were two times higher in the whole-grain group compared to the low-bran group.

Conclusions: *Lactobacillus* is known for its numerous health benefits and may be linked to the benefits of a high-fiber diet.

How Much Fiber Should I Eat?

The majority of people living in industrialized nations don't eat enough fiber daily. Most commonly consumed foods are low in dietary fiber. Generally, foods that are a "source of fiber" will provide 2 to 3 grams of fiber per serving. The average North American typically consumes 10 to 15 grams of fiber daily — well short of the 25 to 35 grams of fiber recommended. Flours, grains and potatoes are the most popular sources of fiber in the American diet, while fruits, legumes and nuts are the least popular sources.

The recommended amounts of fiber are needed to regulate bowel movements, among other health benefits described earlier. If you are not eating enough fiber and are keen on doing so, ramp up your fiber intake slowly. Adding large amounts of fiber-rich foods to your diet all at once may cause abdominal cramping, bloating and perhaps some diarrhea. When you make this adjustment more gradually, your intestines will love you, rather than scream in distress.

Forms of Fiber

Dietary fiber comes in two forms: soluble and insoluble. Most sources of fiber include both soluble and insoluble fibers, although one type of fiber may predominate. Dietary fiber is found mainly in fruits, vegetables, whole-grain products, legumes, nuts and seeds.

Dietary fiber, usually insoluble fiber, is also known as roughage or bulk and includes all the parts of plant foods that your body cannot digest or absorb. In contrast, soluble fibers can be found in some vegetables, fruits and legumes. When water is added to soluble fiber, the fiber thickens into a gel consistency, contributing to many health benefits (see "Benefits of a High-Fiber Diet," page 63).

Unlike other food components such as fats, proteins and carbohydrates, fiber cannot be broken down and absorbed by your body. Fiber passes relatively intact through your stomach, small intestine and colon. It plays many important roles in maintaining health, such as preventing constipation and diarrhea.

Soluble fibers not only help slow digestion but also lower blood cholesterol, control blood sugar levels and reduce IBS symptoms.

Soluble Fiber

Soluble fiber slows down the rate at which food travels through your gut and it increases water absorption in the colon by fecal matter. This action encourages the formation of thickened, gel-like stools while reducing diarrhea. The absorptive properties of soluble fiber also allow the passage of softer, gel-like waste, which softens and encourages the excretion of impacted stool. Soluble fibers not only help slow digestion but also lower blood cholesterol, control blood sugar levels and reduce IBS symptoms.

Fruits and vegetables high in soluble fiber are listed in the table below. People should aim for 10 grams of soluble fiber daily.

Top 10 Soluble Fiber Food Sources

Food Source	Serving Size	Soluble Fiber (grams)
Passion fruit, purple, fresh	$1/2$ cup (125 mL)	6.5
Black beans, cooked	$3/4$ cup (175 mL)	5.4
Lima beans, cooked	$3/4$ cup (175 mL)	5.3
Soy nuts, roasted	$1/4$ cup (60 mL)	3.5
Navy beans, cooked	$3/4$ cup (175 mL)	3.3
Pinto beans, cooked	$3/4$ cup (175 mL)	3.2
Kidney beans, cooked	$3/4$ cup (175 mL)	2.6 to 3.0
Tofu, cooked	5 oz (150 g)	2.8
Bran buds with psyllium	$1/3$ cup (75 mL)	2.7
Beans, canned, with pork and tomato sauce	$3/4$ cup (175 mL)	2.6

Soluble Fiber Supplements

Food is not the only source of beneficial soluble fiber. Over-the-counter soluble fiber supplements are usually made from psyllium (for example, Metamucil) or inulin (for example, Benefibre). Marketers claim the tasteless and odorless supplements can be added to an endless array of foods and beverages, with minimal impact on the consumer.

Guidelines for Taking Soluble Fiber Supplements

1. *When incorporating fiber supplements into your diet, increase the amount gradually.* Despite what package directions recommend, begin with just 1 teaspoon (5 mL) a day for 1 week. After your intestine has adjusted to this dose, gradually increase the frequency of the supplement to twice daily for 1 week, and so on until you reach the maximum recommended dose. If you immediately take them as recommended in the product directions, the supplements can increase your symptoms of gas, bloating, flatulence and abdominal cramping.

Did You Know?

Gradual Doses

A common mistake when starting to take fiber supplements is to start off with a large dose instead of beginning gradually.

2. *Take fiber supplements with adequate water intake.* Aim to drink 6 to 8 glasses of water a day. Water should not be confused with other liquids. Caffeinated liquids have diuretic properties and may serve to dehydrate more than hydrate.

3. *Be patient.* It will take a little while before you see the effects of the supplement, so don't give up if you don't feel better after a few days. It may take 2 to 4 weeks to fully experience the positive side effects of fiber supplementation.

FAQ

 Is taking fiber supplements a good strategy to maintain good health?

 Unequivocally, obtaining fiber through natural sources is the preferred strategy. Besides the fiber content, whole foods also provide other nutrients, such as antioxidants, vitamins, minerals and electrolytes. When you choose fiber-rich foods, you are also cutting down your consumption of harmful foods like simple sugars, high-fat options and processed foods. Relying on fiber supplements to achieve fiber targets deprives you of the opportunity to make healthy food choices and develop habits that help to better manage your health. Nonetheless, fiber supplements offer some benefits, in particular for those who suffer from the common GI symptoms of diarrhea and constipation. Fiber supplements may also be used to help lower cholesterol and maintain more stable blood sugars.

Common Commercial Fiber Supplements

All these supplements are rich sources of soluble fibers and function in a very similar manner. The fiber source in Benefibre is unique — inulin is a prebiotic fiber, which has been shown to have a unique effect on the gut microbiome.

Product	Type of Fiber
Benefibre	Inulin
Konsyl	Psyllium
Metamucil	Psyllium
Normacol	Sterculia
Prodiem	Methylcellulose

Insoluble Fiber

Unlike soluble fiber, insoluble fiber does not dissolve in water. It helps bowel regularity and maintains a healthy digestive system by attracting fluid into the small intestine so stool moves more quickly throughout the intestine. Generally, fruits and vegetables contain both soluble and insoluble fiber, but the part of a plant food that is rough in texture or stringy or the tough skin or outer peel is, in fact, the insoluble fiber portion. Rich sources of insoluble fiber include the bran of whole grains, nuts, seeds, and the skins or peels of fruits and vegetables.

Benefits of a High-Fiber Diet

Increased fiber intake reduces the formation of diverticula, which are pockets of weakness in the large intestine that can perforate, burst or bleed, leading to severe abdominal pain and infection within the abdomen.

The benefits of a diet rich in fiber are numerous, including its effect on the motility of the gut and its influence on metabolic benefits, such as strengthening the barrier in the colon, increasing beneficial short-chain fatty acids and improving immunity — all of which are facilitated through the gut microbes. Here is more detail about certain benefits.

Normalizes Bowel Movements

Dietary fiber increases the weight and size of your bowel movement and softens it. A bulky stool is easier to pass and reduces the risk of straining and pushing. This limits your risk of developing painful hemorrhoids, which may bleed. Increased fiber intake also reduces the formation of diverticula, which are pockets of weakness in the large intestine that can perforate, burst or bleed, leading to severe abdominal pain and infection within the abdomen. In people who suffer from looser stools or diarrhea, dietary fiber often provides relief because it helps to solidify the stool by absorbing water and adding bulk.

Lowers Blood Cholesterol Levels and Blood Pressure

Soluble fibers, such as those found in beans, oats, oat bran and flax seeds, may help lower total blood cholesterol levels by altering low-density lipoprotein (LDL), or "bad," cholesterol levels. Medical studies have shown a link between increased fiber in the diet and a reduction in blood pressure, which is protective of heart health.

Controls Blood Sugar Levels

Fiber, in particular soluble fiber, can slow the absorption of sugar from recently consumed food. In people who suffer from diabetes, this is great news, since blood sugar levels are better controlled when fiber is incorporated into the diet. Studies show fiber is associated with the prevention of type 2 diabetes.

Encourages Weight Loss

High-fiber foods are known to slow the passage of food and fluid through the stomach. This means that fiber-rich foods sit in your stomach slightly longer than other types of foods. When food stays in your stomach longer, there is a sense of fullness or satiety, tricking the brain into believing that you are not hungry. You stay satisfied or full for a greater period of time, reducing the amount of food and calories consumed. Essentially, you minimize the risk of overeating. Fiber-rich foods are generally less "energy-dense" — that is, they have fewer calories for the same volume or portion of food eaten, leading to a more optimal weight.

> Fiber-rich foods are generally less "energy-dense" – that is, they have fewer calories for the same volume or portion of food eaten, leading to a more optimal weight.

What Are Prebiotic Fibers?

Prebiotics are natural non-digestible carbohydrate fibers that change the bacterial composition in the intestine. Prebiotic fibers differ from other fiber sources — medical studies have shown they alter the composition of gut bacteria in a positive way.

We have already discussed fiber in detail, and hopefully the rationale for increasing dietary fiber intake is compelling. Researchers and doctors now understand that certain fibers, such as prebiotic fibers, have unique properties. Not all dietary fibers have "prebiotic potential," or the prebiotic effect, which occurs when a prebiotic-rich food is metabolized in the gut to selectively grow beneficial bacteria in the colon. Other foods, such as probiotics and fermented foods, can achieve the same result. The combined therapeutic approach of optimizing prebiotic fibers and probiotics contributes to the power of altering the microbiome and, therefore, health in a very positive way.

Did You Know?

Prebiotic vs. Probiotic Recap

Prebiotics are non-digestible carbohydrate fibers that influence the composition of gut bacteria in a positive way. Probiotics, which primarily come from fermented foods, are live bacteria that can selectively alter the gut environment to create a beneficial bacterial milieu.

Features of Prebiotics

Prebiotics such as garlic, chicory root, leeks, asparagus and onions, just to name a few, contribute to a gut-friendly microbiome. Prebiotics help grow good bacteria that remain in the gut. Although both insoluble and soluble fibers have many beneficial properties, not all fibers impact the gut bacteria in the same manner. Prebiotics display the following features:

1. *Have an ability to resist stomach acid.* Many substances cannot survive the strong acid environment of the stomach. Therefore, for a substance to pass into the intestines and escape the stomach unchanged, it has to be fairly resilient. To be called a prebiotic, the ingredient must not be absorbed in the upper GI tract and must pass into the colon unchanged.

2. *Are fermented by the intestinal bacteria.* Because fibers are not digested by the small intestine, they pass uninterrupted into the large intestine or colon. The bacteria in the colon then act on the undigested fiber to ferment it. The end products of this fermentation process include fatty acids, vitamins, minerals and energy.

3. *Selectively stimulate the growth and activity of good intestinal bacteria.* Prebiotics encourage certain beneficial bacteria, such as *Lactobacillus*, *Bifidobacterium* and *Faecalibacterium*.

> Prebiotics help grow good bacteria that remain in the gut.

> ➤ Research Spotlight

Prebiotics and Obesity

Background: There is a growing interest in modulating gut microbes using diet to measure its effect on obesity.

Objective: To evaluate the effect of prebiotics (inulin and oligofructose) on the gut microbiome.

Methods: Lean and obese male rats were randomly assigned to various doses of prebiotic fibers. Gut microbiota were measured.

Results: *Bifidobacterium* and *Lactobacillus* increased in the obese high-fiber group compared to the low-fiber group. Microbial species in the Bacteroidetes division decreased, whereas Firmicutes increased in rats exposed to high fiber intake.

Conclusions: Prebiotics alter the gut microbiota in a favorable manner and the efficacy is dependent on dosing.

The History of Prebiotics

The concept of prebiotics is relatively new, although foods rich in prebiotic content have been consumed since prehistoric times. Analyses of well-preserved stool samples from tens of thousands of years ago suggest that dietary intake of prebiotic foods was about 135 grams a day, primarily reflecting a rich consumption of fruits, vegetables, nuts and seeds, as prehistoric times would have demanded. Contrast this to the typical American and European dietary consumption of prebiotic fibers, which amounts to only a few grams a day.

In societies that consume large amounts of fiber, many common GI illnesses are minimized. The underlying mechanisms of prebiotics were not explored until the mid-1990s, when the concept gained popularity among researchers.

Modern Prebiotics: Diet vs. Supplements

The intake of prebiotics is achieved primarily through diet, and it is preferred over supplements. Good-quality prebiotic supplements may be challenging to find, expensive for the consumer and devoid of many other nutrients that tend to accompany fiber-rich foods. Adopting a varied fiber-rich diet will ensure the intake of adequate prebiotics and other nutrient requirements.

An important function for dietary fiber and prebiotics is fermentation in the colon. Recent research showing the health-promoting properties of certain gut microorganisms has encouraged dietary-based strategies to improve the composition and function of gut bacteria. In most countries, prebiotics are accepted as naturally occurring food substances that exert many benefits, similar to prescription medication. Many foods contain small amounts of prebiotics (the list of prebiotic-containing foods is extensive; see the top 10 prebiotic fiber–containing foods, page 108).

Research studies evaluating prebiotics are limited — to date they have used only a powder-based supplement with one of the two major classes of prebiotics: fructo-oligosaccharides (FOS) and galacto-oligosaccharides (GOS). Inulin is the best known type of FOS and has been the most studied. Therefore, since knowledge is limited to the effect of only these two prebiotic supplements, they are the ones most recommended. Most of the prebiotic fibers outlined in the following table fall into one of these two classes.

> Good-quality prebiotic supplements may be challenging to find, expensive for the consumer and devoid of many other nutrients that tend to accompany fiber-rich foods.

Fiber Sources with Prebiotic Effects

Prebiotic Food Source	Prebiotic Effects
Acacia gum	Increases *Bifidobacterium*
Banana	Increases *Bifidobacterium*
Galacto-oligosaccharide (GOS)	Increases *Bifidobacterium*
Inulin	Increases *Bifidobacterium*
Polydextrose	Increases *Bifidobacterium*
Psyllium	Prebiotic potential
Wheat dextrin	Decreases disease-producing bacteria

> ➤ Research Spotlight

Healthy Colons

Background: Change in the gut microbiome could help distinguish individuals with healthy colons from those with either colon polyps (benign growths in the colon) or colon cancer. Changes in gut microbiome between these groups of patients may be a marker for colon cancer, which is the second leading cause of cancer-related deaths in North America.

Objective: To characterize the gut microbiome in three groups of patients: healthy patients, those with colon polyps and those with colon cancer.

Methods: Patients had a colonoscopy (direct examination of the bowel assessing for polyps and cancer). Stool samples were also collected to conduct DNA analysis and gene sequencing.

Results: Individuals with healthy colons had a different gut microbiome than those with polyps and cancers. Larger amounts of the species *Fusobacterium* were seen on the surface of tumors compared with healthy tissue, suggesting that *Fusobacterium* may be a marker for the presence of tumors.

Conclusions: These findings could be important in preventing colon cancer in situations where access to a colonoscopy procedure may be limited, and may provide an alternative to colonoscopy in detecting the early changes of colon cancer.

Effects of Prebiotic Fibers

Prebiotic fibers provide a number of health benefits by altering the composition of the intestinal flora. Currently, there is no consensus regarding an ideal daily serving of prebiotics; however, recommendations range from 3 to 8 grams a day to support good digestive health, and more than 15 grams for those with an active digestive disorder. Total dietary fiber intake should range between 25 and 35 grams a day, depending on age and gender.

Increase Healthy Flora

Prebiotic fibers increase the growth of the two most important gut bacteria to human health, *Bifidobacterium* and *Lactobacillus*. Prebiotics have been shown to increase *Bifidobacterium* content in the stool even when ingested in relatively low doses.

Produce Short-Chain Fatty Acids

Some fermentable fibers, such as psyllium, that don't officially meet the definition for prebiotics still provide health benefits by producing short-chain fatty acids (SCFAs). As previously discussed, the three most abundant SCFAs are acetate, propionate and butyrate, each of which produces unique effects that are important for health. For colonic health, butyrate is the most important, since the colon relies on it for energy (see FAQ, page 25). Butyrate also helps decrease inflammation, improves immunity and may be protective against certain cancers.

Certain fibers have been shown to interact with immune cells, stimulating the immune system directly.

Improve Immune Protection

Some fibers that produce SCFAs may also play a role in improving the immune system. In animal-based studies, adding SCFAs to food improves immune function by increasing the number of white blood cells fighting infections. There is also some evidence of increased resistance to illness and infection with fiber intake. For example, foods with oligofructose, a type of inulin fiber, were found to reduce the frequency of fevers and severe infectious complications associated with diarrhea and respiratory illnesses. Certain fibers have been shown to interact with immune cells, stimulating the immune system directly.

Health Benefits of Prebiotics

- Reduce the prevalence and duration of infections
- Reduce the frequency of antibiotic-associated diarrhea
- Improve the symptoms associated with irritable bowel syndrome
- Exert protective effects to prevent colon cancer by enhancing butyrate production
- Enhance the availability and absorption of essential minerals, such as calcium, magnesium and possibly iron
- Lower the risk factors predisposing toward heart disease
- Improve satiety, thereby decreasing appetite, promoting weight loss and preventing obesity

Treating Disease with Prebiotics

With the knowledge that prebiotic intake produces desirable bacteria, let's examine the role and function of prebiotics in diseases.

Infectious Diarrhea

One traveler's-diarrhea study examined the effect of using 10 grams a day of inulin for 2 weeks before and during travel to a high- or medium-risk destination. The study concluded that this strategy reduced the frequency and severity of diarrhea. Another study using galacto-oligosaccharides replicated these positive findings.

Did You Know?

Prebiotics When Traveling

Consider taking inulin before and during travel. The strategy may be the most natural way of replicating the powerful results of drug-based strategies that prevent diarrhea or limit its severity — without the fear of side effects.

➤ Research Spotlight

Limiting Traveler's Diarrhea

Background: Prebiotics are known for their ability to positively affect the gut microbiome, therefore increasing resistance to infection and diarrheal illness.

Objective: To assess the impact of a prebiotic galacto-oligosaccharide mixture on the severity and incidence of traveler's diarrhea.

Methods: The study involved 159 healthy patients who traveled to a country that was known to be either medium- or high-risk for traveler's diarrhea. Subjects received either prebiotic intervention or a placebo.

Continued on next page...

Results: There was a significant reduction in the incidence and duration of traveler's diarrhea in subjects receiving the prebiotic. Diarrhea duration for the prebiotic group compared to the control group was 2.4 days compared to 4.6 days. Similarly, symptoms of abdominal pain were reduced in the prebiotic group. Duration of abdominal pain in the prebiotic group compared to the control group was 2.0 days compared to 3.5 days.

Conclusions: Consumption of the prebiotic mixture showed significant potential for reducing the incidence and symptoms of traveler's diarrhea.

Irritable Bowel Syndrome

Irritable bowel syndrome (IBS) is an extremely common disorder, affecting more than 20% of the population. It is among the top five reasons why patients seek attention from health-care providers. IBS is characterized by abdominal discomfort or pain that is associated with changes in bowel habits. IBS symptoms are chronic and unsettling and can have a negative effect on the quality of life of those who suffer from it. One research group showed that galacto-oligosaccharide prebiotic fiber enhanced the representation of *Bifidobacterium* in patients with IBS, which improved stool consistency, reduced bloating and gas, and produced an overall sense of well-being.

Intake of inulin-based prebiotics results in increased calcium absorption, thereby improving bone strength in people predisposed to osteoporosis.

Colon Cancer

Prebiotics may modify the risk for colon cancer. Prebiotic fibers selectively enhance the *Bifidobacterium* population in the gut, which may in turn increase the SCFA content in the colon. This is a promising area for future study.

Osteoporosis

Perhaps a lesser-known fact regarding prebiotic fibers surrounds calcium absorption. Research shows that intake of inulin-based prebiotics results in increased calcium absorption, thereby improving bone strength in people predisposed to osteoporosis.

Cardiovascular Disease

Consistent evidence from well-designed clinical research suggests protective effects on the heart from fiber intake. Cereal fibers are highly effective, likely because they help to reduce LDL ("bad") cholesterol and improve inflammation.

The U.S. Food and Drug Administration allows health claims for oats, barley and psyllium fibers.

Obesity and Blood Sugar Control

Medical researchers have found that, in some clinical studies, prebiotic fibers have led to modest weight loss following 3 months of supplementation with oligofructose in overweight and obese adults. This weight loss was achieved without any effort to reduce food intake or increase physical activity. In addition, the hormones that are known to increase appetite and, therefore, encourage greater food intake were suppressed. In fact, when researchers reviewed the study subjects' detailed food journals, those who were taking prebiotic supplements reported less food intake, even though there was no effort to limit intake. There were modest improvements in blood sugar control as well, suggesting a protective effect against developing diabetes, in addition to improvements in a variety of hormones that have been known to influence appetite.

> In some clinical studies, prebiotic fibers have led to modest weight loss following 3 months of supplementation with oligofructose in overweight and obese adults.

➢ Research Spotlight

Beans and the Heart

Background: Dietary strategies are increasingly recognized as essential in combating the current obesity epidemic and related metabolic disorders.

Objective: To evaluate the potential prebiotic effects of Swedish beans in relation to cardiovascular risk.

Methods: Either brown beans or white bread were randomly given to 16 young, healthy adults as an evening meal. Metabolic parameters were measured and colonic fermentation activity was estimated by measuring short-chain fatty acids.

Results: An evening meal of brown beans compared to white bread lowered blood sugar and increased the sensation of feeling full. In addition, butyrate production increased, indicating higher colonic fermentative activity.

Conclusions: An evening meal of brown beans beneficially affected important measures of cardiac risk, likely in part due to bacterial fermentation in the gut.

Nonalcoholic Fatty Liver Disease

The major predisposing factors for nonalcoholic fatty liver disease (NAFLD) are obesity, diabetes, high blood cholesterol and high blood triglyceride levels. While the ill effects of excess alcohol consumption on the liver are well known, you might be surprised to learn that when the liver is analyzed under the microscope, livers from people with alcohol-related liver disease and nonalcoholic liver disease look similar.

In addition to modifying the bacteria in the gut, there is medical evidence that prebiotic fibers reduce the liver's ability to produce fat. NAFLD stems from excessive fat deposited in the liver, which can come from excess dietary fat as well as fat made in the liver. In healthy people without NAFLD, the amount of fat that is naturally made in the liver is relatively low. The opposite is true of people with NAFLD. Prebiotic-rich diets may play a role in changing the genes that control fat metabolism, thereby decreasing the amount of fat made by the liver.

Very few studies have shown what happens to the liver in patients with NAFLD after taking prebiotics for a period of time, but what we do know so far is that there seems to be a significant improvement in liver function tests among people who have received prebiotic fiber supplements. None of these patients underwent a liver biopsy to confirm definite improvement. Nonetheless, with the positive impact on risk factors for NAFLD and possible improvement in liver function tests, it is reasonable to suggest a potential benefit of prebiotic fibers in NAFLD.

Prebiotic Fiber Safety

The North American average daily intake of prebiotic fibers lies between 3 and 8 grams. Recently, prebiotic fibers have been added as ingredients to many common food products, such as bread, cereal bars and ready-to-eat breakfast cereals. Prebiotics are recognized as safe natural food ingredients in most countries. Given that some of the prebiotic fibers are insoluble fibers, there may be some side effects of bloating, gas and abdominal cramping if used in particularly high doses. Therefore, people who are predisposed to these symptoms, such as those who suffer from irritable bowel syndrome, should increase prebiotic intake only after symptoms are tolerated.

Prebiotic Health Claims

National health agencies recognize that the foods we eat can affect our health in different ways. A health claim is any representation in labeling or advertising that states, suggests or implies that a relationship exists between consuming a food or an ingredient and a person's health. Therefore, in order for a prebiotic food to be labeled as such, a specific and measurable health benefit must be demonstrated in humans, and this must be accompanied by a change in gut bacterial composition.

Doc Talk

In North America, if a food product is labeled as a prebiotic, then it likely has some benefit. However, just because a food is labeled as a prebiotic or contains prebiotic ingredients, you cannot jump to the conclusion that you are going to have an immediate health benefit; it is not yet known how much prebiotic is required for good health and disease prevention. The gut microbiome responds to dietary adjustments very rapidly. Just the same, the health benefits associated with these changes to prevent or treat diseases may take longer to materialize, depending on the disease and its severity. In the later sections of this book, you will find recommendations and guidelines for prebiotic doses and dietary sources.

PART II

How to Achieve a Healthy Microbiome

The Vegetarian Diet

📁 Case Study

A Rounded Approach

Teresa, 38 years old, was diagnosed with Crohn's disease and IBS 15 years ago. Fortunately, her symptoms were mild and her disease course relatively quiescent. More recently, however, she was experiencing an increase in abdominal cramping, diarrhea and bleeding through her bowels.

Teresa came to my office most concerned about her family history of colon cancer — her father was diagnosed with colon cancer at age 45 — and was quite concerned that she could also have it. Teresa managed her Crohn's with a standard Crohn's-specific anti-inflammatory medication called Salofalk, which seems effective only in very mild Crohn's cases. Teresa had not lost any significant amount of weight in the past year. Her last colonoscopy was more than 5 years ago and results were normal. Her diet was rich in meat, and she relied frequently on fast food and restaurant meals because of her job's travel demands.

I ordered blood work, a colonoscopy and a specialized MRI to reassess her small bowel. Her blood work and MRI were normal. Her colonoscopy revealed only moderate-size hemorrhoids, with no evidence of cancer or active Crohn's. I told Teresa that some of her symptoms may have been driven by IBS but that we could not predict how active her Crohn's disease might be in the future. Subsequently, she asked me for some dietary strategies to manage her symptoms and prevent her Crohn's from flaring. Although they are still experimental for Crohn's, I advised dietary therapies because of the strong preliminary research that supports reducing inflammatory foods and modifying the gut microbiome in a friendly manner. We discussed introducing a vegetarian diet; increasing dietary fiber, prebiotics and probiotics; and taking a particular probiotic, VSL#3, for 3 months. Teresa was assessed by a registered dietitian who has experience treating patients with Crohn's disease.

At her follow-up visit, she reported that her symptoms had improved significantly; as an added bonus, she had lost 10 pounds (4.5 kg).

I hope by now you are convinced that optimizing your gut microbiome may be the key to improving health and preventing disease. We know about the positive impact of carbohydrates and the effect of starch on the microbiome, the favorable benefits of probiotic-rich foods in shaping the microbiome and the impact of dietary fiber, including prebiotic-rich fiber. We are also more familiar with the less favorable consequences of high-protein diets in shaping a beneficial microbiome. Couple these facts with evidence that plant foods have bioactive compounds like polyphenols and phytochemicals that improve health and prevent disease, and it should be no surprise that more and more people are choosing a vegetarian diet.

History of Vegetarianism

By assessing the anatomy and physiology of carnivores (meat-eaters) and herbivores over time, researchers have determined that humans are omnivores (non-vegetarians) by nature. In ancient times, plants and fruits were readily available and easy to gather. Hunting animals was difficult, often dangerous, and consequently, animal products were likely consumed only sporadically compared to non-animal products, which were eaten more regularly. Many early human civilizations were predominantly vegetarian, with religious and cultural beliefs playing a factor in their nutrition choices. Even in modern times, these beliefs continue to be influential.

> Plant foods have bioactive compounds like polyphenols and phytochemicals that improve health and prevent disease.

The primary staple foods of ancient cultures and modern-day vegetarians are wheat, rice, corn and legumes — fiber-rich vegetarian sources. In contrast, the staples of Westernized nations are animal products (33%) and cereals (26%). The shift to foods that are higher in fat and lower in fiber over the past two to three decades is parallel with a flourishing increase in chronic diseases in the Westernized world.

The following table summarizes the main foods of early cultures.

Staple Foods of Early Civilizations	
China	Sorghum, soy, wheat
Egypt	Barley, wheat
India	Corn, lentils, rice, wheat
Mexico/Mayas	Amaranth, corn, maize
Middle East	Chickpeas, wheat
Peru/Incas	Potatoes, quinoa

Vegetarian diets have increased in popularity, and vegetarianism has been recognized by health professionals as a healthy and potentially therapeutic strategy. A recent survey, for example, of almost 1,500 participants (including 104 vegans) found that a vegan diet received the highest diet-quality score when measured by the Healthy Eating Index (HEI), a measure of diet quality in terms of conformance with U.S. federal dietary guidance. In comparison, an omnivorous diet received the lowest score for quality.

Throughout the 1970s, there were concerns that vegetarians might experience nutritional deficiencies; it seemingly went unnoticed that many Asians had consumed vegetarian diets for millennia without nutrient deficiencies. During the 1980s and 1990s, many nutritional studies began documenting the health benefits of vegetarian diets — in particular the reduction of many chronic diseases. For example, the development of obesity, diabetes and certain cancers declined while longevity increased. Health-protective effects were consistently shown for plant-rich diets compared to diets rich in animal proteins.

In several cases, many observational studies have identified consistent results with certain diet patterns. For example, the Mediterranean diet, which includes primarily fruits, vegetables, legumes, whole grains, nuts, seeds and some dairy, has been confirmed in two randomized controlled clinical trials to lower incidence of both heart diseases and inflammatory-related diseases. Researchers are concluding that a plant-centered diet may be broadly recommended for health prevention, and that many of these benefits are linked to a vegetarian diet and the changes in the gut microbiome that it produces.

What Exactly Is a Vegetarian Diet?

A vegetarian diet is a plant-based diet with lots of fruits, vegetables, legumes, whole grains, nuts and seeds. Red meat, poultry and seafood are excluded. There are different types of vegetarian diets.

The food components of a vegetarian diet that are believed to have health benefits include fiber, phytochemicals and antioxidants.

Type of Vegetarian Diet	Included Foods Aside from Plant-Based Foods
Lacto	Dairy (milk, cheese, yogurt and butter)
Lacto-ovo	Dairy and eggs
Ovo	Eggs
Vegan	No additions; plant-based foods only

➢ Research Spotlight

Vegan vs. Omnivorous

Background: Few studies have rigorously evaluated and compared omnivorous, vegetarian and vegan diets for their impact on health. It is possible that a vegan health advantage may be associated with a unique gut microbiota profile, and the microbiome changes in vegans might be protective against metabolic and inflammatory diseases.

Objective: To compare the biochemical profiles of vegans and omnivores who have similar characteristics, such as age, gender and weight.

Methods: In 24 vegans and 25 omnivores, researchers reviewed the subjects' body composition, a 7-day food diary and their physical activity.

Results: Vegans had significantly lower blood pressure and higher intake of carbohydrates and fiber. Vegans also had lower triglyceride levels.

Conclusions: Vegans have food intake and a biochemical profile that will decrease the risk of developing cardiac illness. This study was designed to compare only a vegan diet to an omnivorous diet; however, it is possible that a similar advantage may be observed in other vegetarian diets.

Health Benefits of the Vegetarian Diet

Body Weight

Our society is obsessed with weight loss, as reflected in the number and variety of diets people follow. Several research studies have now established a relationship between adopting a vegetarian diet and a decrease in the body weight of adults and teenagers. In fact, vegetarian males on average weigh 17 pounds (7.7 kg) less than non-vegetarian males, and vegetarian females are typically 9 pounds (4 kg) lighter than non-vegetarian females. These findings have been replicated in many large clinical studies.

Cardiovascular Disorders

Eating an adequate amount of vegetables and fruits benefits the cardiovascular system. Plant-based foods provide the body with multiple antioxidants — the most active of these are flavonoids, carotenoids and antioxidant vitamins (alpha-tocopherol, also known as vitamin E, and ascorbic acid, also known as vitamin C). Antioxidants exert their helpful effects by inhibiting LDL ("bad") cholesterol, increasing HDL ("good") cholesterol and reducing total cholesterol levels. This results in a lower risk of developing arteriosclerosis, or hardening of the arteries, which is the first step in developing heart disease.

Another heart-related benefit is blood pressure control. On average, the blood pressure of vegetarians is 10 points lower than that of non-vegetarians, thus reducing their risk of heart attack and stroke. Although it isn't clear which factors in the vegetarian diet affect blood pressure levels, it is believed that the higher fiber intake of vegetarians results in better weight control. Vegetarians' higher intake of potassium-rich foods is another factor. Potassium has the opposite effect to sodium, which hardens blood vessels and is a proven risk factor for high blood pressure. Potassium helps excrete sodium through the urine and, therefore, relax the blood vessels.

FAQ

How are observational studies evaluating vegetarianism different from controlled clinical trials?

Studies known as "observational" studies vary in their design from controlled studies. In observational studies, diets are not "tested." They are simply evaluated based on what people are actually doing. Because of this, the researchers cannot control for other lifestyle factors, such as stress, exercise or smoking, that may also play a role in contributing to a certain outcome. Clinical trials, on the other hand, are conducted in clinical settings where participants are asked to comply with specific interventions/therapies, which may include a placebo. Data are then collected to assess the impact of these interventions on certain outcomes, which are generally health related.

Diabetes

A higher incidence of type 2 diabetes occurs in meat-eaters compared to semi-vegetarians, lacto-ovo-vegetarians and vegans, in descending order. Vegetarians are believed to have better insulin sensitivity due to higher fiber intake. Improving insulin sensitivity will improve blood sugar control and reduce the risk of developing diabetes.

Cancer

The research surrounding cancer rates in vegetarians and non-vegetarians has been limited to studies that have simply observed people over the course of time. Keeping this shortcoming in mind, lower rates of cancer, particularly breast, colon and prostate, have been identified in people who follow a vegetarian diet. Breast cancer rates are dramatically lower in countries where diets are typically plant-based. A very large recent study reported that vegans have lower rates of cancer than both meat-eaters and vegetarians. Vegan women had a one-third lower risk of female-specific cancers such as breast, cervical and ovarian cancer. The researchers controlled for other factors that could potentially impact the study findings, such as rates of smoking, alcohol use and family history of cancer.

Despite the findings regarding cancer and vegetarian diets, stronger clinical trials are needed to confirm a cause-and-effect relationship. The body of evidence to date suggests that people should greatly increase the amount of plant-based foods in their diets.

The most recent nutrition guidelines published by both the American Cancer Society and the Canadian Cancer Society recommend eating a balanced diet with an emphasis on plant sources, which includes:

- Eating five or more servings of vegetables and fruits each day (50% of your plate should be vegetables and fruits)
- Choosing whole grains over processed and refined grains (25% of your plate should be whole-grain products)
- Limiting processed meats and red meats (less than 25% of your plate should be meat products)
- Balancing your calorie intake with physical activity to get to or remain at a healthy weight
- Limiting alcohol intake

Did You Know?

Lower Cancer Risk

In studies, vegans were found to have a very low level of the hormone insulin-like growth factor 1 (IGF-1), which promotes cancer in adults. Animal protein intake increases the levels of IGF-1, but within a few short weeks of switching to a plant-based diet, IGF-1 levels in the blood drop. Another group of researchers, including Nobel Prize–winner Dr. Elizabeth Blackburn, showed that a vegan diet resulted in beneficial gene changes that limited the risk of certain cancers and other illnesses.

Vegetarian Influencers

Background: The impact of a vegetarian versus a non-vegetarian diet on the microbiome is not completely understood.

Objective: To investigate the impact of age, genetics and diet on the microbiome composition.

Methods: Ninety-eight healthy volunteers collected diet information using two standardized questionnaires about recent diet and long-term diet. Subsequently, 10 subjects were voluntarily hospitalized for a controlled feeding study and received either a high-fat/low-fiber diet or a low-fat/high-fiber diet. Stool samples were collected for analysis.

Results: Nutrients from the same food groups tended to cluster together. For example, diets high in fat compared to those higher in plant products and fiber had inverse associations with regard to the microbes that dominated in the gut. *Bacteroides* species were highly associated with animal protein and saturated fats. *Prevotella* species were associated with a high carbohydrate intake. Among the subjects who were hospitalized for the feeding experiment, changes in the microbiome were detectable within 24 hours. The study did not measure the stability of the microbiome over the 10 days.

Conclusions: Vegetarian compared to non-vegetarian diets had very different effects on the microbiome, and although changes in the microbiome were noted after 24 hours, a longer dietary intervention period is required to maintain these changes. More studies are needed to determine if a long-term commitment to a plant-based diet could permanently alter an individual's microbiome and provide health benefits.

Vegetarian Diets and the Microbiome

There is growing concern that modern dietary choices, particularly the growing intake of high-fat foods, animal protein and sugar, have altered the genetic composition and metabolic activity of the gut microbiome. These diet-induced changes to the gut microbiome are suspected of contributing to the increasing rates of chronic illness in the developed world. Yet it remains unclear how quickly and reproducibly the gut bacteria respond to dietary change.

Inflammation

Inflammation may be a critical component linking gut microbiota to several conditions, including obesity, metabolic dysfunction and chronic disease.

One research group investigated the role of a vegan diet in influencing obesity and inflammation. Subjects who followed a vegan diet for one month were found to have improved blood sugars, reduced body weight, and lower triglycerides and cholesterol. In addition, the vegan diet altered gut microbiota by reducing the abundance of the Firmicutes class of bacteria and increasing the amount of another group (Bacteroidetes) significantly. Specifically, within the Bacteroidetes class, *Prevotella* species — which are associated with higher carbohydrate intake and vegetarianism — was enriched. Another dominant genus within the Bacteroidetes class is *Bacteroides*, and researchers see a higher proportion of it in subjects whose diets are high in protein and animal fats. For example, a Thai study found that among adult non-vegetarians, a significantly higher amount of *Bacteroides* prevailed, while vegetarian subjects had a higher level of *Prevotella*.

In another study assessing the microbiome in vegan and vegetarian subjects, vegans had an abundance of *Faecalibacterium prausnitzii* (an anti-inflammatory bacterium and a big producer of butyrate). Recall that butyrate is a short-chain fatty acid that is critical for gut health and protects against the development of inflammatory diseases. Vegan and vegetarian diets are higher in carbohydrates and fiber than omnivore diets, and stool samples show a lower pH, which prevents the growth of some disease-predisposing bacteria (like *E. coli*) that do not tolerate a more acidic environment.

> Vegan and vegetarian diets are higher in carbohydrates and fiber than omnivore diets, and stool samples show a lower pH, which prevents the growth of some disease-predisposing bacteria (like *E. coli*) that do not tolerate a more acidic environment.

Obesity

The role of a vegan diet in influencing obesity was explored by one research group. Subjects following a vegan diet showed improved blood sugars and reduced body weight over those following an unrestricted Western diet, along with a marked improvement in cholesterol. The group that followed the vegan diet had altered the state of their microbiome — in particular, showing an increase in the class of Bacteroidetes and a decrease in the Firmicutes class. Notably, the vegan diet was associated with a decrease in pathobionts (bacteria that have the potential to promote disease if circumstances promote a disease-favoring environment) residing in the gut.

Vegan Link

Research in the field of diet and the microbiome is rapidly evolving, but there is strong evidence that vegan and vegetarian diets are associated with improved microbiome health and may be used as a treatment strategy for certain inflammatory-based diseases.

Metabolic Dysfunction

The most recent evidence that a vegan diet promotes gut microbes that reduce metabolic risk is from research linking red meat to a specific protein called carnitine. Metabolism of carnitine, primarily found in meat, by microbes in the gut may promote heart disease. In vegans, the microbiome required for metabolizing carnitine is lacking, minimizing the risk of heart disease and hardening of the arteries. In fact, in the one year that subjects were assessed, they consistently had a favorable microbiome that limited the metabolism of carnitine into undesirable end products. The degree of disease-predisposing bacteria was found to be the lowest in vegans and the highest with non-vegetarian diets, with vegetarian diets falling somewhere in between.

Doc Talk

A substantive body of evidence in recent years makes it very compelling to follow a vegetarian diet. However, I recognize that there can be practical challenges in modifying your lifestyle to support the diet. The broad appeal of a vegetarian diet is often not sustainable, especially for those of us accustomed to a North American diet. I feel that a diet rich in fiber, including prebiotic fibers and probiotic foods, with an abundance of fruits and vegetables and even some consumption of meat, has a greater health benefit than a vegetarian diet that is overrepresented in simple sugars and highly processed foods. There are some benefits to eating fish rich in omega-3 fatty acids. One possible drawback is the potential for mercury ingestion, and its impact on the microbiome is still unknown. Keep in mind that vegetarian diets can vary in quality and composition, and some exposure to meat may still offer health benefits when consumed in moderation.

CHAPTER 6

The Vegetarian Diet in Detail

🗀 Case Study

Embracing Vegetarianism

Jovan is a 35-year-old man with a strong family history of heart disease. His father was diagnosed at the age of 47, after a heart attack, and Jovan's brother was diagnosed at 39. Jovan's uncle on his father's side had recently been experiencing chest pain and difficulty breathing, and his symptoms were under investigation. All three men also have high cholesterol.

Given his family history and his own lack of energy, Jovan decided to visit his doctor for a routine physical. He was shocked to learn that his blood cholesterol levels were 60% higher than the normal range. Jovan's doctor recommended that he make some lifestyle modifications and lose weight. But between his two young children and a full-time job, Jovan felt that he did not have much time for extra activities, including exercise.

Jovan was also experiencing upper abdominal pain and nausea, so his family doctor referred him to me. Jovan was concerned that his stressful job and family life might have led to a stomach ulcer. I explained that, contrary to popular belief, stress does not cause ulcers. Since he did not have any of the usual risk factors, I believed it unlikely that an ulcer was causing his symptoms. Apart from his cholesterol level, his bloodwork was normal. I diagnosed him with non-ulcer dyspepsia — essentially irritable bowel syndrome of the upper digestive system — which is known to be associated with stress and poor dietary choices.

When he learned that improvements in his diet would not only help resolve his digestive issues but would also play a role in reducing his blood cholesterol and increasing his energy, Jovan was eager to make better choices and take control of his health. He had never consumed large amounts of meat and found the idea of a vegetarian diet appealing, especially in light of his risk factors for cardiac disease. We discussed the numerous merits of a vegetarian diet, and I offered some preliminary advice on how he could boost dietary fiber, increase his consumption of fruits and vegetables, and limit sugar-containing beverages and foods. I referred him to a registered dietitian for further counseling.

As we have seen, rapidly emerging findings show that vegan and vegetarian diets are capable of shaping the microbiome to limit chronic diseases and potentially treat them. Historically, there have been many misconceptions regarding the nutritional value of vegetarian diets, among them an increased risk of nutritional deficiencies such as vitamins, iron and protein.

In the following chapter, I dispel the myths surrounding nutritional inadequacy and build strategies to help you implement the vegetarian diet.

FAQ

Q Now that I may be considering a vegetarian diet, how do I ensure that I get proper nutrition and not miss essential nutrients?

A The key to any healthy diet is to choose a wide variety of foods and to consume adequate calories to meet your macronutrient (protein, carbohydrates, fat) and micronutrient (vitamins and minerals) needs. If your diet is varied enough, the risk of nutrient-related deficiencies is low. A diet that is not diverse runs the risk of developing deficiencies of protein, vitamin B_{12}, iron, calcium, vitamin D, zinc and omega-3 fatty acids. The following sections will detail how to ensure that a vegetarian diet meets nutrition targets.

Vitamin B_{12}

Vegetarians, in particular vegans, are at particular risk of vitamin B_{12} deficiency, mainly because vitamin B_{12} is naturally found only in animal food sources and some nutritional yeast. (It is also added to manufactured foods and is available as a dietary supplement and prescription medication.) Vitamin B_{12} is required for proper red blood cell formation, neurological function and cell development. So, how much vitamin B_{12} do we need?

Vegetarian Sources of Vitamin B_{12}

Vitamin B_{12} is generally not found in plant foods, but it can fortify foods such as soy milk, meat alternatives, energy bars and breakfast cereals. Fortified foods vary in formulation, so be sure to read product labels. Tempeh, miso, sea vegetables and other plant-based foods may contain vitamin B_{12} but are not considered reliable sources.

Recommended Daily Allowances for Vitamin B_{12}

Age (Males and Females)	Vitamin B_{12} (mcg/day)
0–6 months	0.4
7–12 months	0.5
1–3 years	0.9
4–8 years	1.2
9–13 years	1.8
14+ years	2.4
During pregnancy	2.6
During lactation	2.8

Vegetarian Sources of Vitamin B_{12}

Food	Serving Size	Vitamin B_{12} (mcg)
Coconut milk, fortified with vitamin B_{12}	1 cup (250 mL)	3.0
Meatless luncheon slices	2$\frac{1}{2}$ oz (75 g)	3.0
Soy burger patty	2$\frac{1}{2}$ oz (75 g)	1.8
Cheese: Swiss/Emmental	1$\frac{1}{2}$ oz (50 g)	1.7
Eggs, cooked	2 large	1.5–1.6
Cottage cheese (1%)	$\frac{3}{4}$ cup (175 mL)	1.5
Milk (nonfat, 1%, 2% or 3.25%)	1 cup (250 mL)	1.2–1.4
Meatless chicken, fish sticks, wieners/ frankfurters or meatballs, cooked	2$\frac{1}{2}$ oz (75 g)	1.0–3.8
Almond, oat or rice beverage, fortified with vitamin B_{12}	1 cup (250 mL)	1.0
Red Star T6635+ Yeast (vegetarian support formula)	2 g (1 tsp/5 mL powder or 2 tsp/10 mL flaked)	1.0
Soy milk, fortified with vitamin B_{12}	1 cup (250 mL)	1.0
Yogurt, plain (low-fat)	$\frac{3}{4}$ cup (175 mL)	1.0
Cheese: Brie, Cheddar, Edam, feta, fontina, Gouda, Gruyère, mozzarella, provolone	1$\frac{1}{2}$ oz (50 g)	0.7–0.9

Did You Know?

Vegan Supplementation

Strict vegans should strongly consider taking a vitamin B_{12} supplement on a daily basis.

Did You Know?

Deficiency Treatment

Vitamin B_{12} deficiency is typically treated with intramuscular vitamin B_{12} injections. In some people, once vitamin B_{12} stores have been replenished, patients maintain adequate levels by taking oral supplements or by following a diet richer in vitamin B_{12}.

Vitamin B_{12} Dietary Supplements

As a dietary supplement, vitamin B_{12} is usually compounded as cyanocobalamin, a form that the body readily converts into active vitamin B_{12}. Current scientific evidence does not highlight any differences among the oral vitamin B_{12} forms available in supplements and food sources when it comes to the body's ability to absorb and use it for various functions. In addition to dietary supplements, vitamin B_{12} is also available as tablets and lozenges that can be placed under the tongue.

Vitamin B_{12} Prescription Medications

Vitamin B_{12} can be administered by injection into the muscle. This route of administration is typically used to treat vitamin B_{12} deficiency caused by a specific autoimmune disease called pernicious anemia, as well as other conditions that may cause malabsorption of vitamin B_{12}.

Vitamin B_{12} Deficiency

Vitamin B_{12} deficiency is characterized by anemia, or low blood counts in hemoglobin, fatigue, weakness and loss of appetite. Neurological changes such as numbness and tingling in the hands and feet can occur and can lead to irreversible nerve damage. Symptoms may also include difficulty maintaining balance, depression, confusion, dementia, poor memory and soreness of the mouth and/or tongue.

FAQ

 Who is most at risk for vitamin B_{12} deficiency?

 Groups at risk for vitamin B_{12} deficiency include strict vegetarians and vegans, who are at greater risk than lacto-ovo-vegetarians and non-vegetarians. Pregnant and lactating women who follow a strict vegetarian diet must keep in mind that a deficiency of vitamin B_{12} in their diet can result in very limited stores of vitamin B_{12} in their breast milk. If this occurs, babies of these mothers may develop vitamin B_{12} deficiency early in life.

Undetected and untreated vitamin B_{12} deficiency in infants can cause negative neurological outcomes, and for this reason, the Academy of Nutrition and Dietetics recommends supplemental vitamin B_{12} for vegans and lacto-ovo-vegetarians during both pregnancy and lactation to ensure that enough vitamin B_{12} is transferred to the fetus and infant. If you are pregnant or lactating, please consult with your pediatrician regarding the optimal dose of vitamin B_{12} supplements.

> Research Spotlight

Arthritis in Vegans

Background: Several researchers are looking at potential strategies to use bacteria as medicine to treat immune disorders such as rheumatoid arthritis. Specialists have observed that some patients with rheumatoid arthritis have benefited from cutting meat from their diet or adopting a Mediterranean diet, which is rich in fish, olive oil and vegetables.

Objective: To evaluate the role of the gut microbiome in patients with rheumatoid arthritis after adopting a vegan diet.

Methods: Detailed clinical assessments, including stool assessments, were performed before and after a dietary intervention. Patients were assigned to one of two groups. The test group received a strict vegan diet and the control group continued their standard omnivorous diet.

Results: Researchers noted a significant change in the gut microbes of the group assigned to the vegan diet, but not in the control group. Further, in the test group there was significant improvement in the severity of disease-related symptoms.

Conclusions: A vegan diet changes the gut microbiome in patients with rheumatoid arthritis and these changes are associated with reduced symptoms.

Iron

Iron is an essential mineral. It is an important component of hemoglobin (found in red blood cells), which helps carry oxygen from your lungs to the rest of your body. If you do not have enough iron, your body cannot make enough healthy oxygen-carrying red blood cells. A lack of red blood cells in this case is called iron-deficiency anemia.

There have been concerns about the adequacy of iron in vegetarian diets. Not all the iron found in food is bioavailable. A vegetarian diet is likely to contain iron in amounts equal to a non-vegetarian diet; however, because of the form of the iron from plant sources, it is less bioavailable. This is called non-heme iron. Heme iron, the form of iron found in meat products, is more bioavailable.

The composition of vegetarian diets can be as varied as that of non-vegetarian diets. Choosing high-fiber foods and whole grains rather than low-fiber foods and refined grains can greatly affect iron absorption. Since non-heme iron is influenced by other dietary factors and nutrients ingested in a meal, vegetarians generally need about twice as much iron as meat-eaters.

Did You Know?

Bioavailability Definition

The term "bioavailability" refers to the amount of a substance that enters the body and is actually absorbed and used.

Iron Under the Microscope

Recent data suggest that iron may influence the gut microbial composition. For example, in two small studies among African children and infants, iron fortification predisposed them to a potentially more harmful gut microbial profile, with the potential to increase the prevalence of inflammatory diseases. Gut microbial changes caused by iron ingestion have the potential to affect the immune responsiveness of the gut; however, more studies are needed to define this relationship further. It is tempting to conclude that an iron-rich non-vegetarian diet may alter the microbiome in a less than desirable manner.

How Much Iron Should I Aim For?

	Non-vegetarian Diet (mg/day)	Vegetarian Diet (mg/day)
Men 19 and older	8	16
Women 19–50	18	32–36
Women 51 and older	8	14–16

Increasing Iron Absorption

Greens and Legumes

A balanced vegetarian diet with legumes, fortified grains and green vegetables can provide adequate iron. Studies confirm that the incidence of iron-deficiency anemia is not greater among individuals who eat a healthy vegetarian diet compared to non-vegetarians.

Dairy Products

Dairy products, including milk and certain forms of calcium, may decrease or inhibit iron absorption. Because milk-based products, including cheese and yogurt, can be an excellent source of important nutrients, vegetarians should aim to enjoy a certain amount of milk or other dairy sources every day, but not to exceed guidelines. For adults, two servings of dairy a day are recommended. One serving of dairy is equal to 1 cup (250 mL) milk or ¾ cup (175 mL) yogurt. Spacing out the times when you eat iron-rich foods and milk-based products will also help enhance iron absorption — aim to eat foods high in iron 2 to 3 hours before or after eating milk products.

Did You Know?

Timed Nutrition

Consume foods with polyphenols at least 2 hours before or after your main iron-rich meal.

Vitamin C

Some nutrients tend to work better when taken together than on their own. The combination of iron and vitamin C is no exception. In particular, fruits and vegetables that contain vitamin C and organic acids improve the absorption of non-heme iron.

Vitamin C is involved in many reactions in the body and plays an important role in the synthesis of collagen, which is responsible for healthy tissue, skin and bones. In its role regarding absorption, vitamin C changes non-heme iron to a form that is easily absorbed in the small intestine. Good sources of vitamin C include bell (sweet) peppers, berries, broccoli, cabbage, cantaloupe, cauliflower, honeydew, kale, kiwifruit, lemons, oranges, potatoes, tomatoes and juices fortified with vitamin C.

> Vitamin C plays an important role in the synthesis of collagen, which is responsible for healthy tissue, skin and bones.

Polyphenols

Polyphenols are plant chemicals that work as antioxidants to protect cells in the body from damage. They are found in tea, coffee, colas and cocoa. There are many benefits to including polyphenols in your diet, but they should not be eaten together with iron-rich foods. If you have an iron deficiency or are at risk of developing one, they compromise iron absorption.

Iron-Deficiency Anemia

A vegetarian diet can predispose you to iron-deficiency anemia unless you are mindful about eating double the amount of iron-rich plant foods. Iron-deficiency anemia can be the result of many other conditions, some of which can be life-threatening, so it's important to determine the cause. If you have been diagnosed with iron-deficiency anemia, your doctor will likely ask you to have additional testing to correctly identify the cause of your anemia.

Blood Loss

Blood contains iron within its red cells. Therefore, if you lose blood, you lose iron. Women with heavy menstrual periods are at risk for iron deficiency because of excessive blood loss. Similarly, chronic blood loss over time, such as from a stomach ulcer, a colon polyp or colon cancer, can cause iron deficiency. The use of over-the-counter pain medication, such as anti-inflammatories like aspirin or ibuprofen, can also increase your chances of iron-deficiency anemia.

Causes of Iron Deficiency
- Celiac disease
- Colon cancer
- Colon polyps
- Crohn's disease (extensive)
- Heavy menstrual bleeding
- Nosebleeds (chronic, uncontrolled)
- Poor dietary intake
- Stomach ulcers
- Ulcerative colitis

FAQ

Q How do you know if you have iron-deficiency anemia?

A The most common symptom of iron-deficiency anemia is fatigue (tiredness). Other signs and symptoms include irregular heartbeat, chest pain, dizziness, cold hands and feet, pale skin, uncomfortable or crawling feeling in your legs, restless legs syndrome, brittle nails, inflammation or soreness of your tongue, weakness, shortness of breath, headache, sores at the corner of your mouth and cravings that include non-nutritive substances, such as dirt, clay or ice. Other nutrient deficiencies can also mimic these symptoms; therefore, it is important to see your health-care professional to confirm a diagnosis and/or rule out other possible causes. Your health-care professional may assess your condition by using blood work and laboratory testing.

Did You Know?

Anemia and Advanced Age

If you are around or over the age of 50, iron-deficiency anemia could be indicative of serious medical problems, such as colon polyps or colon cancer, even in the absence of any other symptoms.

Inability to Absorb Iron

Iron from food is absorbed into your bloodstream through your small intestine. Intestinal disorders, such as celiac disease, can lead to iron-deficiency anemia. An autoimmune condition, celiac disease occurs with a higher frequency in people of northern European descent. People with celiac disease may have gastrointestinal symptoms, such as bloating, abdominal cramping, diarrhea and/or constipation. However, some people don't experience any gastrointestinal symptoms and are diagnosed through a simple blood test. Undiagnosed celiac disease can lead to nutritional problems and — in rare cases — cancer.

Lack of Iron in Your Diet

We discussed earlier the impact of a vegetarian diet on the risk for iron deficiency. If you consume too little iron, whether in the context of a vegetarian or a non-vegetarian diet, you can become iron deficient over time. Pay particular attention if you are restricting certain dietary sources for purposes of weight loss or to control other symptoms.

Vegetarian Sources of Iron

Food	Serving Size	Iron (mg)
Vegetables and Fruits		
Tomato purée	1/2 cup (125 mL)	2.4
Lima beans, cooked	1/2 cup (125 mL)	2.2
Asparagus, raw	6 spears	2.1
Spinach, cooked	1/2 cup (125 mL)	2.0–3.4
Swiss chard, cooked	1/2 cup (125 mL)	2.0
Snow peas, cooked	1/2 cup (125 mL)	1.7
Apricots, dried	1/4 cup (60 mL)	1.6
Prune juice	1/2 cup (125 mL)	1.6
Potato, with skin, cooked	1 medium	1.3–1.9
Kale, cooked	1/2 cup (125 mL)	1.3
Green peas, cooked	1/2 cup (125 mL)	1.3
Asparagus, cooked	1/2 cup (125 mL) chopped	1.0
Figs, dried	5	1.0
Grain Products		
Cream of wheat	3/4 cup (175 mL)	5.7–5.8
Oatmeal, instant, cooked	3/4 cup (175 mL)	4.5–6.6
Cold cereal, enriched	1 oz (30 g)	4.0
Amaranth	1/2 cup (125 mL)	3.0
Bagel	1/2	2.0
Pasta or egg noodles, enriched, cooked	1/2 cup (125 mL)	2.0
Granola bar (oat, fruits and nut)	1 bar (1 oz/32 g)	1.2–2.7
Quinoa	1/2 cup (125 mL)	1.0

continued on next page...

Vegetarian Sources of Iron (continued)

Food	Serving Size	Iron (mg)
Meat Alternatives		
Soybeans, mature, cooked	³⁄₄ cup (175 mL)	6.5–7.0
Lentils, cooked	³⁄₄ cup (175 mL)	4.1–5.0
Tofu, cooked	³⁄₄ cup (175 mL)	3.0–4.0
Beans, cooked: black, kidney, navy, pinto, white	³⁄₄ cup (175 mL)	3.0–4.0
Chickpeas, cooked	³⁄₄ cup (175 mL)	2.0–3.5
Peas, cooked: black-eyed, split	³⁄₄ cup (175 mL)	2.0–3.5
Pumpkin or squash seeds	¹⁄₄ cup (60 mL)	2.0–3.0
Lima beans, cooked	¹⁄₂ cup (125 mL)	2.0
Hummus	¹⁄₄ cup (60 mL)	1.4
Nuts, shelled: almonds, cashews, hazelnuts, macadamias, pistachios	¹⁄₄ cup (60 mL)	1.3–2.2
Almond butter	2 tbsp (30 mL)	1.2
Egg, cooked	1 large	0.6–0.9
Other		
Molasses, blackstrap	1 tbsp (15 mL)	4.0

Iron Supplements

It is not advisable to take iron supplements without a formal assessment and proper diagnosis by your health-care professional. Excessive iron can be dangerous and may damage your liver and cause other complications. Iron supplements can also cause side effects such as stomach upset, nausea, vomiting and constipation. If your doctor believes you need an iron supplement, based on your blood work, he or she will prescribe appropriate iron formulations, advise on dosing requirements and monitor your progress.

Protein

Amino acids are the building blocks of protein. Humans need 20 different amino acids for normal functioning. Nine of these amino acids are considered essential because your body is unable to synthesize them; therefore, they must be obtained from your diet. The remaining, nonessential amino acids can be sourced from your diet and can be made by your body as needed. Plant-based foods, with the exception of soybeans, soybean products and quinoa, are incomplete sources of protein because they contain inadequate amounts of one or more of the essential amino acids. However, by combining a variety of plant proteins over several meals throughout the day, you can ensure that you are getting all the essential amino acids in your diet.

If you are worried about not getting enough protein on a vegetarian diet, you might be surprised to learn that most North Americans eat far too much protein. Vegetarians are, in fact, not particularly at risk for inadequate protein intake. Unfortunately, the idea that meat is the only main source of protein still prevails — even though there are many excellent non-meat sources of protein.

> Humans need 20 different amino acids for normal functioning.

FAQ

Are there types of protein that are more beneficial/harmful to the gut microbiome?

Scientifically, it's difficult to answer this question, because study participants would need to receive either animal-based protein or plant-based protein with all other dietary intake being equal. In other words, to assess the microbiome, a researcher would need to extract animal-based protein and plant-based protein while keeping all other factors neutral. Animal-based protein sources are accompanied by other nutrients, such as saturated fats, that are known to negatively impact health. Similarly, plant-based protein sources are accompanied by many other favorable nutrients, in particular fiber. Researchers would be required to control for the fiber effects on the microbiome findings before any direct impact could be attributed to plant proteins. This type of research has not yet been conducted. Practically speaking, plant-based proteins are preferred over animal-based proteins because of their numerous benefits, not only as a protein source but also for their inherent nutrients.

Vegetarian Sources of Protein

Legumes

Legumes include all beans, lentils and peas and are an excellent vegetarian source of protein.

Food	Serving Size	Protein (g)
Lentils, cooked	1 cup (250 mL)	18
Chickpeas, cooked	1 cup (250 mL)	15
Beans, cooked: black, kidney, lima, pinto	1 cup (250 mL)	15
Peas, black-eyed, cooked	1 cup (250 mL)	13
Peas, green, cooked	1 cup (250 mL)	8

Did You Know?

Soy Boost

Many of the soy-based foods, such as tofu, tempeh and other soy products, are also fortified with nutrients that are important for health, such as calcium, iron and vitamin B_{12}.

Tofu, Tempeh and Soy Products

Tofu, tempeh and other soy products are excellent sources of protein for vegetarians. Options include soy milk, which can be found in many flavors, as well as edamame, soy yogurt, soy ice cream, soy nuts and soy-style cheese.

Food	Serving Size	Protein (g)
Tempeh	1 cup (250 mL)	31
Soybeans, cooked	1 cup (250 mL)	22
Tofu, firm or regular	4 oz (125 g)	10–11
Soy milk, plain	1 cup (250 mL)	7
Soy yogurt, plain	1 cup (250 mL)	6

Spirulina

Spirulina is a highly nutritious blue-green algae. It is noteworthy for protein and B vitamins.

Food	Serving Size	Protein (g)
Spirulina, dried	1–2 tsp (5–10 mL)	1–3

Quinoa

Quinoa is loosely considered the world's most popular "superfood." Quinoa is a good source of protein. It also provides 5 grams of fiber, 15% of your iron needs, and micronutrients such as folate, zinc, potassium, manganese and phosphorus. It is often viewed as a complete protein, but there is a catch. The amount of protein in quinoa is less than the amount in meat-based sources, eggs, milk and most legumes. For example, 1 cup (250 mL) quinoa contains 8 grams of protein; contrast that to the 25 grams of protein found in 100 grams of steak. This is why quinoa is classified in the grain category rather than as a meat and alternative food.

> The amount of protein in quinoa is less than the amount in meat-based sources, eggs, milk and most legumes.

Food	Serving Size	Protein (g)
Quinoa, cooked	1 cup (250 mL)	6 to 8

Whole Grains and Grain Products

A whole grain is the entire seed of a plant. This seed is made up of the bran, germ and endosperm. Refining grains removes the bran and germ, leaving only the endosperm. The bran and germ contain 25% of a grain's protein as well as at least 17 key nutrients.

Food	Serving Size	Protein (g)
Seitan (meat substitute made of wheat)	2 oz (60 g)	21
Bagel	1 medium (3$\frac{1}{2}$ oz/ 100 g)	10
Whole-grain spaghetti, cooked	1 cup (250 mL)	8
Whole wheat bread	2 slices	7
Bulgur, cooked	1 cup (250 mL)	6
Brown rice, cooked	1 cup (250 mL)	5

Veggie Burgers and Meat Substitutes

Most commercial products in this category are made from either soy protein or wheat protein. These burgers are great for barbecues and can be combined with a side of whole grains and/or vegetables. Add some kimchi or sauerkraut to your veggie dog for an added boost of prebiotics — it will enhance your gut microbiome to maintain a healthy immunity and prevent inflammatory-mediated diseases.

Food	Serving Size	Protein (g)
Veggie burger	1 patty	13
Veggie dog	1 link	8

Nuts and Seeds

In addition to being excellent sources of protein, nuts and seeds also contain vitamins, minerals, fiber and other helpful nutrients that may help prevent cancer and heart disease. Many people resist eating nuts because of their fat content, but they can provide a sense of fullness and satisfaction that may actually help you reduce your intake of other, high-caloric and less nutritious foods. Because nuts are high in essential amino acids and healthy fats, they are an important part of any vegetarian diet.

- Almonds are a good source of protein, vitamin E, manganese, copper and vitamin B_2. The majority of the fat in almonds is monounsaturated fat, which is known to protect against heart disease and high cholesterol.
- Cashews are another good source of protein. They are high in antioxidants and have a lower fat content than most other nuts. Three-quarters of the fat in cashews is unsaturated.
- Pumpkin seeds are a good source of protein, essential fatty acids and a number of micronutrients, such as magnesium. They promote good prostate health for men and anti-inflammatory benefits for those with arthritis, and they help lower cholesterol.

Food	Serving Size	Protein (g)
Peanut butter	2 tbsp (30 mL)	8
Almonds	$\frac{1}{4}$ cup (60 mL)	8
Hemp seeds	2 tbsp (30 mL)	7–11
Almond butter	2 tbsp (30 mL)	7
Sunflower seeds	$\frac{1}{4}$ cup (60 mL)	6
Cashews	$\frac{1}{4}$ cup (60 mL)	5
Chia seeds	2 tbsp (30 mL)	5
Pumpkin seeds	$\frac{1}{4}$ cup (60 mL)	3

Vegetables

Vegetables are not typically known for their protein content, but spinach and broccoli are two of the better sources.

Food	Serving Size	Protein (g)
Spinach, cooked	1 cup (250 mL)	5
Broccoli, cooked	1 cup (250 mL)	4

Eggs

Eggs contain all 9 essential amino acids and many minerals and essential vitamins (vitamins A, B_6, B_{12}, D, E, riboflavin, thiamin, choline, niacin, folate).

Food	Serving Size	Protein (g)
Eggs	2 medium	12

Protein from Dairy and Dairy Substitutes
Milk Products

Milk contains two types of protein: whey (20%) and casein (80%). Both are high-quality proteins and contain all the essential amino acids needed to support the multiple roles of protein in the body. One cup (250 mL) milk contains 8 grams of protein, while ¾ cup (175 mL) yogurt has a similar protein load. Compare this to ½ cup (125 mL) cottage cheese, which provides 15 grams of protein. It is pretty convincing that milk products are rich sources of protein, and vegetarians need not look too far to obtain their protein sources.

FAQ

How do I know if I have a lactose intolerance? If so, how should I modify my diet?

Lactose intolerance is typically seen in patients of specific ethnicities and from certain geographical regions and who have had previous medical issues; however, lactose intolerance is on the rise and between 25% and 35% of people may now be diagnosed as lactose intolerant.

Lactose is the main source of sugar from milk and milk products. Lactase is an enzyme and it digests lactose. It is produced by the cells lining the small intestine. In lactose intolerance, lactase is deficient, either partially or completely, which results in malabsorption of the lactose sugar. In this circumstance, lactose bypasses absorption in the small intestine and passes into the colon (large intestine), causing diarrhea, bloating and abdominal distention, all of which are common symptoms — although these symptoms may also be seen in other conditions.

Formal testing, such as breath and blood tests, can confirm a diagnosis. The treatment of lactose intolerance should be aimed at improving digestive symptoms. Frequently, reduction of lactose is recommended — rather than complete exclusion. The quantity of lactose found in yogurt, hard cheeses and pills or tablets is very unlikely to cause gastrointestinal symptoms. If symptoms persist despite these small doses, there could be another, underlying problem.

Alternative lactose substitutes include lactose-free dairy products and lactase enzyme replacement. Although restricting dietary lactose may improve gastrointestinal symptoms, the long-term effects of a diet deficient in dairy products may deprive the body of calcium and put it at higher risk of fractures and incidence of obesity.

Dairy Benefits

Dairy products are an important component of human nutrition and are associated with potential health benefits. Some research suggests that intake of dairy can have a weight-lowering effect. The high calcium content in dairy may facilitate weight loss by suppressing the formation of fat and increasing the excretion of fat. In addition, the whey protein found in milk can contribute to a feeling of fullness and reduce appetite.

Interestingly, high dairy intake has also shown a positive effect with certain diseases. For example, it has been associated with lower rates of developing diabetes. The mechanism behind the impact of dairy consumption on type 2 diabetes can likely be explained in part by the weight-lowering effect of dairy intake. The intake of milk and low-fat dairy has also been associated with lower rates of developing high blood pressure. This is in part related to weight-lowering effects, but also from the impact of dairy on maintaining blood vessel tone in the body. Other minerals found in dairy foods, such as magnesium, calcium and potassium, may also lower blood pressure. Dairy also has an important role to play in preventing bone diseases like osteoporosis.

Dairy-Free Options

Foods that are dairy-free are generally recommended for people who are lactose intolerant. Because these foods do not contain lactose, they should not cause gastrointestinal symptoms if a patient is lactose intolerant. Dairy-free options do not require the lactase enzyme for digestion of these foods. Just the same, patients who are lactose intolerant can still tolerate lactose/dairy in small quantities. Alternatives for lactose-intolerant individuals include yogurt and low-lactose cheeses, in addition to the following dairy-free options:

- **Soy milk:** The term "soy milk" is perhaps misleading, since it isn't technically a milk product. It consists of a liquid extract of soybeans. Soy milk contains a wealth of protein, with 6 to 10 grams a cup (250 mL). Soy milk is fortified with calcium, riboflavin and additional vitamins, making it a nutritious food source. Notably, soy foods are the only plant-based complete protein source and, therefore, are the preferred non-dairy source when needed.

Did You Know?

Probiotics in Dairy

An added benefit of dairy, particularly with fermented dairy products (such as yogurt and dairy-based probiotics), is that it improves the gut bacteria in a favorable manner.

The whey protein found in milk can contribute to a feeling of fullness and reduce appetite.

Did You Know?

Yogurt

One of the advantages of eating yogurt is the positive impact it has on the microbiome, since it is rich in probiotics.

- **Rice milk:** Rice milk is made from boiled rice, brown rice syrup and rice starch. This is also a popular alternative for a vegan lifestyle or those with a dairy intolerance. Compared to traditional dairy milk, the rice variety has less protein (only 1 gram per cup/250 mL) and only a small amount of natural calcium and may or may not be fortified with vitamin D. Most brands, however, are fortified with calcium and are enriched with other vitamins. Because of the lower protein content in rice milk, you would need to lean on other foods to meet protein requirements.

- **Almond milk:** This is another milk alternative, made from ground almonds, water and a small amount of sweetener. Although it can be formulated to have a taste and texture similar to cow's milk, it may be lacking in other nutrients. The protein content in almond milk is lower and generally devoid of the B family of vitamins. Although there is a role for almond milk in the vegan/vegetarian diet, these factors must be considered. Many people prefer the taste of almond milk over other milk substitutes.

- **Coconut milk:** This milk is higher in calories and fat than most milk and milk substitutes. It contains fiber and iron, two notable and beneficial differences in the nutritional profile when compared to cow's milk. Coconut milk is a rich source of protein, containing 6 grams per cup (250 mL).

Omega-3 Sources

Omega-3 fatty acids are essential fatty acids that can be obtained only from your diet. The best-known role for omega-3 fatty acids is in supporting optimal cardiovascular health, but they also help in brain and eye development. Plant-based sources highest in omega-3 fatty acids are sea vegetables, such as arame, dulse, nori, kelp, kombu and wakame. Vegetarians can also find omega-3 fatty acids in flax seeds, flaxseed oil and walnuts. Omega-3 fatty acids keep gaining in popularity and can now be found in fortified foods such as eggs, yogurt, soy beverages and margarine.

Calcium and Vitamin D

Calcium and vitamin D are vital for growth and the maintenance of bones and teeth. Limiting alcohol, caffeine and salt will help keep your bones strong. Here is how much calcium and vitamin D you need.

Calcium and Vitamin D Recommendations

Age (Years)	Calcium RDA (mg/day)	Calcium Upper Limit (mg/day)	Vitamin D RDA (IU/day)	Vitamin D Upper Limit (IU/day)
19–50	1000	2500	600	4000
51–70 (men)	1000	2000	600	4000
51–70 (women)	1200	2000	600	4000
70 and older	1200	2000	800	4000

Calcium from foods is much better absorbed than calcium from supplements. Natural sources of vitamin D are hard to find. While our skin can make vitamin D, the best food sources for lacto-ovo-vegetarians are milk and eggs. Other sources include vitamin D–fortified breakfast cereals and fortified plant-based beverages such as soy milk, rice milk, almond milk and orange juice.

Vegetarian Sources of Calcium

Food	Serving Size
Best sources: 300 mg calcium or more	
Cheese: ricotta	1/2 cup (125 mL)
Cheese: Swiss, Cheddar, Gouda, mozzarella	1 1/2 oz (50 g)
Collard greens, cooked	1 cup (250 mL)
Goat's milk, fortified	1 cup (250 mL)
Milk, lactose-reduced milk and buttermilk	1 cup (250 mL)
Skim milk powder	3 tbsp (45 mL)
Soy, rice or almond beverage, fortified	1 cup (250 mL)
Tofu	5 oz (150 g)
Yogurt, plain	3/4 cup (175 mL)

continued on next page...

Vegetarian Sources of Calcium (continued)

Food	Serving Size
Good sources: 200 to 300 mg of calcium	
Cheese: Parmesan	2 tbsp (30 mL)
Cheese: feta, Camembert	1$\frac{1}{2}$ oz (50 g)
Kale, cooked	1 cup (250 mL)
Molasses, blackstrap	1 tbsp (15 mL)
Mustard greens, cooked	1 cup (250 mL)
Pudding made with milk	$\frac{1}{2}$ cup (125 mL)
Yogurt, flavored	$\frac{3}{4}$ cup (175 mL)
Sources: Less than 200 mg of calcium	
Beans, cooked: navy, white, soy	$\frac{3}{4}$ cup (175 mL)
Bok choy, cooked	$\frac{1}{2}$ cup (125 mL)
Broccoli, cooked	1 cup (250 mL)
Cheese: Brie	1$\frac{1}{2}$ oz (50 g)
Chinese cabbage, cooked	1 cup (250 mL)
Cottage cheese	1 cup (250 mL)
Nuts: almonds, Brazil	$\frac{1}{4}$ cup (60 mL)
Oats, instant	$\frac{3}{4}$ cup (175 mL)
Okra, cooked	$\frac{1}{2}$ cup (125 mL)
Orange juice, fortified	$\frac{1}{2}$ cup (125 mL)
Spinach, cooked	$\frac{1}{2}$ cup (125 mL)
Turnip greens, cooked	$\frac{1}{2}$ cup (125 mL)

Zinc

Zinc is a mineral required daily in small amounts. Its main functions include helping the body use carbohydrates, protein and fat, strengthening the immune system and healing wounds.

Zinc Recommendations

	Recommended Daily Amount (mg/day)	Upper Limit (mg/day)
Men 19 and older	11	40
Women 19 and older	8	40
Pregnant women 19 and older	11	40
Breastfeeding women 19 and older	23	40

Meats provide two to four times the amount of zinc per serving when compared to plant-based sources, so vegetarians need to add more zinc-rich sources to their diet. Also, vegetarian diets can be high in phytates and fiber, which bind zinc and reduce absorption. The best vegetarian sources of zinc are pumpkin and squash seeds, baked beans, wheat germ and tempeh.

Vegetarian Sources of Zinc

Food	Serving Size	Zinc (mg)
Vegetables and Fruits	This food group contains very little zinc.	
Grain Products		
Wheat germ	2 tbsp (30 mL)	2.4
Cereal, bran	1 oz (30 g)	1.8–2.4
Wild rice, cooked	½ cup (125 mL)	1.2
Dairy Products		
Cheese: Brie, Cheddar, Gouda, mozzarella, Swiss	1½ oz (45 g)	1.2–2.2
Yogurt, plain or fruit on the bottom	¾ cup (175 mL)	1.1–1.6
Milk	1 cup (250 mL)	1.0–1.1

continued on next page...

Vegetarian Sources of Zinc (continued)

Food	Serving Size	Zinc (mg)
Meat Alternatives		
Baked beans, cooked	¾ cup (175 mL)	4.3
Seeds: pumpkin, squash	¼ cup (60 mL)	2.7–4.4
Tempeh	¾ cup (175 mL)	2.4
Lentils, cooked	¾ cup (175 mL)	1.9
Cashew butter	2 tbsp (30 mL)	1.7
Soy nuts	¼ cup (60 mL)	1.4
Tahini or sesame butter	2 tbsp (30 mL)	1.4
Soy burger	1 patty (2½ oz/70 g)	1.3
Tofu	¾ cup (175 mL)	1.2–1.7
Eggs, cooked	2 large	1.2–1.3
Peanuts and nuts, shelled: pine nuts, cashews, almonds	¼ cup (60 mL)	1.1–2.2
Chickpeas, cooked	¾ cup (175 mL)	1.1–1.9
Peas, cooked: black-eyed, split	¾ cup (175 mL)	1.1–1.9
Seeds, sunflower, shelled	¼ cup (60 mL)	0.6–1.8

CHAPTER 7

Optimizing Dietary Fiber and Prebiotics

🗁 Case Study

Preventing Obesity and Diabetes

Ben is a 44-year-old male who came to me with concerns about fatty liver disease and diabetes. Ben has experienced some gradual weight gain over the past 5 years. At age 35, his weight was 160 lbs (72 kg); he now weighs 180 lbs (82 kg). Since he was laid off from his job involving heavy physical labor, he has been less motivated to engage in physical activities. The quality of his diet had deteriorated since separating from his wife, 5 years before he was laid off, and he has not made healthy living a priority.

Ben's father was recently diagnosed with liver cirrhosis from fatty liver disease, even though he did not drink alcohol. He was told the cirrhosis was related to obesity and diabetes, and now Ben fears the same for himself.

In the clinic, no significant GI or liver-related symptoms were identified; however, the results showed moderately elevated liver tests and an abnormal fasting sugar, indicating early diabetes. Ben was very keen to avoid medications and was committed to managing his health problems through dietary interventions.

I asked Ben to keep a 7-day food diary. On his follow-up visit, I noted the frequency of packaged and frozen foods, the lack of fruits and vegetables, and the reliance on canned soups for dinner. There were some healthy habits too, though: he enjoyed stir-fries and a morning fruit-rich smoothie, which was notably absent from the diary he brought in for review. Consequently, I referred Ben to a registered dietitian for more counseling on enriching his fiber intake. I discussed how boosting fiber was perhaps the single most important strategy to prevent obesity, improve blood pressure and reduce dependency on medications for diabetes. We discussed how fiber increases the feeling of fullness and slows down the rate of sugar absorption. I also told him about the beneficial impact of fiber on the microbiome. Ben left the clinic motivated to take charge of his health.

Dietary Fiber Through the Ages

In earlier sections of this book, we discussed the benefits of dietary fiber and a vegetarian diet. During prehistoric times, our ancestors lived off the land and consumed between 50 and 100 grams of fiber a day. All fiber came from plant sources, such as berries, other fruits and root vegetables. With sociocultural development and more organized societies came villages with farming and livestock. Over time, fiber intake gradually decreased and, in industrialized nations, fiber was removed from grains because it was not thought to have nutritional value, leaving us with white bread with no fiber and the absence of many important minerals and vitamins. This was accompanied by an increase in processed and ready-made foods designed for convenience and busy lifestyles.

Prebiotic Fibers

We learned earlier that prebiotics are dietary fibers that are non-digestible in the GI tract. Once eaten, prebiotic fibers selectively alter the bacterial composition in the intestine. There are two main categories of prebiotic fibers: fructo-oligosaccharides (FOS) and galacto-oligosaccharides (GOS). Inulin is the most well-known type of FOS and is naturally found in plant foods. Vegetables and fruits rich in inulin include Jerusalem artichokes, asparagus, bananas, leeks and onions. Grains rich in inulin are barley, rye and whole-grain products. Rich root sources of inulin are chicory, dandelion and the herb elecampane. Maximizing prebiotic fibers in the diet will result in many beneficial health effects, as discussed previously. Here is a list of the top 10 prebiotic fiber–containing foods:

1. Asparagus (raw)
2. Chicory root (raw)
3. Jerusalem artichokes (raw)
4. Dandelion greens (raw)
5. Garlic (raw)
6. Onions (raw and cooked)
7. Leeks (raw)
8. Bananas (raw)
9. Wheat bran (raw)
10. Whole wheat flour

This subset of fiber has very specific effects on the bacteria in the gut and may assist in disease prevention and treatment (see "Treating Disease with Prebiotics," page 69). A prebiotic effect occurs when there is an increase in the activity of healthy bacteria in the intestine — that is, prebiotics stimulate the growth of healthy bacteria, such as *Bifidobacterium* and *Lactobacillus*, and thus increase their resistance against bad bacteria.

Adding Prebiotic-Rich Foods to Your Diet

In this section, you will learn about the many health benefits of some prebiotic fiber–rich foods beyond their impact of fiber on health. Remember that in Chapter 4 we reviewed how fiber-rich foods modify the microbiome to reduce the risk of heart disease, diabetes and inflammatory disorders. The beauty of many fiber-rich foods lies in their versatility. Whether eaten fresh or cooked, there are multiple ways to enjoy the richness of nutrients in these prebiotic foods.

Asparagus

Asparagus contains anti-inflammatory nutrients in addition to antioxidant nutrients, including vitamin C, beta-carotene, vitamin E and the minerals zinc, manganese and selenium. Asparagus is a good source of fiber, providing about 3 grams per cup (250 mL), and is also rich in inulin. Cooking asparagus affects the inulin content, potentially reducing the availability of the prebiotic.

Preparation Tips

Raw asparagus is not as palatable, so gently steaming or sautéing it is a good way to balance the inulin and fiber benefits while enhancing taste. You can grate raw asparagus into a salad or gently steam it and toss into a favorite pasta recipe. Chopped asparagus adds flavor and color to omelets. Make asparagus a complete meal by sautéing it with garlic and mushrooms and pairing it with tofu.

Chicory Root

Chicory root is an herb that is available worldwide. It is rich in inulin and has more recently been making an appearance in organic baked snacks, granola bars, yogurts and ice cream. It has little taste and a smooth and creamy texture. Chicory root is also used as a coffee substitute in many parts of the world; the roasted roots are ground and brewed. Like other high-fiber foods, chicory root prevents constipation, helps maintain a healthy balance of good bacteria in the gut and lowers cholesterol levels. Consuming too much chicory root can result in bloating, gas, nausea and abdominal cramping.

Jerusalem Artichoke

The Jerusalem artichoke is the tuber of a variety of perennial flower in the aster family. Its flowers resemble small yellow sunflowers and its roots are similar to gingerroot in appearance. These tubers have a potato-like texture and are often recommended as a potato substitute for diabetics. Interestingly enough, the Jerusalem artichoke is not an artichoke and does not have a Jerusalem connection. Today, the term "Jerusalem artichoke" is used interchangeably with its less-known name "sunchoke." The Jerusalem artichoke is exceptionally rich in inulin, which contributes to its slightly sweet flavor.

Preparation Tips

Very thinly sliced Jerusalem artichokes are a great addition to salads. Puréed Jerusalem artichokes are excellent in risottos and soups. Drizzled in oil and roasted along with potatoes, these tubers make a delicious side dish.

Dandelion Greens

Like other leafy greens, these bitter greens are rich in fiber and include a host of other nutrients such as phytochemicals; vitamins A, K and C; and minerals such as iron and calcium.

Preparation Tips

Use dandelion greens in salads or substitute them in recipes that call for kale, spinach or collard greens.

Garlic

The health benefits of garlic are well known. Native to central Asia, garlic is one of the oldest cultivated plants in the world, grown for more than 5,000 years. Garlic is an herb and is best known for flavoring food. Over the years, it has also been used as a medicine to prevent or treat a wide range of diseases and conditions.

Preparation Tips

Eating raw garlic is the best way to derive its health benefits. Purée it in a dip or toss it into a fresh pesto or salsa. If you cannot tolerate eating it raw, adding chopped garlic toward the end of cooking may maximize its nutritive inulin content and taste.

FAQ

 What are some of the health benefits of garlic?

 Garlic is used by a variety of different cultures around the world and is one of the oldest medicinal plants for the treatment and prevention of disease. Its benefits are vast and include antimicrobial activity similar to some antibiotics. Garlic also has immune-stimulating properties that give it the ability to fend off harmful bacteria. Garlic is known to have antioxidant properties, which may reduce the impact of toxic metabolic products that could find their way into the body from the environment or that are produced naturally. When it comes to protecting against heart disease, garlic delays hardening of the arteries, a condition known as atherosclerosis. In animal studies, it has been shown that garlic reduces cholesterol and triglycerides, which are significant risk factors for heart disease and heart attacks. Last, garlic has been known to have anti-inflammatory and anticancer effects. The magnitude of these effects is not entirely known, but studies continue to investigate the health benefits of garlic.

Garlic in the Gut

Background: Many health benefits of garlic are known but the effect of garlic on the microbiome is not well defined.

Objectives: To describe the influence of garlic on the body's gut microbiota.

Methods: This study was conducted in vitro: either in test tubes or in a culture dish, outside the human body. Multiple bacterial cultures were used and test tubes were inoculated with bacterial strains. Subsequently, garlic powder was added to the test tubes. A control test tube was also used — bacterial cultures were inoculated but did not receive garlic.

Results: Garlic powder killed multiple bacterial strains in the test tubes. Particularly, strains of *Bacteroides* and *Clostridium* bacteria showed a significant reduction in numbers in the tubes infused with garlic. A number of other bacterial strains, such as *Lactobacillus* species, were not as affected by garlic. In the control tube, the bacterial numbers proliferated.

Conclusions: Garlic had an inhibitory effect on some species of bacteria. The impact of these test-tube findings in the human body is still unknown but deserves further study. It is conceivable that with long-term exposure, garlic may promote a favorable microbiome composition.

Did You Know?

Onion Potency

Onions have been shown to have a blood sugar–lowering action. They also have potent antibacterial activity, perhaps because of their inulin prebiotic properties, which have the ability to destroy many disease-causing pathogens.

Onions/Leeks

More than just a tasty culinary plant, the onion contains natural sugar; vitamins A, B_6, C and E; minerals such as sodium, potassium and iron; dietary fiber; and inulin. Raw onions are exceptionally powerful. In their raw state, they contain an abundance of organic sulfur compounds that are partially destroyed when exposed to heat. For people who have trouble eating raw onions, cooking them will make them more palatable while still conserving most of their health benefits.

Preparation Tips

Onions and leeks can be eaten raw (in salads, appetizers or cold soups) or steamed, boiled or roasted. Sautéed chopped onions can be added to almost any vegetable dish to enhance its nutritional content and taste. So be liberal with your onion intake and enjoy the many health advantages.

Raw Bananas

"Raw banana" refers to the green banana, before it ripens. Nutritionally, the green banana is a source of fiber, vitamin B_6 and potassium. The high fiber content in raw bananas has been shown to regulate blood sugar and manage weight.

Wheat Bran/Whole Wheat Flour

Wheat bran is the hard outer layer of the wheat berry. Raw wheat bran has the most prebiotic fibers. In addition to a whopping amount of fiber, wheat bran is also a good source of iron, magnesium and vitamin B_6.

Whole wheat flour is derived from the whole grain and contains all its components.

Incorporate both wheat bran and whole wheat flour as often as possible in everyday meals.

Incorporate both wheat bran and whole wheat flour as often as possible in everyday meals.

Tips to Increase Your Fiber Intake

1. Aim to eat 5 to 10 servings of fruits and vegetables daily. Eat at least one dark green vegetable and one orange vegetable daily. Choose vegetables and fruits prepared with little or no added fat, sugar or salt. Minimize juices and eat the whole fruit when possible.
2. Include legumes in your diet on a regular basis. Eat them on their own and use them in stews, salads and dips.
3. Eat at least 6 servings of whole-grain products daily. Choose whole-grain breads, breakfast cereals, pastas and baked goods made with oats, barley, quinoa, amaranth, millet, brown rice or whole wheat.
4. Add 1 tablespoon (15 mL) ground flax seeds (flaxseed meal) or wheat bran to your cereal in the morning.
5. Aim to eat high-fiber foods throughout the day.
6. Increase the fiber in your diet gradually, as rapid increases may cause gas, bloating and diarrhea.
7. Read food labels. Compare products and choose the ones with the most fiber. Become knowledgeable about comparing similar serving sizes. Check for grams of fiber. Look for ingredients that include wheat bran or whole wheat flour, as these are especially rich in prebiotic content.
8. Replace at least half of the white (all-purpose/cake) flour in your recipes with whole-grain flour.

Fiber Claims on Food Labels	
Standardized Definitions	**Grams of Fiber Per Serving**
Source of fiber	2
High source of fiber	4
Very high source of fiber	6

Prebiotic Supplements

Apart from diet, prebiotics may be found in the following forms:

- On their own as a prebiotic supplement
- In a probiotic supplement
- In a nutritional supplement
- In a meal replacement
- In a fiber supplement
- In a vitamin, mineral or herbal supplement (typically as inulin or fructo-oligosaccharides)

Prebiotic Claims

Recommended intakes for dietary fiber, with attention to prebiotic-rich fibers, should be sufficient to meet requirements.

Many countries have no standards or recommendations for the consumption of prebiotics because there has been no established system for health claims. In the United States, the Dietary Guidelines for Americans Committee (DGAC) stated that the gut microbiota plays a role in health and recognizes that consumer interest in altering the microbiota is high. However, the DGAC currently feels that there is insufficient evidence to make blanket recommendations for Americans about prebiotics or probiotics. The committee has noted, however, that although not all fibers are prebiotics, all prebiotics are fibers. Therefore, recommended intakes for dietary fiber, with attention to prebiotic-rich fibers, should be sufficient to meet requirements. In the U.S., health claims attributed to prebiotics are not used because the Food and Drug Administration (FDA) has not yet approved such claims.

Similarly, nutrient claims cannot be made because a daily value has not been established for prebiotics.

In Canada, Health Canada is in the process of developing guidelines to clarify acceptable use of the term "prebiotic." In Europe, the French Agency for Food, Environmental and Occupational Health and Safety has approved both inulin and FOS as prebiotics at 5 grams a day. There are two allowable claims: First, a bifidogenic effect at a daily dose of 5 grams oligofructose stimulates *Bifidobacterium* in the gut. Second, native inulin from chicory at a daily dose of 5 grams is prebiotic. Similarly, in the Netherlands, inulin was approved as a prebiotic at 5 grams a day.

Doc Talk

How can all of this information be interpreted? A large part of my clinical practice focuses on nutrition. For a gastroenterologist, it may seem intuitive that nutrition and GI health and treatment go together. However, there are many challenging aspects to the practice of nutrition in the field of gastroenterology, and this is because there is a lack of well-established scientific evidence for many nutrition-based therapies. This is not to say that nutrition is unimportant or that it does not have a role in the prevention of disease and maintenance of health. Quite the contrary. I truly believe that nutrition is the cornerstone of good health and disease prevention. Researchers tend to focus efforts on discovering the next blockbuster drug to cure cancer or fight AIDS or Ebola virus. Because of limited resources, nutrition-related research has often taken a back seat to other pressing global health concerns, resulting in smaller studies that may be applicable to larger populations. With the limited amount of evidence for the role of prebiotic fiber in health, the evidence has to be interpreted based on the body's biology — in other words, what we know the body is capable of doing.

I remind my patients that the average North American diet contains barely one-third of the recommended amount of fiber. You might assume that if this is the case, any potential health benefit from prebiotic fiber is lost, since it falls short of the recommended amounts. Taking a fiber supplement may seem like an easy way to make up for the shortfall and incorporate fiber in your diet, but I recommend rethinking your daily dietary routine and your approaches to food and nutrition instead. While fiber supplements can boost fiber intake, they cannot provide you with the wealth of nutrients that accompany the fiber found in naturally occurring food sources. There is a place for fiber supplements in your diet, but only in conjunction with a well-balanced diet. Your doctor may have other reasons to recommend fiber supplements; if they are recommended, be sure to follow your doctor's directions. In the context of health and prevention, there is no substitute for a nutritionally balanced diet.

CHAPTER 8

How to Optimize Dietary Probiotics

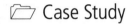 Case Study

Managing IBS

Param is a 48-year-old woman who had been experiencing abdominal bloating and cramping for 10 years. In a routine visit to her family physician, she reported that she was constipated for most of the week and had only three semi-formed bowel movements each week. Her abdominal pain and bloating usually improved following a bowel movement. She had no family history of gastrointestinal illness, nor did she have any concerning associated symptoms, such as weight loss or bloody bowel movements.

The colonoscopy ordered by her doctor came back normal, and her blood work was reassuring. Her doctor diagnosed her with irritable bowel syndrome, reassuring her that IBS is a benign diagnosis, and quite prevalent. He recommended dietary modification and a trial of probiotic supplements, explaining that probiotics are important in the management of IBS.

Param subsequently decreased her intake of lactose-containing products, simple sugars, caffeine and higher-fat foods, all of which are known triggers for IBS. However, she decided not to take supplemental probiotics, because she believed she could consume enough probiotics simply by eating more yogurt.

When she returned to see her physician at her follow-up appointment, Param reported symptom improvement thanks to her dietary changes, and wondered whether he still recommended probiotic supplements. Her doctor assured her that yogurt is, indeed, rich in probiotics when refrigerated appropriately and used by the expiry date stated on the label. He agreed that her increased consumption of yogurt would likely be sufficient to maintain her goals of symptom control and improved quality of life. However, he also passed along some reading material on other natural sources of probiotics, so that she could add some variety to her diet as desired.

As noted earlier in the book, probiotics are organisms (such as bacteria) that improve health. They should not be confused with prebiotics, which are a subset of dietary fibers that are metabolized in the gut to specifically grow bacteria that are beneficial to health. Just the same, both are used for the same reason. Adding a full variety of prebiotic- and probiotic-friendly foods to your diet will improve your health tremendously.

Probiotics can help replace good bacteria in your body after you lose them, as in the case of taking antibiotics. Probiotics can also lower the numbers of harmful gut bacteria that may predispose you to infections and inflammation; they do this by stimulating your immune system in a helpful manner. In addition, probiotics can help balance your good and bad bacteria to maintain health.

Probiotics are available in foods and supplements. Below are some probiotic-friendly foods.

> Adding a full variety of prebiotic- and probiotic-friendly foods to your diet will improve your health tremendously.

Top 8 Probiotic-Rich Foods

Yogurt

One of the best probiotic foods is live-cultured yogurt. There are several benefits to eating yogurt, including relief of symptoms from constipation, diarrhea and inflammatory bowel disease. Yogurt with active cultures may prevent vaginal infections. It is also believed to boost the immune system, a probiotic consequence. Yogurt is good for the heart too — intake may reduce the risk of high blood pressure. One study confirmed a 50% reduction in the risk of developing high blood pressure in people who ate two to three servings of low-fat yogurt daily compared to those who ate no yogurt. Beyond the probiotic benefits, yogurt is a source of calcium, which is best known to have beneficial effects on bone mass in people of all ages. For vegetarians, note that yogurt is a rich source of protein and a staple of the lacto-vegetarian diet.

Did You Know?

Fighting Candida
Candida infections, or vaginal yeast infections, are a particular problem in women with diabetes. A small study assessing women with chronic vaginitis who consumed 6 ounces (175 mL) of yogurt per day for 6 months reported a decrease in the frequency of candida infections.

FAQ

Q **What types of yogurt should I purchase and what are the differences between the many brands available?**

A Yogurt is available in regular-fat, low-fat or fat-free varieties. If you have been diagnosed with any cardiac risk factors (such as high blood pressure) or high cholesterol, or if you are overweight or smoke, a better choice for you would be a lower-fat yogurt option. Some brands have higher sugar content than others, in some cases to replace the fat in their fat-free options — compare the labels for sugar content per serving size. Plain yogurt is a better choice. Simply add fruit, chia seeds or cereal. Look for "active cultures" and "probiotic" on the label. Most brands will have a label that says "live and active cultures," which refers to the living organisms *Lactobacillus delbrueckii* subsp. *bulgaricus* and *Streptococcus salivarius* subsp. *thermophiles*, which convert pasteurized milk into yogurt during the fermentation process. But since all yogurts are required to be made with these two cultures, the labels only reveal the obvious. Some yogurts, however, contain additional probiotics, particularly *Lactobacillus acidophilus* and *Bifidobacterium*, which can offer greater benefit to gut health.

Kefir

Like yogurt, kefir is a cultured milk product with a tart and sour taste. Kefir is made with bacteria and yeast. It is prepared by exposing cow's, goat's or sheep's milk to kefir grains or bacteria. As with yogurt, several varieties of probiotic bacteria are found in kefir, including *Lactobacillus acidophilus*, *Bifidobacterium* and *Streptococcus thermophilus*, among others. These beneficial strains of probiotic bacteria can shape the gut microbiome to maintain health and fight infections and inflammatory diseases. There are few scientifically validated studies exploring the health benefits of kefir. Similarly to milk, several dietary minerals are found in kefir, such as calcium, iron, phosphorus, magnesium, potassium and zinc. Their values have not yet been accurately captured, making it impossible to enter kefir's profile into nutritional databases. Kefir can be used to make sourdough bread or as a buttermilk substitute in baking, or it can be enjoyed on its own as a drink. It is available for purchase or can be made at home.

Sauerkraut

In addition to being a probiotic star, sauerkraut is rich in vitamins B_1, B_6, folic acid and C and in minerals, including iron, magnesium, manganese, phosphorus and potassium. Sauerkraut is finely cut cabbage that has been fermented by various bacteria. It has a distinctive sour flavor and is typically used as a condiment with various foods, although many enjoy it as a side dish with meals. Raw sauerkraut can be homemade and is preferable to store-bought sauerkraut. Many food manufacturers can or jar their sauerkraut using heat, which extends shelf life; however, this process may compromise the probiotic effect. In contrast, raw sauerkraut is fermented over days or weeks at room temperature, packed into jars at room temperature and then refrigerated to preserve the probiotic effect.

Miso Soup

Miso soup is one of the staples of the Japanese diet, dating back more than 2,500 years, and is used in macrobiotic cooking as a remedy for digestive ailments. Miso is a paste made from soybeans, sea salt and a mold starter, often mixed with rice, barley or other grains. By adding 1 tablespoon (15 mL) of miso to some hot water, a probiotic-rich soup full of *Lactobacillus* and *Bifidobacterium* is created, which enriches the microbiome. For those individuals who abstain from milk-based products, consider miso an excellent probiotic source.

By adding 1 tablespoon (15 mL) of miso to some hot water, a probiotic-rich soup full of *Lactobacillus* and *Bifidobacterium* is created, which enriches the microbiome.

Sour Pickles

Pickles are another source of dairy-free probiotics. If you choose not to eat dairy foods or cannot tolerate them, finding dairy-free probiotics can pose a challenge. Sour pickles are the traditional alternative to vinegar pickles and are prepared using sea salt and chlorine-free water. Sour pickles are raw after culturing, unlike vinegar-based cucumber pickles, which are cooked during the canning process, reducing the probiotic effect.

Tempeh

Tempeh is a fermented food that has its origins in Indonesia several centuries ago. Traditionally, this food is made by adding a yeast-based starter to legumes, whole grains, vegetables and other types of beans. During the fermentation process, the yeast starter binds with the base ingredients to give the tempeh a cake-like form. Tempeh is a good source of micronutrients, including magnesium, manganese, calcium and iron. In addition, the fermentation process increases the probiotic effect and provides yet another non-dairy-based probiotic alternative.

Kimchi

The health benefits of kimchi — in addition to the positive impact on the microbiome — include anticancer properties, immune promotion, a reduction in cholesterol and improvement of constipation.

Kimchi is a traditional Korean food manufactured by fermenting vegetables with probiotic lactic acid bacteria. Kimchi can be considered a vegetable probiotic food that contributes health benefits in a similar way to yogurt or other dairy probiotic foods. Furthermore, the major ingredients of kimchi are cruciferous vegetables and other healthy, fiber-rich foods, such as garlic and ginger, which all undergo fermentation by the lactic acid bacteria. Because kimchi is tasty and so beneficial for the microbiome, it is used very frequently as a dietary staple in Korean meals. The health benefits of kimchi — in addition to the positive impact on the microbiome — include anticancer properties, immune promotion, a reduction in cholesterol and improvement of constipation.

Kombucha Tea

Kombucha tea is a sweetened black tea fermented by a colony of bacteria and yeast. The bacterial components of kombucha tea cultures have not been studied extensively but are known to consist of several species, including acetic acid bacteria and lactic acid bacteria.

To date, there have been very few scientific studies endorsing the health benefits of kombucha tea. However, the same can be said for a number of common or less common foods. Emerging data suggest that kombucha tea has antioxidant effects and can promote the detoxification of toxic metabolites and improve states of depressed immunity. Collectively, these factors make kombucha tea an attractive fermented beverage for health maintenance. Consult a registered dietitian for further information regarding kombucha tea and methods of preparation.

Tips for Probiotic Living

1. Aim to eat one to two servings of yogurt daily. Milk and yogurt have similar health benefits, but yogurt has the clear probiotic advantage. Remember that people who have been diagnosed with lactose intolerance can also enjoy and tolerate yogurt, since it is low in lactose. You can add yogurt to smoothies, to your morning cereal and to fruit as a dessert.
2. Need a break from yogurt? Consider adding a glass of kefir to your morning routine once a week.
3. Add some sour pickles to your salad. Or pack some sour pickles for your mid-afternoon snack at work to keep those salt cravings at bay.
4. Enjoy sauerkraut as a side dish with your main meal.
5. Soup fan? Try miso soup.
6. Limit antibiotics to conditions that require them, and comply with your doctor's suggestions with regard to duration.

Doc Talk

A frequent question that I receive in my practice relates to the superiority of natural probiotic sources compared to probiotic supplements. I typically respond to these questions on a case-by-case basis, taking into consideration the medical history, concurrent medical diagnoses and current medications. No single answer fits all patients. In general, if you are a healthy individual looking to maintain your good health and prevent diseases, probiotic-rich foods from naturally occurring sources are adequate, more economical and perhaps healthier, since natural foods are loaded with other beneficial nutrients that are not found in supplements. If you have a GI medical diagnosis or have been exposed to antibiotics and are experiencing GI side effects from them, or are planning to travel and wish to prevent traveler's diarrhea, then arguably probiotic supplements are a more appropriate choice for you.

PART III

The 8-Step Biotic-Balanced Program

CHAPTER 9

Nutrition Prescription for Healthy Living

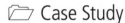 Case Study

Balanced Living

Mariah is a 52-year-old woman who came to my clinic 5 years ago with low hemoglobin and a concern about the potential for iron-deficiency anemia. She complained about some mild constipation and generalized fatigue. She expressed some anxiety about developing colon cancer, since her mother was diagnosed at age 50 with the disease. She was also newly diagnosed with type 2 diabetes.

I recommended a colonoscopy, given her family history and evidence of iron-deficiency anemia. Fortunately, we discovered only one polyp, which was benign, and I recommended a follow-up colonoscopy in 5 years.

Mariah also requested a nutrition prescription to improve the course of her diabetes, lower the risk of developing colon cancer and prevent further metabolic diseases, such as high cholesterol and heart disease. I prescribed an eight-step biotic-balanced program (see "Overview of the 8-Step Biotic-Balanced Program," page 125). I referred her to a registered dietitian to reinforce these principles and to learn about recording her intake in a food diary.

Five years later, I saw Mariah on a follow-up visit. She was a completely new person. She had lost 18 lbs (8 kg). Her diabetes was controlled, her cholesterol was within normal limits, her fatigue had cleared up and she was following a very active and healthy lifestyle. Her bowel movements were regular and she had just completed her first marathon. Mariah ascribed her new health status to adopting a vegetarian diet and to reducing her intake of foods that are processed, high in sugar and high in salt. She particularly emphasized the benefits of a high-fiber diet in helping her with weight loss and reducing her dependency on medications to maintain good blood-sugar control.

The premise of this book has been to present and interpret the scientific evidence for the microbiome's impact on health and disease. A crucial factor in shaping the microbiome is no doubt diet. As this field continues to emerge and explode in research labs, more robust data will allow health-care professionals to refine and prescribe nutrition practices with greater clarity. In the meantime, incorporating what we know about both diet and disease will shape the optimal nutrition prescription for microbiome-friendly health.

Overview of the 8-Step Biotic-Balanced Program

1. Follow a balanced diet rich in plant-based foods. Determine which vegetarian foods you enjoy and eat them regularly.

2. Choose vegetarian foods from all food groups:
   - Whole grains
   - Fruits
   - Vegetables
   - Legumes
   - Nuts and seeds
   - Eggs
   - Dairy (milk, yogurt, cheese)
   - Vegetable oils

3. Include probiotic-rich foods in your diet on a daily basis.
   - Incorporate 1 to 2 cups (250 to 500 mL) yogurt into your diet daily.
   - Add kefir and sauerkraut to your regular routine.
   - Enjoy miso soup.

4. Strive for 25 to 35 grams of dietary fiber daily through the intake of:
   - Whole grains
   - Fruits and vegetables
   - Legumes
   - Nuts and seeds

5. Keep your pantry stocked with prebiotic-rich foods.

6. Consider fiber supplements if fiber intake is still lacking despite these suggestions.

7. Ensure adequate intake of iron-rich foods, and eat or drink vitamin C with them.

8. Consider a vitamin B_{12} supplement if you are a vegan. If you eat eggs and drink milk, you likely do not need a vitamin B_{12} supplement.

The 8 Steps Expanded

① Follow a Balanced Diet Rich in Plant-Based Foods

Before following any nutrition program, it makes sense to identify the foods that you naturally tend to enjoy, eat frequently and have at home on a regular basis. However, you might be surprised to hear that when people are asked to provide a food diary from memory, or are asked to recall foods they've eaten in the past 24 hours, they often miss many foods. Therefore, start a food diary to document your natural eating patterns, without making any modifications to your usual pattern of eating. The food diary should capture 7 days of eating patterns, with attention to meals, snacks, beverages, portion sizes, frequency of restaurant meals, and mode of preparation. You should complete the food diary in real time, not at the end of the day, for greater accuracy.

Once you have kept a food diary for 7 days, it should be critically reviewed, with attention to the sources and frequency of your food choices. Count your servings of whole grains, fruits and vegetables. Compare your intake of these foods to reliable recommendations for healthy living, such as the United States Department of Agriculture's (USDA's) MyPlate guidelines (www.choosemyplate.gov) or Eating Well with Canada's Food Guide (http://www.hc-sc.gc.ca/fn-an/food-guide-aliment/index-eng.php). Attempt to eat at least one dark green vegetable and one orange vegetable a day. This will help ensure an optimal variety of nutrients. Prepare vegetables and fruits with little or no added fat, sugar or salt. Limit juices in favor of whole fruits and vegetables. Choose whole grains from a variety of sources, such as barley, brown rice, oats, quinoa and wild rice. Think about whole wheat or whole-grain pasta instead of white pasta.

Next, consider your sources of milk and milk alternatives. Milk products are rich sources of calcium and protein. Compare your intake of milk products with the recommendations in MyPlate or Canada's Food Guide. Both guides provide very general guidelines on food intake patterns based on aspects of nutritional science believed to maintain health and reduce the

> Attempt to eat at least one dark green vegetable and one orange vegetable a day. This will ensure an optimal variety of nutrients.

rates of chronic diseases. Select lower-fat milk alternatives, such as nonfat, 1% or 2%, and enjoy them every day. Look for reduced-fat and lower-sodium cheese options. Limit cream cheese, ice cream, half-and-half (10%) cream and heavy or whipping (35%) cream, since these are rich in calories and predispose you to obesity and chronic diseases.

Next, look at your protein sources. If you are a non-vegetarian and enjoy meat products, your biggest protein sources are likely animal-based. While reviewing your food diary, assess your proportion of animal sources compared to vegetable protein sources. If you were to reduce animal-based proteins in your diet, which plant-based proteins would you choose? Figure out which vegetarian protein sources you enjoy most. Are there vegetarian sources of protein you haven't previously tried but are interested in trying? Remember that beans, eggs, hummus, lentils, nuts, nut butters and tofu are just a few excellent vegetarian sources of protein. Consult the earlier chapters in this book regarding a more comprehensive strategy to integrate vegetarian sources of protein into your diet. Not ready to give up meat just yet? Changing your diet and lifestyle are incredibly difficult steps to take. Consider reducing your meat-based servings gradually, and consider cutting out animal protein even just one day a week.

Remember that the quantity of food eaten is as important as the quality of food choices. One of the most important decisions we make about food is how much to eat. Many people struggle with understanding the appropriate portion sizes to eat. First, it is important to understand that *serving size* and *portion size* refer to two different concepts. A serving size is a reference amount of food as defined by a health body, such as Health Canada or the Food and Drug Administration (FDA). The recommended servings for common foods are itemized in the USDA's MyPlate and Canada's Food Guide. In contrast, a portion size is the amount of food that you actually put on your plate, the portion that you plan to eat in a single meal. In most cases, people's portion sizes are very different from recommended serving sizes. When keeping a food diary, and subsequently when reviewing it, remember this fact, as it will determine your current intake and provide insight about remaining needs.

Beans, eggs, hummus, lentils, nuts, nut butters and tofu are just a few excellent vegetarian sources of protein.

② Choose Vegetarian Foods from All Food Groups

We have covered aspects of this guideline in the previous section. Four food groups are required for healthy living. These food groups are vegetables/fruits, whole-grain products, milk/alternatives, and meat/alternatives. Increasing variety, even within one food group, is important to health. Variety increases the likelihood that you will obtain all the nutrients and minerals that are required for good health. For example, some foods are rich sources of vitamin A or C, while others are excellent sources of folate or iron. Also, increasing variety will make your meals more interesting.

③ Include Probiotic-Rich Foods in Your Diet on a Daily Basis

Review your food diary to assess the frequency and portion sizes of probiotic-rich foods documented. Remember that people with lactose intolerance can enjoy most probiotic-rich foods without fear of symptoms. Aim to eat one to two servings of yogurt daily. Be creative and don't be afraid to experiment with blended yogurt smoothies or protein shakes — a delicious start to your day. Try a glass of kefir or make some homemade traditional sauerkraut. Add a hot bowl of miso soup to your dinner on a chilly evening. Miso is an indispensable seasoning found in most Japanese kitchens, and the soup's ease of preparation and simplicity of taste make it a popular probiotic-rich food.

Slowly increasing your probiotic-rich food intake to four servings a day will result in a very favorable gut microbiome. Most probiotic-rich foods are vegetarian in nature, and this fits in nicely with the idea of optimizing plant-based foods in your diet.

④ Strive for 25 to 35 Grams of Dietary Fiber Daily

It is important to become proficient in reading food labels. This is particularly true when it comes to understanding the sources of fiber. For foods that are packaged, the Nutrition Facts table can help you make food choices that are optimal for you. The top of the Nutrition Facts table shows the serving size and the servings per container, which is key to understanding the rest of the table.

Slowly increasing your probiotic-rich food intake to four servings a day will result in a very favorable gut microbiome. Most probiotic-rich foods are vegetarian in nature, and this fits in nicely with the idea of optimizing plant-based foods in your diet.

Sample Nutrition Facts Tables

American Table

Nutrition Facts

Serving Size 1 cup (228 g)

Amount Per Serving

Calories 250   **Calories** from Fat 110

	% Daily Value
Total Fat 12 g	**18%**
Saturated Fat 3 g	**15%**
Trans Fat 3 g	
Cholesterol 30 mg	**10%**
Sodium 470 mg	**20%**
Total Carbohydrate 31 g	**10%**
Dietary Fiber 3 g	**12%**
Sugars 5 g	
Protein 5 g	

Vitamin A 4%	•	Calcium 20%
Vitamin C 2%	•	Iron 4%

* Percent Daily Values are based on a 2,000 calorie diet. Your Daily Values may be higher or lower depending on your calorie needs.

	Calories	2,000	2,500
Total Fat	Less than	65 g	80 g
Sat Fat	Less than	20 g	25 g
Cholesterol	Less than	300 mg	300 mg
Sodium	Less than	2,400 mg	2,400 mg
Total Carbohydrate		300 g	375 g
Dietary Fiber		25 g	30 g

Canadian Table

Nutrition Facts

Per 250 mL (228 g)

Amount	% Daily Value
Calories 250	
Fat 12 g	18%
Saturated 3 g + Trans 3 g	15%
Cholesterol 30 mg	
Sodium 470 mg	20%
Carbohydrate 31 g	10%
Fibre 3 g	12%
Sugars 5 g	
Protein 5 g	

Vitamin A	4%	Vitamin C	20%
Calcium	2%	Iron	4%

The nutrition information about the food is based on one serving. If you eat two servings, you are getting double the calories and nutrients described in the table. Take every opportunity to increase dietary fiber to a target of 25 to 35 grams a day. Assess your current food choices and determine which ones you could substitute with a higher-fiber item. Remember, as previously discussed, that there are two types of fiber — soluble and insoluble fiber — and both offer various benefits (see "Forms of Fiber," page 60). Note that the nutrition table will not break down the types of fiber found in a product.

Compare labels and choose the foods with higher fiber, in particular when evaluating whole-grain products such as whole-grain breads, cereals, pastas, brown rice and whole wheat couscous, among others. Similarly, compare the fiber content in canned and frozen fruits and vegetables.

Although the focus is on fiber intake, keep in mind that the fiber in packaged foods may be accompanied by sugar and fats. Ultimately, a comparison of labels for fat and sugar content is critical to making optimal health choices. For example, a food with 10 grams of fiber that is rich in simple sugar may not be as beneficial as a food with 8 grams of fiber that is lower in simple sugar content. With more awareness and practice interpreting food labels, you will find this task becomes less daunting and actually more enjoyable, knowing that you are in control of your health.

⑤ Keep Your Pantry Stocked with Prebiotic-Rich Foods

If you consistently eat the suggested fiber amounts, chances are good that your prebiotic fiber intake will be adequate. Many high-fiber foods are also prebiotics. Review the contents of your refrigerator and pantry to ensure that you have the highest concentration of prebiotic foods — raw chicory root, raw Jerusalem artichokes, raw dandelion greens, raw garlic, raw leeks, raw and cooked onions, raw asparagus, raw wheat bran, whole wheat flour and raw bananas. View this as your opportunity to try new foods, be creative with recipes and enjoy new flavors while remodeling your gut microbiome. Presently, the quantity of prebiotic fiber needed for optimal health is unknown; however, a diet that includes a diverse variety of high-fiber fruits and vegetables has the greatest potential for obtaining sufficient amounts of prebiotics.

⑥ Consider Fiber Supplements in Some Cases

The best way to meet your fiber requirements is to eat whole natural foods. Natural foods that are rich in fiber are robust in many other nutrients, such as antioxidants and inflammation-fighting agents. However, meeting daily fiber requirements consistently may remain a challenge for even the most well-intentioned person. Once you have completed a comprehensive week-long food diary, you will have a good idea of your fiber

Fiber Boost

Tips to increase fiber intake:
- Enjoy a high-fiber breakfast cereal.
- Add nuts, dried fruits and seeds to cereals, and enjoy them for snacks.
- Choose whole-grain products.
- Eat fresh fruits and vegetables with skins, where possible.
- Enjoy legumes and lentil dishes for supper.

intake. If you still struggle to eat 25 to 35 grams of fiber daily, it is reasonable to consider a fiber supplement. Fiber supplements are usually made from functional fibers, which are fibers that are extracted from plants. They are packaged as powders, capsules and tablets. Common fiber supplements include psyllium, inulin and oligofructose. Inulin and oligofructose are prebiotic fibers, whereas psyllium is a soluble fiber without documented prebiotic properties, although it does have other health benefits. Consider choosing a prebiotic-rich fiber supplement to close the fiber gap as a first step.

⑦ Ensure Adequate Intake of Iron-Rich Foods, and Eat or Drink Vitamin C with Them

Review your food diary for iron-rich food sources (see "Vegetarian Sources of Iron," page 93, for more details). Remember to double your amount of iron-rich sources if you're a vegetarian, as plant-based sources of iron are not as well absorbed. The good news, though, is that dietary iron is absorbed best when coupled with a rich source of vitamin C. Consider drinking a glass of orange juice, adding some grapefruit to your meal or having a side salad rich in broccoli, kiwis, tomatoes or peppers with your iron-rich foods.

Some foods and nutrients, such as calcium, coffee and tea, reduce iron absorption. Tea, coffee and calcium supplements should be consumed several hours before or after a meal that is high in iron.

While reviewing your food diary, pay attention to the timing of foods and nutrients in addition to the contents and portion sizes. Remember that if you have been diagnosed with iron-deficiency anemia and your dietary iron intake is adequate, you must see your doctor for additional testing.

> Dietary iron is absorbed best when coupled with a rich source of vitamin C.

Did You Know?

Mother Nature Knows Best

Fortunately, many iron-containing vegetarian foods are also rich in vitamin C, which must be Mother Nature's strategy to assist with better iron absorption in the body.

⑧ Consider a Vitamin B₁₂ Supplement if You Are a Vegan

The only reliable vegan sources of vitamin B_{12} are foods fortified with vitamin B_{12} and B_{12} supplements. To ensure adequate vitamin B_{12} intake as a vegan, eat fortified foods two to three times daily to get at least 3 micrograms of vitamin B_{12} a day. To do this, review your current food diary for estimates of vitamin B_{12}–fortified foods. Reading and interpreting food labels is an asset when doing this calculation. If you are relying on fortified foods, check the food labels carefully to ensure that you understand what a serving size is and how much vitamin B_{12} is offered in each serving. There are very minimal risks or side effects if your intake of vitamin B_{12} exceeds the recommended amounts. If you are not meeting these recommendations, take a vitamin B_{12} supplement daily and notify your doctor that you are doing so.

A vegetarian's risk of developing vitamin B_{12} deficiency is lower than a vegan's, as long as cheese, yogurt, eggs and milk are included in the diet.

CHAPTER 10

Changing Your Eating Habits

📁 Case Study

Developing Goals

Malia is a busy mother of three. She works part-time as a nurse, picking up a variety of shifts at the local hospital. Her husband works full-time as a contractor and often comes home late. Between all the demands of long and variable working hours and three school-age children involved in after-school sports and music, Malia ends up picking up takeout or relying on convenience meals to feed herself and her family.

After coming home yet again to no groceries in the fridge and hungry children, she vows to make a change. She and her husband decide to put some time aside on the weekend to come up with a plan. With some online research, she learns that SMART goals are a practical approach that will help her feed her family healthy meals despite their busy schedules.

Malia is inspired and comes up with the following SMART goal:

- **Specific:** She and her family will plan their meals on Sunday mornings using an online meal planner and create a shopping list of items needed to stock their pantry, fridge and freezer.

- **Measurable:** The meal plan will include three meals a day for a week, and will rely on quick and easy recipes.

- **Action-oriented:** Each meal will be prepared from fresh or frozen ingredients. Every Sunday, each family member will be assigned a food preparation task. Vegetables will be chopped and ingredients will be portioned for each recipe for the week ahead.

- **Realistic:** Every Saturday, Malia and her family will discuss what worked and what didn't work that week, how they can adjust their schedules and assigned tasks the following week, and what their favorite recipes from that week's meal plan were.

- **Time-framed:** Malia and her family will plan weekly meals for the next 3 months, to allow time for meal planning and family meal preparation to become new habits.

Old habits die hard. Habits are stronger than willpower. No matter how badly you want to make a change, it will not "stick" until the behavior becomes second nature. Developing new habits requires time and commitment, so be patient.

It is important to reflect, replace and reinforce. Create a list of your eating habits by tracking your food intake for a week and look for patterns or trends. The secret to success is to break down your healthy living goals into smaller goals that are easy to master. Start with one small, clear goal that is important to you. This is the idea behind setting SMART goals.

Setting a SMART Goal

Use this checklist to set a SMART goal. Make sure your goal is:

- **Specific:** When will you start? What will you focus on? How will you do it?
- **Measurable:** How often will you do this? How much will you do? What will you track, and how?
- **Action-oriented:** Which eating behavior will you alter? It is important to focus on a behavior that you can change rather than a feeling or a thought.
- **Realistic:** Can you see yourself completing this goal? Be honest! Setting small goals that are achievable is a powerful motivator and a positive way for you to track your progress.
- **Time-framed:** How long will it take you to reach your goal?

The goal "I am going to add more prebiotics to my diet" is not specific enough; it is hard to measure and is not time-framed. Here are some better examples of SMART goals:

- Example #1: I will drink kefir once a week at breakfast.
- Example #2: I will eat a "top 10 prebiotic fiber–containing food" once a day at lunch.

Other tips for success when changing your eating habits are:

- Plan! Plan! Plan! Use the 14-day meal plan included in this book as a guide (see pages 136–39).
- Stock your pantry with fiber-rich, probiotic-rich, prebiotic-rich, vegetarian-friendly foods.
- Keep a shopping list.
- Keep a food diary for the first week.
- Reward your progress and be kind to yourself as you overcome barriers to success and embrace each new food habit.

Introduction to the 14-Day Meal Plan

You may find that adopting a diet that is focused on prebiotics and probiotics presents some initial challenges. It can take some time to consciously plan for lifestyle changes and find ways to successfully incorporate new foods and recipes into your day-to-day life. If you are able to stick with these changes, they will eventually become automatic and a part of your usual eating pattern.

To increase your likelihood of success, make up a weekly grocery list that includes foods rich in probiotics and prebiotics and stock your kitchen regularly with these items.

The following meal plan, which includes many of the recipes found in Part IV of this book, will guide you in planning your daily meals and snacks and help ensure that your diet is well rounded and nutritionally complete.

The meal plan is based on the range of daily food-group servings recommended by the USDA's MyPlate guidelines and Eating Well with Canada's Food Guide for average adults between the ages of 19 and 50. We have not included portion sizes or number of servings, as these will vary based on your age, sex and activity level.

You will note that the meal plan is vegetarian. Omnivores who are hoping to adopt a more plant-based diet or to fully adopt vegetarianism can use it as a guide. From a nutritional point of view, any diet, vegetarian or not, must provide balance, variety and moderation. It must meet special nutrient needs that arise through the life cycle and must accommodate special considerations for individuals with certain health issues. Ultimately, it should reduce the risk of diet-related diseases. There is a general consensus among health experts that a predominantly plant-based diet reduces the risk of contracting various chronic diseases. In the case of a biotic-balanced diet, the goal is to influence the human gut microbiome in a positive way.

> To increase your likelihood of success, make up a weekly grocery list that includes foods rich in probiotics and prebiotics and stock your kitchen regularly with these items.

Week 1

Meal	Monday	Tuesday	Wednesday	
Breakfast	• ¹/₂ grapefruit • Super Health Bread (page 174) • Sunflower Seed Miso Butter (page 160)	• Sweet Tart Smoothie (page 163) • Superpower Breakfast Cookies (page 186)	• Orange-Flavored Breakfast Barley with Cranberries and Pecans (page 149)	
Morning Snack	• Carrot and celery sticks • Low-fat cheese		• Double Cheese, Apple and Maple Bagel (page 155)	
Lunch	• Lean vegetarian sausage • Sauerkraut • Whole wheat bun • Tabbouleh (page 236)	• Jerusalem Artichoke Soup (page 214) • Grilled cheese sandwich (on whole-grain bread) • Spicy Kimchi (page 288)	• Greek Bean Salad (page 242) • Spinach Artichoke Bread (page 179) • Almond milk	
Afternoon Snack	• Apple • Soy milk	• Pear		
Supper	• Stir-Fried Mixed Vegetables (page 300) • Teriyaki Tempeh Satay with Peanut Sauce (page 284) • Steamed rice	• Stir-Fried Shiitakes with Garlic (page 293) • Baked Orzo and Beans (page 277)	• Green Thai Curry with Spinach and Sweet Potatoes (page 304) • Basmati rice	
Evening Snack	• Spiced Banana Walnut Pudding (page 312) • Easy Root Coffee (page 172)	• Cocoa Banana Mini Muffins (page 182) • Milk	• Gazpacho Smoothie (page 165)	

Thursday	Friday	Saturday	Sunday
• Apricot Bran Bread (page 176) • Low-fat cheese	• Pantry Muesli (page 147) • Yogurt	• Banana Flapjacks (page 157) • Vegetarian "bacon" • Milk	• Spicy Tomato Curry with Poached Eggs (page 152) • Cheesy Grits (page 262)
• Banana	• Grapes	• Melon	• Triple B Health Muffin (page 181)
• Barbecued Tofu Nuggets (page 196) • Dandelion Salad with Citrus Dressing (page 232)	• Lentil Soup Italian-Style (page 222) • Sourdough bread	• Green salad dressed with Tomato Basil Dressing (page 244) • Hummus with Roasted Red Peppers (page 208) • Whole wheat pita	• Warm Pear and Snow Pea Salad with Miso Dressing (page 230) • Couscous Bake (page 258)
• Orange	• Artichoke and White Bean Spread (page 209) • Grilled Herbed Crostini (page 199)		• Kiwifruit • Kefir
• Veggie Kabobs (page 301) • Cilantro Black Bean Burger (page 276) • Whole-grain bun • Tomato slices • Finely chopped onion • Pickle	• Penne with Mushrooms, Sun-Dried Tomatoes and Artichokes (page 250) • Tomato Mozzarella Salad (page 233)	• Barbecue Barley and Sweet Potato Chili (page 279) • Cornbread	• Grilled Vegetable Lasagna (page 252) • Soy milk
• Fruity Oatmeal Cookie (page 323) • Milk	• Asparagus Salsa (page 206) • Whole-grain crackers	• Homemade Yogurt (page 159) • Wheat bran • Berries	• Caramel Lime Bananas (page 310)

Week 2

Meal	Monday	Tuesday	Wednesday	
Breakfast	• Banana Bread (page 177) • Peanut butter • Milk	• Kefir yogurt with wheat bran and berries	• Coconut Quinoa Oat Granola (page 146) • Banana • Soy milk	
Morning Snack	• Apple	• Tropical Smoothie (page 164)	• Boiled egg • Whole wheat toast	
Lunch	• Classic French Onion Soup (page 217) • Whole wheat croutons • Toasted Tofu with Onion Miso Jam (page 194)	• Bulgur Asparagus Salad (page 237) • Cheese Straws (page 190)	• Stuffed Zucchini (page 299) • Pasta Salad with Yellow Tomato Sauce (page 240)	
Afternoon Snack	• Sugar Snap Peas with Cherry Tomatoes (page 296)	• Tofu and Chickpea Garlic Dip (page 197) • Flax crackers	• Peaches	
Supper	• Green salad dressed with Creamy Miso Dressing (page 244) • Spaghetti and Soyballs (page 247)	• Baked Curried Tofu with Tomato Masala (page 282) • Saffron rice • Garlic naan	• Vegetarian Pad Thai (page 255)	
Evening Snack	• Avocado tempeh dip • Whole-grain chips	• Cheesy Shoestring Jicama Fries (page 291) • Spring Tonic (page 169)	• Banana Orange Yogurt (page 315)	

Thursday	Friday	Saturday	Sunday
• Crispy Buckwheat Tempehacon Waffles (page 158) • Plain yogurt with sliced kiwi and strawberries	• Asparagus Mango Smoothie (page 165) • Whole wheat toast	• Whole Wheat Buttermilk French Toast (page 155) • Yogurt • Strawberries	• Garden Vegetable Frittata (page 151) • Potato wedges
• Greek Honey Cake (page 318)	• Orange Apricot Oatmeal Scone (page 180)	• Buttermilk Oat-Branana Cake (page 319) • Kiwifruit	• Apple Cranberry Bread (page 175) • Pineapple
• Mushroom Barley Soup with Miso (page 221) • Gouda cheese	• Green salad dressed with "Roasted" Garlic, Hemp and Parsley Dressing (page 243) • Baked tempeh	• Summer Artichoke Salad (page 231) • Tasty Chickpea Cakes (page 273)	• Smoked Gouda Mac and Cheese (page 248) • Creamed Garlic Spinach (page 297) • Green salad with oil and vinegar dressing
• French Lentil Dip with Herbed Crostini (page 201)	• Strawberry Freeze (page 311)	• High-fiber cold cereal • Milk • Raspberries	• Yogurt with cashews and blueberries
• Green Pea and Asparagus Curry (page 295) • Roasted sweet potatoes	• Spicy Tofu with Vegetables (page 281) • Couscous Bake (page 258)	• Squash-Laced Wild Rice and Barley Casserole (page 268) • Barbecue Baked Beans (page 275)	• Jerusalem Artichoke Stew (page 286) • Easy Black Beans (page 274) • Rice
• Brocco-Artichoke (page 170)	• Whole-Grain Power Bar (page 185) • Milk	• Strawberry Sesame Banana Chews (page 322) • Soy milk	• Sweet Vanilla Buckwheat Almond Clusters (page 188)

PART IV

Recipes for a Healthy Microbiome

Introduction
to the Recipes

Hippocrates once said, "Let your food be your medicine and your medicine be your food." We live in a fast-paced society. We work long hours and/or have children with multiple hobbies. We are constantly pulled in different directions and fall into the habit of buying processed and refined convenience foods from grocery stores.

Eating well involves initial effort until it becomes second nature. It's about choosing whole foods and learning what's in your food. Are you eating enough of each nutrient, or too much?

The recipes in this book will help get you back in the kitchen and will transform meal planning and cooking into a fun and time-saving experience.

Should We All Be Vegetarians?

Vegetarianism is a lifestyle choice. You decide if it's right for you. Our intent is not to convince you to become a vegetarian, but instead to encourage you to focus on eating a diet rich in high-fiber plant sources.

Prebiotics are essentially food for probiotics, found in dairy products. In this book you'll find some recipes with raw prebiotics to give you more bang for your buck, and some with cooked prebiotic plants, such as garlic, onions and leeks, for improved palatability and flavor.

Today, prebiotics are gaining more and more in popularity — so much so that we now find them used to fortify breads, breakfast cereals, snack bars, yogurts, soups and sports drinks.

Did You Know?

Natural Prebiotic Sources

Prebiotics are naturally found in plant sources such as artichokes, asparagus, bananas, tomatoes, whole grains and root vegetables, but also in fermented dairy products.

If I'm a New Vegetarian, How Do I Eat a Healthy, Balanced Diet?

A healthy vegetarian lifestyle is not just about cutting out meat; you also need to educate yourself about your body's needs and make sure all of the required nutrients are represented in your diet. Eat a diet abundant in fruits and vegetables, whole grains and protein-rich foods such as soy products, legumes, nuts, seeds and, if desired, eggs and dairy products. Do this and you'll nourish your body with enough protein, vitamin B_{12}, iron, zinc, omega-3 fatty acids, calcium, vitamin D, prebiotics and probiotics — all the nutrients that are sometimes under-represented in the vegetarian diet.

The recipes that follow will make it easy to include these foods on a regular basis in meals and snacks, and even when you're entertaining, so you can make sure you are not missing out on any of these vital nutrients while on the vegetarian path.

About the Nutrient Analysis

The nutrient analysis done on the recipes in this book was derived from the Food Processor SQL Nutrition Analysis Software, version 10.9, ESHA Research (2011). Where necessary, data were supplemented using the following references:

1. USDA National Nutrient Database for Standard Reference, Release #27 (2015). Retrieved July 2015 from the USDA Agricultural Research Service: www.nal.usda.gov/fnic/foodcomp/search/.
2. Hemp Seed Oil Nutrition Facts (2015). Retrieved July 2015 from CHII Naturally Pure Hemp: www.chii.ca/hemp-products/hemp-seed-oil/?gclid=CNazmIGUjscCFYwYHwo deikOeg.

Recipes were evaluated as follows:

- The larger number of servings was used where there is a range.
- Where alternatives are given, the first ingredient and amount listed were used.
- The smaller quantity of an ingredient was used where a range is provided.
- Optional ingredients and ingredients that are not quantified were not included.
- Calculations were based on imperial measures and weights.
- Nutrient values were rounded to the nearest whole number.
- Unsalted butter, 1% milk and calcium-fortified all-purpose flour were used where these ingredients are listed as butter, milk and all-purpose flour.
- Canola oil was used where the type of fat is not specified.
- Recipes were analyzed prior to cooking.

Breakfast and Brunch

Coconut Quinoa Oat Granola 146

Pantry Muesli 147

Mixed Fruit, Chia and Flaxseed Porridge. 148

Orange-Flavored Breakfast Barley
   with Cranberries and Pecans. 149

Malibu Tofu Scramble 150

Garden Vegetable Frittata 151

Spicy Tomato Curry with Poached Eggs 152

Artichoke Quiche 154

Double Cheese, Apple and Maple Bagels. 155

Whole Wheat Buttermilk French Toast. 155

Buckwheat Toast. 156

Banana Flapjacks. 157

Crispy Buckwheat Tempehacon Waffles. 158

Homemade Yogurt 159

Sunflower Seed Miso Butter 160

Coconut Quinoa Oat Granola

Makes about 4¹/₂ cups (1.125 L)

The dynamic whole-grain duo of oatmeal and quinoa is tasty and provides two sources of prebiotics.

- Preheat oven to 300°F (150°C)
- Large rimmed baking sheet, lined with parchment paper

2 cups	large-flake (old-fashioned) rolled oats	500 mL
1 cup	quinoa, rinsed	250 mL
1 cup	unsweetened flaked coconut	250 mL
³/₄ cup	almonds, coarsely chopped	175 mL
1¹/₂ tsp	ground cardamom or ginger	7 mL
¹/₂ cup	virgin coconut oil, warmed	125 mL
¹/₂ cup	liquid honey or brown rice syrup	125 mL
²/₃ cup	chopped dried apricots or golden raisins	150 mL

1. In a large bowl, combine oats, quinoa, coconut, almonds and cardamom.

2. In a medium bowl, whisk together oil and honey until well blended.

3. Add the honey mixture to the oats mixture and stir until well coated. Spread mixture in a single layer on prepared baking sheet.

4. Bake in preheated oven for 20 to 25 minutes or until oats are golden brown. Let cool completely on pan.

5. Transfer granola to an airtight container and stir in apricots. Store at room temperature for up to 2 weeks.

Nutrients per ¹/₄ cup (60 mL)

Calories	250
Fat	13 g
Saturated Fat	8 g
Cholesterol	0 mg
Sodium	3 mg
Carbohydrate	30 g
Fiber	4 g
Sugars	11 g
Protein	6 g
Calcium	31 mg
Iron	2 mg

Pantry Muesli

Makes about 8 cups (2 L)

This is a very simple muesli made from ingredients you are likely to have in your pantry. It's fun to get creative, adding nuts, cereal flakes, dried fruit or seeds to your liking.

Tips

Make small batches of muesli, experimenting with various whole-grain flakes, such as spelt, barley and rye, to discover your favorites.

Flax seeds are available in grocery or natural food stores either raw or toasted, sometimes referred to as roasted. Raw flax seeds may be toasted in a heavy-bottomed skillet over medium-high heat, stirring or shaking the pan constantly to prevent burning, until seeds turn a golden brown. Store in an airtight container in the refrigerator for up to 3 weeks.

2 cups	large-flake (old-fashioned) rolled oats	500 mL
1 cup	oat bran	250 mL
1 cup	whole-grain spelt, barley and/or rye flakes	250 mL
1 cup	chopped almonds	250 mL
1 cup	dried apple slices	250 mL
1/2 cup	unsweetened flaked coconut	125 mL
1/2 cup	dried cranberries	125 mL
1/2 cup	dried apricots	125 mL
1/4 cup	toasted flax seeds (see tip, at left)	60 mL
1/4 cup	green pumpkin seeds (pepitas)	60 mL
	Nut, rice, hemp or soy milk, cold or warmed	

1. In a large airtight container, combine oats, oat bran, cereal flakes, almonds, apple slices, coconut, cranberries, apricots, flax seeds and pepitas. Store at room temperature for up to 2 months.

2. To serve hot, bring equal amounts of muesli and nut, rice, hemp or soy milk to a gentle boil and simmer for 3 to 5 minutes. Alternatively, soak 1/2 cup (125 mL) muesli in warmed or cold nut, rice, hemp or soy milk for 5 minutes to overnight, depending on desired consistency.

Nutrients per 1/2 cup (125 mL)	
Calories	242
Fat	9 g
Saturated Fat	2 g
Cholesterol	0 mg
Sodium	9 mg
Carbohydrate	37 g
Fiber	7 g
Sugars	9 g
Protein	9 g
Calcium	46 mg
Iron	3 mg

Mixed Fruit, Chia and Flaxseed Porridge

This simple mixture is quick to prepare and will leave you feeling well satisfied throughout the morning. Raw bananas are a great prebiotic source.

Tips

To soak flax seeds, submerge them in double the amount of liquid. Set aside for 30 minutes. Drain and rinse under cold running water.

To remove the membrane from an orange, use a chef's knife to remove a bit of the skin from the top and the bottom. Using the tip of the knife, remove the skin and as much of the white pith as possible without losing flesh. Cut the orange in half and then cut into $\frac{1}{2}$-inch (1 cm) cubes for this recipe.

Nutrients per serving (1 of 3)	
Calories	237
Fat	17 g
Saturated Fat	9 g
Cholesterol	0 mg
Sodium	12 mg
Carbohydrate	19 g
Fiber	9 g
Sugars	8 g
Protein	5 g
Calcium	110 mg
Iron	1 mg

3 tbsp	whole flax seeds, soaked (see tip, at left)	45 mL
$\frac{1}{2}$ cup	Coconut Milk (page 167)	125 mL
$\frac{1}{4}$ cup	chopped apple	60 mL
$\frac{1}{4}$ cup	chopped banana	60 mL
$\frac{1}{4}$ cup	chopped orange, skin and membrane removed (see tip, at left)	60 mL
$\frac{1}{4}$ cup	chopped hulled strawberries	60 mL
$\frac{1}{4}$ cup	blueberries	60 mL
3 tbsp	chia seeds	45 mL
$\frac{1}{2}$ tsp	raw vanilla extract	2 mL

1. In a bowl, toss together coconut milk, apple, banana, orange, strawberries, blueberries, soaked flax seeds, chia seeds and vanilla. Set aside for 5 minutes so the chia seeds can swell and absorb some of the liquid.

Variation

Use $\frac{1}{3}$ cup (75 mL) chia seeds and 1 tbsp (15 mL) flax seeds soaked in 2 tbsp (30 mL) water. The result will have a very similar texture and flavor but a higher content of omega-3 fatty acids, because the chia seeds contain more omega-3 fats than the flax seeds.

Orange-Flavored Breakfast Barley with Cranberries and Pecans

Makes 6 servings

Although it's extremely nutritious, whole barley takes a long time to cook. Fortunately, this isn't a problem if you're making it overnight in a slow cooker. Wake up to a delicious, nutritious breakfast and enjoy.

Tips

Whole (hulled) barley is the most nutritious form of the grain, but if you prefer you can use pot or pearled barley instead.

When making whole-grain cereals in the slow cooker, be aware that stirring encourages creaminess. If you have time, let the cereal sit on Warm for at least 15 minutes before serving, and stir it several times, if possible.

- Small to medium (1½- to 3½-quart) slow cooker, stoneware lightly greased

3 cups	water	750 mL
½ cup	whole (hulled) barley, rinsed and drained (see tip, at left)	125 mL
½ cup	dried cranberries	125 mL
1 tbsp	finely grated orange zest	15 mL
Pinch	salt	Pinch
¼ cup	toasted chopped pecans	60 mL
	Milk or nondairy alternative (optional)	
	Natural cane sugar, liquid honey or pure maple syrup (optional)	

1. In prepared slow cooker stoneware, combine water, barley, cranberries, orange zest and salt. Stir well. Place a clean tea towel, folded in half (so you will have two layers), over top of stoneware to absorb moisture. Cover and cook on Low for 8 hours or overnight or on High for 4 hours. Stir well. Garnish with pecans. Serve with milk or nondairy alternative and/or sugar (if using).

Nutrients per serving	
Calories	118
Fat	4 g
Saturated Fat	0 g
Cholesterol	0 mg
Sodium	7 mg
Carbohydrate	20 g
Fiber	4 g
Sugars	7 g
Protein	2 g
Calcium	14 mg
Iron	1 mg

Malibu Tofu Scramble

Makes 4 to 6 servings

A veritable garden of vegetables, from golden sautéed mushrooms, ripe tomatoes and breakfast potatoes to tangy sprouts and creamy avocado, is about all the yumminess one scramble can hold.

Tip

To bake a medium-size russet potato, scrub it well and slice $\frac{1}{8}$ inch (3 mm) off each end. Bake directly on the middle rack of a preheated 375°F (190°C) oven until potato feels soft when gently squeezed, 45 to 60 minutes.

3 tbsp	olive oil, divided	45 mL
2	cloves garlic, minced	2
$\frac{1}{2}$	onion, chopped	$\frac{1}{2}$
1 lb	cremini mushrooms, sliced	500 g
1	zucchini, diced	1
1	russet (Idaho) potato, baked, peeled and chopped (see tip, at left)	1
1 lb	firm tofu, drained and crumbled	500 g
1 tbsp	ground turmeric	15 mL
1	ripe tomato, seeded and chopped	1
1 cup	fresh basil leaves	250 mL
2 tbsp	champagne vinegar	30 mL
1 tsp	salt	5 mL
$\frac{1}{2}$ tsp	freshly ground black pepper	2 mL
1 cup	broccoli sprouts	250 mL
1	avocado, sliced	1
$\frac{3}{4}$ cup	vegan sour cream alternative (optional)	175 mL

1. Place skillet over medium heat and let pan get hot. Add 1 tbsp (15 mL) oil and tip pan to coat. Add garlic, onion, mushrooms and zucchini and cook, stirring occasionally, until vegetables start to soften, 5 to 6 minutes. Transfer vegetables to a bowl and set aside.

2. Increase heat to medium-high. Add the remaining oil and heat for 30 seconds. Add potato and cook, stirring frequently, until beginning to brown, about 6 minutes. Reduce heat to medium. Add tofu and turmeric and cook, stirring frequently, until potato is golden brown and tofu is warmed through, 6 to 8 minutes. Add tomato, basil, vinegar, salt, pepper and cooked mushroom mixture. Cook, stirring frequently, until tomato is heated through, 3 to 5 minutes. Stir in sprouts and serve topped with avocado slices. Add a dollop of sour cream, if using.

Variations

Substitute apple cider vinegar for the champagne vinegar, if desired.

Any favorite sprout can easily replace the broccoli sprouts.

Nutrients per serving (1 of 6)	
Calories	242
Fat	16 g
Saturated Fat	2 g
Cholesterol	0 mg
Sodium	407 mg
Carbohydrate	18 g
Fiber	5 g
Sugars	4 g
Protein	12 g
Calcium	134 mg
Iron	3 mg

Garden Vegetable Frittata

Makes 6 servings

This makes a beautiful main course or side dish on a buffet, especially during spring and summer, when vegetables are at their peak of ripeness and flavor.

Tip

Shocking vegetables in ice water stops the cooking process after blanching and sets the color, so you will have brightly colored vegetables even after baking.

- Preheat oven to 350°F (180°C)
- 11- by 7-inch (28 by 18 cm) glass baking dish, greased

1 lb	asparagus, trimmed and cut into 1-inch (2.5 cm) pieces	500 g
	Ice water	
1 tbsp	olive oil	15 mL
4 oz	mushrooms, sliced	125 g
1	clove garlic, minced	1
1	shallot, minced	1
1	small zucchini, cut in half lengthwise and thinly sliced	1
6	large eggs	6
⅓ cup	milk	75 mL
1 tbsp	chopped fresh chives	15 mL
1 tsp	salt	5 mL
½ tsp	freshly ground black pepper	2 mL
⅛ tsp	ground nutmeg	0.5 mL
2	tomatoes, thinly sliced	2
¼ cup	freshly grated Parmesan cheese	60 mL

1. In a large pot of boiling water, blanch asparagus for 1 to 2 minutes. Immediately plunge into ice water; let stand until chilled. Drain and place in prepared baking dish.

2. In a skillet, heat oil over medium heat. Sauté mushrooms for about 10 minutes or until tender. Add garlic and shallot; sauté for 2 minutes. Spread over asparagus. Arrange zucchini on top.

3. In a large bowl, whisk eggs until blended. Whisk in milk, chives, salt, pepper and nutmeg. Pour evenly over vegetable mixture. Arrange tomatoes on top. Sprinkle evenly with cheese.

4. Bake in preheated oven for 40 to 45 minutes or until set.

Nutrients per serving	
Calories	143
Fat	8 g
Saturated Fat	3 g
Cholesterol	190 mg
Sodium	22 mg
Carbohydrate	7 g
Fiber	2 g
Sugars	4 g
Protein	11 g
Calcium	111 mg
Iron	3 mg

Spicy Tomato Curry with Poached Eggs

Makes 2 to 4 servings

Here's huevos rancheros, curry-style. It's a superb egg dish that works with toast for a festive breakfast or as part of a multi-dish Indian meal.

Tips

If a flavorful ripe tomato is not available, substitute 1½ cups (375 mL) canned diced tomatoes, with juice, and omit the water. Add the canned tomatoes after the gravy.

Cracking each egg into a separate bowl may seem tedious, but it helps you get them into the sauce quickly, allowing them to cook at the same time.

Be generous with the probiotic-rich yogurt! Your gut will thank you for it.

1 tbsp	vegetable oil	15 mL
1	small onion, finely chopped	1
2 or 3	hot green chile peppers, minced	2 or 3
1	large ripe tomato, chopped	1
1 cup	Basic Gravy (see recipe, opposite)	250 mL
½ cup	water	125 mL
4	large eggs	4
	Salt	
	Chopped fresh cilantro	
¼ tsp	garam masala	1 mL
	Plain yogurt	

1. In a nonstick skillet, heat oil over medium heat. Add onion and cook, stirring, until starting to soften, about 2 minutes. Reduce heat to medium-low and cook, stirring often, until very soft and golden brown, about 5 minutes.

2. Increase heat to medium and add chiles and tomato. Cook, stirring, until tomato is starting to soften, about 2 minutes. Add gravy and cook, stirring, for 2 minutes. Stir in water and bring to a boil. Reduce heat and boil gently, stirring often, until slightly thickened and flavorful, about 5 minutes.

3. Crack each egg into a separate small bowl. Carefully drop eggs into simmering sauce, leaving as much space as possible between each. Reduce heat to low, cover and simmer just until whites are set and yolks are cooked to desired doneness, 5 to 8 minutes. Season to taste with salt. Serve sprinkled with cilantro and garam masala and topped with yogurt.

Nutrients per serving (1 of 4)	
Calories	167
Fat	10 g
Saturated Fat	2 g
Cholesterol	186 mg
Sodium	441 mg
Carbohydrate	12 g
Fiber	2 g
Sugars	5 g
Protein	8 g
Calcium	74 mg
Iron	2 mg

Basic Gravy

This generic curry sauce enhancer, courtesy of Chef Prasannan of the Lonely Planet restaurant in Kovalam Beach, Kerala, speeds up curry recipes and works every time.

Tips

If you don't have a food processor, you can use a blender. Just add enough of the tomato purée to the onion mixture to help the blender purée more easily.

Let extra gravy cool completely, then transfer to an airtight container, cover and refrigerate for up to 1 week. Or divide into ½-cup (125 mL) and/or 1-cup (250 mL) portions in airtight containers and freeze for up to 2 months. Thaw overnight in the refrigerator or defrost in the microwave.

Nutrients per ¼ cup (60 mL)	
Calories	41
Fat	2 g
Saturated Fat	0 g
Cholesterol	0 mg
Sodium	364 mg
Carbohydrate	6 g
Fiber	1 g
Sugars	2 g
Protein	1 g
Calcium	32 mg
Iron	1 mg

- Food processor

1	can (28 oz/796 mL) tomatoes, with juice	1
2 cups	coarsely chopped onions	500 mL
⅓ cup	garlic cloves (about 12), peeled	75 mL
⅓ cup	thinly sliced gingerroot	75 mL
2 tbsp	vegetable oil	30 mL
¼ cup	ground coriander	60 mL
1 tbsp	ground turmeric	15 mL
1 tbsp	garam masala	15 mL
2 tsp	salt	10 mL
1 tsp	cayenne pepper	5 mL

1. In food processor, purée tomatoes until smooth. Pour back into the can or into a bowl and set aside.

2. Add onions, garlic and ginger to food processor and pulse until very finely chopped but not juicy.

3. In a skillet, heat oil over medium heat. Add onion mixture and cook, stirring, until onions start to release their liquid, about 3 minutes. Stir in coriander, turmeric, garam masala, salt and cayenne. Cook, stirring, until well blended and mixture is starting to dry and get thick and paste-like, about 3 minutes.

4. Stir in puréed tomatoes and bring to a simmer, scraping up bits stuck to pan. Reduce heat and boil gently, stirring often, until slightly thickened and flavors are blended, about 5 minutes. Use as directed in recipes.

Artichoke Quiche

Makes 8 servings

This quiche is particularly delightful for brunch, but let's face it: it's good anytime. Artichokes are a source of prebiotics.

Tips

As the quiche bakes, you may need to cover the edges of the crust with foil to prevent excess browning.

Squeeze thawed and drained spinach several times to remove excess moisture.

- Preheat oven to 425°F (220°C)

1	9-inch (23 cm) unbaked pie shell	1
6	large eggs	6
1	package (10 oz/300 g) frozen chopped spinach, thawed and squeezed dry	1
1	can (14 oz/398 mL) artichoke hearts, drained and chopped	1
1	small onion, finely chopped	1
1	clove garlic, minced	1
2 cups	shredded Cheddar cheese	500 mL
1/2 cup	chopped mushrooms	125 mL
1/4 cup	dry bread crumbs	60 mL
1/2 tsp	salt	2 mL
1/4 tsp	freshly ground black pepper	1 mL
1/4 tsp	dried oregano	1 mL
1/4 tsp	hot pepper sauce	1 mL

1. Prick pie shell all over with a fork. Bake in preheated oven for 5 to 10 minutes or until lightly browned. Let cool slightly. Reduce oven temperature to 350°F (180°C).

2. In a large bowl, whisk eggs until blended. Stir in spinach, artichokes, onion, garlic, cheese, mushrooms, bread crumbs, salt, pepper, oregano and hot pepper sauce. Pour into pie crust.

3. Bake for 55 to 60 minutes or until a knife inserted in the center comes out clean.

Nutrients per serving	
Calories	286
Fat	13 g
Saturated Fat	4 g
Cholesterol	145 mg
Sodium	607 mg
Carbohydrate	29 g
Fiber	6 g
Sugars	12 g
Protein	16 g
Calcium	206 mg
Iron	2 mg

Double Cheese, Apple and Maple Bagels

Makes 4 servings

Choose a whole wheat bagel to add prebiotics.

Nutrients per serving	
Calories	280
Fat	14 g
Saturated Fat	9 g
Cholesterol	44 mg
Sodium	451 mg
Carbohydrate	25 g
Fiber	1 g
Sugars	6 g
Protein	14 g
Calcium	244 mg
Iron	2 mg

- Preheat broiler

2	bagels, halved	2
1/4 cup	unsweetened applesauce	60 mL
4 oz	Cheddar cheese, cut into slices	125 g
2 oz	Brie cheese, cut into slices	60 g
4 tsp	pure maple syrup	20 mL

1. Toast bagel halves; spread each with 1 tbsp (15 mL) applesauce. Top each with one-quarter of the Cheddar and the Brie.
2. Broil until the cheese melts, about 5 minutes.
3. Drizzle each half with 1 tsp (5 mL) maple syrup.

This recipe courtesy of the Dairy Farmers of Canada.

Variation

For a change of taste, substitute Havarti and Oka cheeses.

Whole Wheat Buttermilk French Toast

Makes 4 servings

This quick and easy meal packs a nutrition punch of pre- and probiotics! Enjoy.

Nutrients per serving	
Calories	505
Fat	22 g
Saturated Fat	12 g
Cholesterol	230 mg
Sodium	461 mg
Carbohydrate	56 g
Fiber	4 g
Sugars	17 g
Protein	22 g
Calcium	365 mg
Iron	2 mg

4	large or extra-large eggs	4
1 cup	buttermilk	250 mL
2 tbsp	granulated sugar	30 mL
1 tsp	vanilla extract	5 mL
Pinch	salt	Pinch
8	thick slices slightly stale whole wheat bread	8
1/4 cup	butter, divided	60 mL
2 cups	fruit-flavored yogurt	500 mL

1. In a wide, shallow bowl, beat eggs, buttermilk, sugar, vanilla and salt. Soak bread in this mixture, in batches if necessary, until all the liquid is absorbed.
2. In a large skillet, melt half the butter over medium heat. Add soaked bread, in batches, and cook, turning once, until browned on both sides. Transfer to a plate and keep warm. Repeat with the remaining soaked bread, melting the remaining butter between batches. Serve with yogurt.

Buckwheat Toast

Makes 8 slices

This crunchy favorite is great served as a breakfast side with a healthy scoop of almond butter. It's also just perfect on its own.

Tip

To soak the buckwheat for this recipe, combine 4 cups (1 L) groats and 8 cups (2 L) water. Cover and set aside for 2 hours, changing the water every 30 minutes. Drain, discarding soaking water. Rinse under cold running water until the water runs clear.

- Food processor
- Electric food dehydrator

4 cups	buckwheat groats, soaked (see tip, at left)	1 L
1/4 cup	filtered water	60 mL
2 tbsp	cold-pressed extra virgin olive oil	30 mL
1 tsp	nutritional yeast	5 mL
1 tsp	fine sea salt	5 mL
1/2 cup	ground flax seeds (flaxseed meal)	125 mL
2 tbsp	sesame seeds	30 mL

1. In food processor, in batches as necessary, process soaked buckwheat, water, olive oil, nutritional yeast and salt until smooth, stopping the motor and scraping down the sides of the work bowl once, adding more water 1 tbsp (15 mL) at a time, if necessary, to facilitate puréeing. Transfer to a bowl.

2. Add flax seeds and sesame seeds and stir well. Set aside for 10 to 15 minutes, until the flax absorbs the liquid and swells up.

3. Transfer to nonstick dehydrator sheets. Using the palm of your hand, spread the dough evenly in a thin layer approximately 1/2 inch (1 cm) thick. Cut into 8 pieces. Dehydrate at 105°F (41°C) for 10 to 12 hours or until bread is firm enough to handle.

4. Flip bread onto mesh sheets and dehydrate at 105°F (41°C) for 5 to 6 hours or until dry and crisp like toast. Serve warm or allow to cool. Transfer to an airtight container and store at room temperature for up to 5 days.

Tips for Successful Dehydrating

When dehydrating raw breads, you have options in terms of the texture produced. For crispier, firm bread, dehydrate until all the moisture has been removed. This will make storage easier — because it doesn't contain moisture, it can't spoil. For softer, more chewy bread, retain moisture in the middle of the bread by reducing the dehydrating time. Make sure to store breads that contain moisture in the refrigerator. Because they contain water, bacteria have the potential to grow.

When spreading out raw breads or crackers on a dehydrator sheet, keep a small bowl of room-temperature water off to the side. Use this to wet your hands intermittently to prevent the dough from sticking to your hands.

Nutrients per slice	
Calories	364
Fat	10 g
Saturated Fat	1 g
Cholesterol	0 mg
Sodium	362 mg
Carbohydrate	64 g
Fiber	11 g
Sugars	0 g
Protein	11 g
Calcium	54 mg
Iron	3 mg

Banana Flapjacks

These pancakes are guaranteed to leave you smiling, both from the great taste and because the prebiotic-rich bananas contain a high level of tryptophan, which is converted into serotonin, the good-mood neurotransmitter.

Tips

You can peel and freeze very ripe bananas in a sealed plastic bag or airtight container and thaw when ready to use.

Refrigerate pancakes between sheets of waxed paper, tightly covered in plastic wrap, for up to 2 days or freeze, enclosed in a sealable plastic bag, for up to 1 month. Let thaw at room temperature or defrost in the microwave.

$1/2$ cup	chickpea flour	125 mL
$1/4$ cup	coconut flour	60 mL
1 tbsp	potato starch	15 mL
$2 1/4$ tsp	baking powder	11 mL
$1/2$ tsp	ground cinnamon	2 mL
$1/4$ tsp	fine sea salt	1 mL
1 tbsp	coconut sugar	15 mL
$2/3$ cup	mashed very ripe bananas	150 mL
$1/2$ cup	well-stirred coconut milk (full-fat)	125 mL
$1/2$ cup	coconut water or water	125 mL
2 tbsp	melted virgin coconut oil	30 mL
2 tsp	cider vinegar	10 mL
	Additional melted virgin coconut oil	

1. In a large bowl, whisk together chickpea flour, coconut flour, potato starch, baking powder, cinnamon and salt.

2. In a medium bowl, whisk together coconut sugar, bananas, coconut milk, coconut water, 2 tbsp (30 mL) coconut oil and vinegar until blended.

3. Add the banana mixture to the flour mixture and stir until just blended.

4. Heat a griddle or skillet over medium heat. Brush with coconut oil. For each pancake, pour about $1/4$ cup (60 mL) batter onto griddle. Cook until bubbles appear on top. Turn pancake over and cook for about 1 minute or until golden brown. Repeat with the remaining batter, brushing griddle and adjusting heat as necessary between batches.

Variations

Pumpkin Spice Flapjacks: Replace the bananas with an equal amount of pumpkin purée (not pie filling). Replace the cinnamon with $1 1/4$ tsp (6 mL) pumpkin pie spice and increase the coconut sugar to 2 tbsp (30 mL).

Applesauce Flapjacks: Replace the bananas with an equal amount of unsweetened applesauce. Increase the coconut sugar to 2 tbsp (30 mL).

Nutrients per pancake	
Calories	79
Fat	5 g
Saturated Fat	4 g
Cholesterol	0 mg
Sodium	64 mg
Carbohydrate	7 g
Fiber	1 g
Sugars	3 g
Protein	1 g
Calcium	41 mg
Iron	1 mg

Crispy Buckwheat Tempehacon Waffles

Makes about 16 waffles

These rich yet crispy waffles are loaded with prebiotics, thanks to the savory tempeh bacon bits. On the slim chance any are left over, waffles freeze beautifully for up to 1 month. To make a quick flavored syrup, thin a favorite fruit jam with a little orange juice.

Tip

Cook waffle batter promptly, because commercial egg replacer loses its ability to make batters rise shortly after it is mixed with liquids.

Nutrients per waffle

Calories	244
Fat	15 g
Saturated Fat	10 g
Cholesterol	0 mg
Sodium	241 mg
Carbohydrate	24 g
Fiber	2 g
Sugars	5 g
Protein	7 g
Calcium	125 mg
Iron	2 mg

- Preheat oven to 200°F (100°C)
- Waffle iron, preheated

2 cups	buckwheat flour	500 mL
1 cup	all-purpose flour	250 mL
2 tbsp	granulated sugar	30 mL
2 tsp	baking powder	10 mL
1/2 tsp	baking soda	2 mL
1/4 tsp	salt	1 mL
2 3/4 cups	soy milk (store-bought or see recipe, page 166)	675 mL
3/4 cup	virgin coconut oil, melted	175 mL
1 tbsp	powdered egg replacer	15 mL
1/4 cup	warm water	60 mL
1/2 cup	Crunchy Tempehacon Bits (see recipe, opposite) or store-bought vegan bacon bits	125 mL

1. In a large bowl, combine buckwheat flour, all-purpose flour, sugar, baking powder, baking soda and salt. Set aside.

2. In another bowl, whisk together soy milk and coconut oil (it is okay if coconut oil hardens into small chunks). In a small bowl, thoroughly mix egg replacer with warm water and whisk into soy milk mixture. Add soy milk mixture to dry ingredients and stir just until blended. Stir in tempehacon bits.

3. Fill preheated waffle iron with batter, spreading evenly with a heatproof spatula and cook until waffles are browned and crisp, according to manufacturer's instructions. Transfer cooked waffles to a baking sheet and hold in warm oven. Repeat process with the remaining batter. Serve hot with your favorite syrup.

Crunchy Tempehacon Bits

Makes 8 oz (250 g)

Great as a topping for vegetables or tossed into pasta or grain dishes.

Nutrients per 1 oz (30 g)	
Calories	103
Fat	6 g
Saturated Fat	1 g
Cholesterol	0 mg
Sodium	284 mg
Carbohydrate	7 g
Fiber	0 g
Sugars	3 g
Protein	6 g
Calcium	38 mg
Iron	1 mg

1/4 cup	soy sauce	60 mL
2 tbsp	pure maple syrup	30 mL
1 tsp	liquid smoke	5 mL
8 oz	tempeh, well crumbled	250 g
2 tbsp	grapeseed oil	30 mL

1. In a small, shallow container, whisk together soy sauce, maple syrup and liquid smoke until well combined. Add tempeh crumbles and toss to coat. Cover and refrigerate, stirring occasionally, for at least 4 hours or overnight.

2. Spread marinated crumbles on a plate and let air-dry for 10 minutes.

3. Place a large skillet over medium-high heat and let pan get hot. Add oil and tip pan to coat. Transfer crumbles to skillet, reduce heat to medium and cook, stirring frequently, until bits are very crisp and browned, 4 to 6 minutes.

Homemade Yogurt

Makes 4 cups (1 L)

Here's a simple and pleasurable way to eat your probiotics.

Nutrients per 1/2 cup (125 mL)	
Calories	71
Fat	1 g
Saturated Fat	1 g
Cholesterol	7 mg
Sodium	83 mg
Carbohydrate	9 g
Fiber	0 g
Sugars	9 g
Protein	6 g
Calcium	219 mg
Iron	0 mg

4 cups	low-fat milk	1 L
1/2 cup	powdered milk	125 mL
1/4 cup	plain yogurt	60 mL

1. In a saucepan, heat low-fat milk until bubbles form around the edges. Let cool until warm to the touch (about 100°F/38°C) and remove any skin from the surface. Stir in powdered milk and yogurt.

2. Cover with plastic wrap and set in a location with a constant temperature of about 100°F (38°C), such as a closed oven with a pilot light or near a warm radiator or hot-water heater, for 4 to 6 hours. When done, yogurt will be thickened like custard. Refrigerate for several hours and it will become thicker.

Sunflower Seed Miso Butter

Makes 4 cups (1 L)

This delicious probiotic alternative to butter is so rich and creamy, no one will be able to tell the difference if someone asks you to pass the butter. It's perfect on whole wheat toast. With the addition of chopped fresh herbs, you can also use this recipe as the base for a raw butter to use as a dip for breads and crackers or carrot and celery sticks, or with a plate of crudités.

Tip

To soak the sunflower seeds for this recipe, place in a bowl and add 2 cups (500 mL) water. Cover and set aside for 30 minutes. Drain, discarding water and any shells or unwanted particles.

- **Food processor**

1 cup	raw sunflower seeds, soaked (see tip, at left)	250 mL
½ cup	filtered water	125 mL
3 tbsp	apple cider vinegar	45 mL
2 tbsp	brown rice miso paste	30 mL
2 cups	cold-pressed extra virgin olive oil	500 mL

1. In food processor, process soaked sunflower seeds, water, vinegar and miso paste for 3 to 4 minutes or until sunflower seeds have been completely broken down and mixture is smooth.

2. With the motor running, add olive oil through the feed tube in a slow, steady stream until mixture is emulsified. Transfer to a container, cover and refrigerate for up to 4 days.

Variation

Add any fresh or dried herb in step 1 for additional flavor. Try 1 tbsp (15 mL) dried dillweed and 2 tsp (10 mL) freshly squeezed lemon juice.

Nutrients per 1 tbsp (15 mL)	
Calories	70
Fat	8 g
Saturated Fat	1 g
Cholesterol	0 mg
Sodium	8 mg
Carbohydrate	1 g
Fiber	0 g
Sugars	0 g
Protein	0 g
Calcium	2 mg
Iron	0 mg

Smoothies, Juices and Other Beverages

Banana Berry Kefir 162

Purple Power Shake. 162

Apple Mint Smoothie 163

Sweet Tart Smoothie. 163

Tropical Smoothie 164

Green Goddess. 164

Asparagus Mango Smoothie 165

Gazpacho Smoothie 165

Soy Milk 166

Coconut Milk 167

Green Barley Water 168

Spring Tonic 169

C-Blend. 169

Artichoke Eight. 170

Brocco-Artichoke 170

Root Coffee Blend. 171

Easy Root Coffee. 172

Banana Berry Kefir

Start your day with a simple yet nutritious recipe for your gut. Making your own probiotic drink has never been so easy!

Nutrients per serving

Calories	188
Fat	2 g
Saturated Fat	1 g
Cholesterol	7 mg
Sodium	84 mg
Carbohydrate	39 g
Fiber	2 g
Sugars	33 g
Protein	6 g
Calcium	195 mg
Iron	0 mg

• Blender

2	bananas, sliced	2
1 cup	low-fat vanilla-flavored yogurt	250 mL
1 cup	low-fat raspberry-flavored yogurt	250 mL
1 cup	apple-raspberry juice	250 mL
1 tbsp	liquid honey	15 mL

1. In blender, combine bananas, vanilla yogurt, strawberry yogurt, juice and honey; purée until smooth.

2. Pour into a pitcher, cover and chill.

Purple Power Shake

Each sip of this deep purple smoothie delivers prebiotics and probiotics.

Nutrients per serving

Calories	224
Fat	2 g
Saturated Fat	1 g
Cholesterol	5 mg
Sodium	50 mg
Carbohydrate	50 g
Fiber	4 g
Sugars	37 g
Protein	4 g
Calcium	130 mg
Iron	1 mg

• Blender

1½ cups	mixed frozen berries	375 mL
½ cup	sliced frozen ripe banana	125 mL
¾ cup	plain coconut yogurt	175 mL
¾ cup	unsweetened grape juice	175 mL

1. In blender, combine berries, banana, yogurt and grape juice; purée until smooth.

2. Pour into 2 glasses and serve immediately.

Apple Mint Smoothie

Makes 3 to 4 servings

Enjoy this twist on a classic smoothie recipe. It's perfect for a summer day!

Nutrients per serving (1 of 4)	
Calories	52
Fat	0 g
Saturated Fat	0 g
Cholesterol	1 mg
Sodium	14 mg
Carbohydrate	12 g
Fiber	2 g
Sugars	9 g
Protein	1 g
Calcium	43 mg
Iron	0 mg

- Blender

3 tbsp	chopped fresh peppermint leaves (or 2 tsp/10 mL dried), divided	45 mL
1/2 cup	boiling water	125 mL
1/4 cup	plain or frozen yogurt	60 mL
1	apple, quartered	1
1	kiwifruit, quartered	1
1/4 tsp	fennel seeds	1 mL
1/4 cup	unsweetened applesauce	60 mL

1. Place 2 tbsp (30 mL) peppermint in a teapot and pour in boiling water. Cover and steep for 10 minutes. Let cool (no need to strain).

2. In blender, combine mint-infused water, yogurt, apple, kiwi, the remaining peppermint, fennel seeds and applesauce; blend (from low to high if using a variable-speed blender) until smooth.

Sweet Tart Smoothie

Makes 2 servings

Jump-start the day with a unique blend of sweet and tart.

Nutrients per serving	
Calories	382
Fat	4 g
Saturated Fat	0 g
Cholesterol	0 mg
Sodium	25 mg
Carbohydrate	83 g
Fiber	5 g
Sugars	65 g
Protein	7 g
Calcium	357 mg
Iron	2 mg

- Blender

1 1/2 cups	pitted frozen cherries	375 mL
1	frozen banana, cut into 6 pieces	1
2 cups	vanilla-flavored soy yogurt	500 mL
3 tbsp	agave nectar	45 mL
2 tbsp	freshly squeezed lime juice	30 mL

1. In blender, combine cherries, banana, yogurt, agave and lime juice; blend until smooth.

2. Divide between 2 glasses and serve.

Tropical Smoothie

Makes 6 servings

A refreshing drink for breakfast, brunch or a snack.

Nutrients per serving	
Calories	120
Fat	1 g
Saturated Fat	0 g
Cholesterol	2 mg
Sodium	48 mg
Carbohydrate	27 g
Fiber	2 g
Sugars	22 g
Protein	3 g
Calcium	141 mg
Iron	0 mg

- Blender

1 cup	mango pieces	250 mL
1 cup	papaya pieces	250 mL
1 cup	pineapple chunks	250 mL
1 cup	rice, soy or regular milk	250 mL
1 cup	plain yogurt	250 mL
1/2 cup	mango or pineapple juice	125 mL
2 tbsp	liquid honey	30 mL
6	lime slices	6

1. In blender, combine mango, papaya, pineapple, milk, yogurt, juice and honey. Blend until smooth.
2. Pour into glasses. Garnish with lime.

Variation

Replace any of the fruit with other favorites such as strawberries or blueberries.

Green Goddess

Makes 4 servings

Bananas don't have to be boring! Enjoy this citrus-spiked banana beverage.

Nutrients per serving	
Calories	94
Fat	0 g
Saturated Fat	0 g
Cholesterol	0 mg
Sodium	7 mg
Carbohydrate	23 g
Fiber	3 g
Sugars	13 g
Protein	1 g
Calcium	21 mg
Iron	0 mg

- Blender

1/3 cup	kiwi or grapefruit juice	75 mL
	Juice of 1 lime	
1/4	musk melon, cubed	1/4
2	kiwifruits, quartered	2
2	banana chunks	2
1 tbsp	chopped fresh peppermint leaves	15 mL

1. In blender, combine kiwi juice, lime juice, melon, kiwis, banana and peppermint. Secure lid and blend (from low to high if using a variable-speed blender) until smooth.

Variation

You can substitute cantaloupe for the musk melon in this recipe and the result will be a Goddess, just not a green one.

Asparagus Mango Smoothie

Makes 2 servings

Having trouble getting enough vegetables in your diet? Asparagus is one of the best sources of prebiotics!

Nutrients per serving	
Calories	218
Fat	8 g
Saturated Fat	1 g
Cholesterol	0 mg
Sodium	24 mg
Carbohydrate	38 g
Fiber	8 g
Sugars	26 g
Protein	4 g
Calcium	55 mg
Iron	2 mg

• Blender

1/2 cup	carrot juice	125 mL
1	mango, quartered	1
1 cup	cooked chopped asparagus	250 mL
1/2	avocado	1/2
2	ice cubes	2

1. In blender, combine carrot juice, mango, asparagus, avocado and ice. Secure lid and process using the chop or pulse function until smooth.

Gazpacho Smoothie

Makes 2 servings

This vegetable smoothie is fresh and pungent.

Nutrients per serving	
Calories	59
Fat	0 g
Saturated Fat	0 g
Cholesterol	0 mg
Sodium	94 mg
Carbohydrate	12 g
Fiber	3 g
Sugars	9 g
Protein	2 g
Calcium	39 mg
Iron	1 mg

• Blender

2	fresh tomatoes, peeled	2
1	small clove garlic, smashed	1
1 cup	chopped seeded peeled cucumber	250 mL
1 cup	tomato juice	250 mL
2 tsp	freshly squeezed lemon juice	10 mL
Pinch	salt	Pinch
Pinch	freshly ground black pepper	Pinch
6	ice cubes	6

1. In blender, on high speed, purée tomatoes, garlic, cucumber, tomato juice, lemon juice, salt, pepper and ice.

Soy Milk

Makes about 2³⁄₄ cups (675 mL)

A few good reasons to make your own soy milk include the incredible fresh taste not found in store-bought, the low cost and, of course, the bragging rights.

Tip

A nut milk bag, available in most kitchen or natural food stores, makes straining nut or soy pulp easy. If you do not have one, line the sieve with two layers of cheesecloth.

- Blender
- Large wire-mesh strainer
- Nut milk bag (see tip, at left)

1 cup	dried soybeans, picked through and rinsed	250 mL
	Water	

1. Place soybeans in a bowl and add water to cover by 3 inches (7.5 cm). Cover bowl and let soak for 10 to 12 hours.

2. Drain beans and rinse well. Place half of the beans and 1¹⁄₃ cups (325 mL) warm water into blender and blend into a thin, smooth paste, 3 to 4 minutes. Transfer mixture to a bowl. Add the remaining beans to blender, add 1¹⁄₃ cups (325 mL) warm water and repeat process.

3. In a heavy-bottomed saucepan, bring 1 cup (250 mL) water to a boil over high heat. Stir in puréed mixture and bring to a boil, stirring frequently and watching constantly, as mixture will quickly froth over. Remove from heat and let cool slightly.

4. Place nut milk bag in strainer set over a large bowl and pour soy mixture into bag. Close bag and use the bottom of a mug to gently press liquid from soy pulp. When pulp appears dry, pour 1 cup (250 mL) warm water into nut bag and press again. Discard soy pulp.

5. Pour soy milk from bowl into a clean saucepan and bring to a boil over medium heat. Reduce heat and simmer, stirring occasionally, until bitterness has cooked out, 10 to 20 minutes. Let cool completely and transfer to a glass airtight container and refrigerate for up to 5 days.

Variation

Add 2 tbsp (30 mL) or more, to taste, of a sweetener such as agave nectar, brown rice syrup or pure maple syrup, or a flavoring such as vanilla extract or almond extract to taste.

Nutrients per ¹⁄₄ cup (60 mL)	
Calories	30
Fat	2 g
Saturated Fat	0 g
Cholesterol	0 mg
Sodium	0 mg
Carbohydrate	2 g
Fiber	1 g
Sugars	1 g
Protein	3 g
Calcium	17 mg
Iron	1 mg

Coconut Milk

Makes 4 cups (1 L)

Coconut milk is higher in fat than other raw milks, which makes it perfect for adding to tea and other warm beverages.

Tips

To soak the coconut for this recipe, place in a bowl and add 2 cups (500 mL) water. Cover and set aside for 30 minutes. Drain and rinse under cold running water until the water runs clear.

If you do not have a nut milk bag, line a sieve with two layers of cheesecloth and place it over the pitcher. Add the puréed coconut mixture and strain. Use a wooden spoon to press out the liquid, extracting as much of it as possible. Collect the corners of the cheesecloth and twist them to form a tight ball. Using your hands, squeeze out the remaining liquid.

- Blender
- Nut milk bag (see tip, at left)

1 cup	unsweetened dried shredded coconut, soaked (see tip, at left)	250 mL
4 cups	filtered water	1 L
Pinch	fine sea salt	Pinch

1. In blender, combine water, coconut and salt. Blend at high speed for 1 minute or until the liquid becomes milky white and no visible pieces of coconut remain.

2. Pour into a nut milk bag placed over a pitcher large enough to accommodate the liquid, and strain. Starting at the top of the bag and using your hands, squeeze in a downward direction to extract the remaining milk. Cover and refrigerate the milk for up to 3 days. Discard the pulp.

Variation

Strawberry Chocolate Coconut Milk: After straining the coconut milk, return it to the blender. Add 1/2 cup (125 mL) chopped hulled strawberries, 3 tbsp (45 mL) agave nectar and 2 tbsp (30 mL) cacao powder and blend again until smooth.

Nutrients per 1/4 cup (60 mL)	
Calories	20
Fat	2 g
Saturated Fat	2 g
Cholesterol	0 mg
Sodium	2 mg
Carbohydrate	1 g
Fiber	0 g
Sugars	0 g
Protein	0 g
Calcium	1 mg
Iron	0 mg

Green Barley Water

Quench your thirst with barley! Did you know it has prebiotics?

Tip

Store, tightly covered, in the refrigerator for up to 3 days.

3 tbsp	bruised fresh oregano leaves	45 mL
2 cups	boiling water	500 mL
1/4 cup	pot barley	60 mL
1 tbsp	liquid honey (or to taste)	15 mL
2 tbsp	freshly squeezed lemon juice (or to taste)	30 mL
2 cups	noncarbonated mineral water	500 mL

1. In a nonreactive teapot, combine oregano and boiling water. Cover tightly and steep for 5 minutes.

2. Strain off and discard oregano. Reserve and set aside 1 cup (250 mL) of the infusion. Combine the other cup (250 mL) of infusion in a saucepan with barley. Cover and bring to a boil over medium-high heat. Reduce heat and simmer gently, stirring occasionally, for 10 minutes or until barley is soft.

3. Turn heat off, stir in honey and reserved oregano infusion. Cover and let cool. Strain liquid into a glass jug and discard barley solids. Stir in lemon juice and mineral water. Taste and add more honey and lemon juice, if required. This water is meant to be drunk at room temperature but may be chilled.

Nutrients per 1 cup (250 mL)	
Calories	21
Fat	0 g
Saturated Fat	0 g
Cholesterol	0 mg
Sodium	7 mg
Carbohydrate	6 g
Fiber	0 g
Sugars	5 g
Protein	0 g
Calcium	22 mg
Iron	0 mg

Spring Tonic

Dandelion roots and greens are a fantastic source of prebiotics any time of the year!

Nutrients per ½ cup (125 mL)	
Calories	1
Fat	0 g
Saturated Fat	0 g
Cholesterol	0 mg
Sodium	3 mg
Carbohydrate	0 g
Fiber	0 g
Sugars	0 g
Protein	0 g
Calcium	15 mg
Iron	0 mg

1	fresh dandelion root, coarsely chopped	1
1	fresh burdock root, coarsely chopped	1
1	fresh ginseng root, coarsely chopped (optional)	1
2 tbsp	chopped fresh parsley	30 mL
2 tbsp	chopped fresh dandelion leaf	30 mL
1 cup	fresh maple sap or pure filtered water	250 mL

1. In a saucepan, combine 2 cups (500 mL) water and dandelion, burdock and ginseng (if using). Cover and bring to a boil over medium heat. Reduce heat and simmer gently for 10 minutes. Remove from heat and stir in parsley and dandelion leaf. Let stand, covered, for 20 minutes.

2. Strain into a clean jar, pressing on solids to extract all liquid. Discard solids and pour into a glass jar with a lid. Add maple sap, if available, or water.

3. Store, tightly covered, in the refrigerator for up to 1 day.

C-Blend

Nutrients per serving	
Calories	257
Fat	1 g
Saturated Fat	0 g
Cholesterol	0 mg
Sodium	5 mg
Carbohydrate	68 g
Fiber	13 g
Sugars	28 g
Protein	4 g
Calcium	158 mg
Iron	1 mg

• Juicer

2	oranges	2
1	grapefruit, cut to fit juicer tube	1
1	lime	1
½ cup	whole cranberries (fresh or frozen)	125 mL
1 tbsp	liquid honey (optional)	15 mL

1. Using juicer, process oranges, grapefruit, lime and cranberries. Whisk and pour into a glass. Whisk in honey, if desired.

Artichoke Eight

Drink your veggies! This recipe includes two of the best sources of prebiotics: raw Jerusalem artichoke and raw leek. Your healthy gut will thank you.

Nutrients per serving	
Calories	199
Fat	1 g
Saturated Fat	0 g
Cholesterol	0 mg
Sodium	347 mg
Carbohydrate	47 g
Fiber	13 g
Sugars	18 g
Protein	6 g
Calcium	170 mg
Iron	3 mg

- Juicer

1	handful Jerusalem artichoke roots	1
2	stalks celery	2
2	carrots	2
1	parsnip	1
1/4	head cabbage, cut to fit juicer tube	1/4
1 cup	fresh spinach leaves	250 mL
1	apple	1
1/2	leek	1/2

1. Using juicer, process artichoke roots, celery, carrots, parsnip, cabbage, spinach, apple and leek. Whisk and pour into glasses.

Brocco-Artichoke

Jerusalem artichoke roots are especially high in prebiotics.

Nutrients per serving	
Calories	106
Fat	1 g
Saturated Fat	0 g
Cholesterol	0 mg
Sodium	195 mg
Carbohydrate	24 g
Fiber	11 g
Sugars	2 g
Protein	7 g
Calcium	119 mg
Iron	3 mg

- Juicer

1	spear broccoli	1
2	Jerusalem artichoke roots	2
3	sprigs fresh parsley	3
1/4	fennel bulb	1/4

1. Using juicer, process broccoli, artichoke roots, parsley and fennel. Whisk and pour into a glass.

Root Coffee Blend

Makes 2½ cups (625 mL)

This coffee alternative will give your gut a boost!

Tips

Do not use licorice if you have high blood pressure.

To make root coffee, grind a small amount of the root blend and use 1 tbsp (15 mL) for every 1 cup (250 mL) boiling water. Stir and allow solids to settle on the bottom (or strain) before drinking.

- Preheat oven to 300°F (150°C)
- Large rimmed baking sheet, ungreased
- Mortar and pestle, food processor or blender

6 to 8	fresh dandelion roots, chopped	6 to 8
4 to 6	fresh burdock roots, chopped	4 to 6
3 to 4	fresh chicory roots, chopped	3 to 4
1	2-inch (5 cm) piece cinnamon stick	1
¼ cup	chopped fresh or dried licorice (see tip, at left)	60 mL
1 tbsp	ground ginseng	15 mL

1. Spread dandelion, burdock and chicory roots on baking sheet. Bake in preheated oven, stirring after 20 minutes, for 45 minutes or until golden. Reduce oven temperature to 200°F (100°C) and roast for 45 minutes to 1 hour or until thoroughly dry, stirring every 20 minutes. Set aside to cool.

2. Meanwhile, using mortar and pestle, food processor or blender, crush cinnamon stick.

3. In a bowl, combine roasted roots, crushed cinnamon, licorice and ginseng. Transfer to an airtight jar to store. (Roots must be thoroughly dried before storing.)

Nutrients per 1 tbsp (15 mL)	
Calories	13
Fat	0 g
Saturated Fat	0 g
Cholesterol	0 mg
Sodium	3 mg
Carbohydrate	3 g
Fiber	1 g
Sugars	1 g
Protein	0 g
Calcium	9 mg
Iron	0 mg

Easy Root Coffee

Makes 1¼ cups (300 mL)

Using the powdered form of roots makes them easy to blend — an "instant" coffee substitute.

Tip

To make 1 cup (250 mL) Easy Root Coffee, measure 1 tbsp (15 mL) root blend into a mug and pour in 1 cup (250 mL) boiling water. Stir and allow solids to settle on the bottom (or strain) before drinking.

½ cup	powdered chicory root	125 mL
¼ cup	powdered dandelion root	60 mL
¼ cup	powdered burdock root	60 mL
¼ cup	powdered carob	60 mL
1 tbsp	ground ginseng	15 mL

1. In a mixing bowl, combine chicory, dandelion, burdock, carob and ginseng. Transfer to an airtight jar to store.

Nutrients per 1 tbsp (15 mL)	
Calories	26
Fat	0 g
Saturated Fat	0 g
Cholesterol	0 mg
Sodium	9 mg
Carbohydrate	6 g
Fiber	1 g
Sugars	1 g
Protein	1 g
Calcium	34 mg
Iron	1 mg

Baked Goods

Super Health Bread 174

Apple Cranberry Bread 175

Apricot Bran Bread 176

Banana Bread 177

Peanut Butter and Banana Bread 178

Spinach Artichoke Bread 179

Orange Apricot Oatmeal Scones 180

Triple B Health Muffins 181

Cocoa Banana Mini Muffins 182

Artichoke Cheddar Squares 184

Whole-Grain Power Bars 185

Superpower Breakfast Cookies 186

Super Health Bread

Makes 16 slices

This nutrition-packed bread can help you to "eat right anytime." It is very easy to make and tastes great served with milk, juice or coffee.

Tip

Wheat germ, the embryo of the wheat berry, is very high in fiber. Use it to replace some of the bread crumbs in recipes such as meat loaf, or when breading meats such as turkey cutlets. Because it contains oils that go rancid quickly, it should be stored in the refrigerator.

- Preheat oven to 350°F (180°C)
- 9- by 5-inch (23 by 12.5 cm) loaf pan, lightly greased

½ cup	boiling water	125 mL
1 cup	raisins	250 mL
1	large egg, beaten	1
1 cup	lightly packed brown sugar	250 mL
1 cup	buttermilk	250 mL
1 cup	whole wheat flour	250 mL
1 cup	large-flake (old-fashioned) rolled oats	250 mL
1 cup	high-fiber bran cereal	250 mL
¼ cup	wheat germ	60 mL
1½ tsp	baking soda	7 mL
½ tsp	salt	2 mL

1. Pour boiling water over raisins; cool. Stir in egg, sugar and buttermilk.

2. In a medium bowl, combine flour, oats, cereal, wheat germ, baking soda and salt. Stir in egg mixture until thoroughly combined. Pour into prepared loaf pan.

3. Bake in preheated oven for about 45 minutes or until tester inserted in center comes out clean. Let cool before removing from pan.

This recipe courtesy of Alma R. Price.

Nutrients per slice	
Calories	183
Fat	2 g
Saturated Fat	1 g
Cholesterol	13 mg
Sodium	237 mg
Carbohydrate	40 g
Fiber	4 g
Sugars	22 g
Protein	5 g
Calcium	53 mg
Iron	3 mg

Apple Cranberry Bread

This delicious bread makes a great snack or a nutritious dessert, and can even be eaten for breakfast.

Tips

This bread can be made in almost any kind of baking dish that will fit in your slow cooker: a small loaf pan (about 8 by 4 inches/20 by 10 cm) makes a traditionally shaped bread; a round (6-cup/1.5 L) soufflé dish or square (7-inch/18 cm) baking dish produces slices of different shapes.

Natural cane sugar contains some nutrients, but if you don't have it, substitute packed brown sugar.

- 8- by 4-inch (20 by 10 cm) loaf pan, greased (see tip, at left)
- Large (minimum 5-quart) oval slow cooker

1 cup	all-purpose flour	250 mL
1 cup	whole wheat flour	250 mL
1/4 cup	ground flax seeds (flaxseed meal)	60 mL
2 tsp	baking powder	10 mL
1/2 tsp	salt	2 mL
1/2 tsp	ground cinnamon	2 mL
3/4 cup	natural cane sugar (such as Demerara or other evaporated cane sugar)	175 mL
1/4 cup	olive oil	60 mL
1	large egg	1
2 tbsp	finely grated orange zest	30 mL
3/4 cup	freshly squeezed orange juice	175 mL
1 tsp	vanilla extract	5 mL
1 cup	finely chopped peeled cored apple	250 mL
1 cup	fresh or frozen cranberries	250 mL

1. In a bowl or on a sheet of waxed paper, combine all-purpose and whole wheat flours, flax seeds, baking powder, salt and cinnamon. Mix well.

2. In a separate bowl, beat sugar, oil, egg, orange zest and juice and vanilla until thoroughly blended. Add dry ingredients, stirring just until blended. Fold in apple and cranberries.

3. Spoon batter into prepared pan. Cover pan tightly with foil and secure with a string. Place pan in slow cooker stoneware and pour in enough boiling water to come 1 inch (2.5 cm) up the sides of the dish. Cover and cook on High for 4 hours, until a tester inserted in the center comes out clean. Unmold and serve warm or let cool.

Nutrients per slice	
Calories	294
Fat	9 g
Saturated Fat	1 g
Cholesterol	23 mg
Sodium	158 mg
Carbohydrate	48 g
Fiber	4 g
Sugars	22 g
Protein	5 g
Calcium	125 mg
Iron	3 mg

Apricot Bran Bread

Makes 14 slices

This tasty and nutritious quick bread freezes well. Keep some in the freezer for unexpected guests.

Tip

Freeze this and other quick breads as individually wrapped single slices. Pop them into lunch bags. They will be defrosted by the time lunch comes around.

- Preheat oven to 350°F (180°C)
- 8- by 4-inch (20 by 10 cm) loaf pan, lightly greased

2 cups	bran cereal flakes	500 mL
1/2 cup	all-purpose flour	125 mL
1/2 cup	whole wheat flour	125 mL
1/2 cup	packed brown sugar	125 mL
2 tsp	baking powder	10 mL
1/2 tsp	salt	2 mL
1/2 tsp	ground nutmeg	2 mL
3/4 cup	chopped dried apricots	175 mL
1 tsp	grated orange zest	5 mL
1	large egg, lightly beaten	1
1/2 cup	skim milk	125 mL
1/2 cup	freshly squeezed orange juice	125 mL
1/4 cup	vegetable oil	60 mL

1. Crush cereal to make 3/4 cup (175 mL) crumbs. In a large bowl, combine cereal, flours, sugar, baking powder, salt, nutmeg, apricots and orange zest.

2. In a second bowl, beat together egg, milk, orange juice and oil; stir into dry ingredients until well combined. Pour into prepared loaf pan.

3. Bake in preheated oven for about 55 minutes or until tester inserted in center comes out clean. Let cool for 10 minutes before removing from pan. Let cool completely on a wire rack.

This recipe courtesy of Maryanne Cattrysse.

Nutrients per slice	
Calories	143
Fat	5 g
Saturated Fat	0 g
Cholesterol	13 mg
Sodium	141 mg
Carbohydrate	25 g
Fiber	2 g
Sugars	14 g
Protein	3 g
Calcium	71 mg
Iron	4 mg

Banana Bread

Everybody needs a great banana bread recipe in their repertoire, and this one fits the bill, with fantastic flavor and a tender, moist texture. As a bonus, you'll reap the prebiotic benefits of the bananas.

Tips

A glass pan of the same dimensions may also be used. Add 4 to 8 minutes to the baking time.

Store the cooled bread, wrapped in foil or plastic wrap, in the refrigerator for up to 5 days. Alternatively, wrap it in plastic wrap, then foil, completely enclosing bread, and freeze for up to 3 months. Let thaw at room temperature for 4 to 6 hours before serving.

- Preheat oven to 350°F (180°C)
- 9- by 5-inch (23 by 12.5 cm) metal loaf pan, greased with virgin coconut oil

¾ cup	chickpea flour	175 mL
6 tbsp	coconut flour	90 mL
1½ tbsp	potato starch	22 mL
1 tsp	baking soda	5 mL
½ tsp	baking powder	2 mL
¼ tsp	fine sea salt	1 mL
¼ tsp	ground nutmeg	1 mL
⅓ cup	coconut sugar	75 mL
2 tbsp	psyllium husk	30 mL
1 cup	mashed very ripe bananas	250 mL
½ cup	well-stirred coconut milk (full-fat)	125 mL

1. In a large bowl, whisk together chickpea flour, coconut flour, potato starch, baking soda, baking powder, salt and nutmeg.

2. In a medium bowl, combine coconut sugar, psyllium, bananas and coconut milk until well blended. Let stand for 5 minutes to thicken.

3. Add the banana mixture to the flour mixture and stir until just blended.

4. Spread batter evenly in prepared pan.

5. Bake in preheated oven for 45 to 50 minutes or until top is golden brown and a tester inserted in the center comes out clean. Let cool in pan on a wire rack for 10 minutes, then transfer to the rack to cool completely.

Nutrients per slice	
Calories	90
Fat	4 g
Saturated Fat	3 g
Cholesterol	0 mg
Sodium	130 mg
Carbohydrate	14 g
Fiber	2 g
Sugars	8 g
Protein	1 g
Calcium	16 mg
Iron	1 mg

Peanut Butter and Banana Bread

Makes 16 slices

The nut butter provides some protein in this tasty bread.

Tips

Store bread, tightly covered, in the refrigerator for up to 1 week.

Two bananas will provide enough for this moist and nutritious breakfast or snacking bread. The sugar is adjusted for natural nut butter. If using a commercial peanut butter, reduce the amount of sugar to 2 tbsp (30 mL).

- Preheat oven to 375°F (190°C)
- 9- by 5-inch (23 by 12.5 cm) loaf pan, lightly oiled

1 cup	whole wheat flour	250 mL
1 cup	whole-grain granola	250 mL
3 tbsp	natural cane sugar	45 mL
1 tbsp	baking powder	15 mL
$1/2$ tsp	salt	2 mL
$3/4$ cup	mashed ripe banana	175 mL
$1/4$ cup	natural peanut or cashew butter	60 mL
2	large eggs, lightly beaten	2
2 tbsp	soy or rice milk	30 mL
2 tbsp	olive oil	30 mL

1. In a large bowl, combine flour, granola, sugar, baking powder and salt and stir to mix well. Make a well in the center.

2. In a bowl, using a fork, beat banana with peanut butter. Beat in eggs, milk and oil. Pour liquid ingredients into dry ingredients and stir just until mixed. Scrape into prepared loaf pan.

3. Bake in center of preheated oven for 35 to 45 minutes or until a tester comes out clean. Transfer to a wire rack and let cool.

Nutrients per slice	
Calories	130
Fat	6 g
Saturated Fat	1 g
Cholesterol	23 mg
Sodium	105 mg
Carbohydrate	16 g
Fiber	2 g
Sugars	5 g
Protein	4 g
Calcium	58 mg
Iron	1 mg

Spinach Artichoke Bread

The leek, garlic and artichoke hearts in this bread will keep your gut happy!

- Preheat oven to 400°F (200°C)
- Baking sheet, greased

2 tsp	olive oil	10 mL
1	leek (white part only), finely chopped	1
1	clove garlic, minced	1
5 oz	frozen chopped spinach, thawed and drained	150 g
Pinch	ground mace	Pinch
	Salt and freshly ground black pepper	
2	marinated artichoke hearts, chopped	2
8 oz	white bread dough (homemade or frozen, thawed)	250 g
	Ice water	

1. In a large skillet, heat oil over medium heat. Sauté leek and garlic until tender. Add spinach and sauté until almost dry. Season with mace and with salt and pepper to taste. Remove from heat and add artichoke hearts.

2. Pat dough into an 8- by 6-inch (20 by 15 cm) rectangle. Spread artichoke mixture over dough and, starting with one long side, roll up jelly roll–style. Pinch ends closed and place seam side down on prepared baking sheet. Cover with a damp towel and let rise until doubled in bulk.

3. Slash top of loaf and brush with ice water.

4. Bake in preheated oven for 35 to 40 minutes, until crisp and golden on top and bottom. Let cool on a rack for 15 minutes. Serve warm.

Nutrients per serving	
Calories	210
Fat	5 g
Saturated Fat	0 g
Cholesterol	0 mg
Sodium	375 mg
Carbohydrate	33 g
Fiber	4 g
Sugars	3 g
Protein	8 g
Calcium	60 mg
Iron	3 mg

Orange Apricot Oatmeal Scones

Makes 12 scones

These tasty scones are delicious with a relaxing cup of tea.

Tip

Sour milk can be used instead of buttermilk. To prepare, combine 2 tsp (10 mL) lemon juice or vinegar with 1 cup (250 mL) milk and let stand for 5 minutes.

- Preheat oven to 375°F (190°C)
- Baking sheet, greased

2 cups	all-purpose flour	500 mL
1½ cups	quick-cooking rolled oats	375 mL
¼ cup	granulated sugar, divided	60 mL
1 tbsp	baking powder	15 mL
2 tsp	grated orange zest	10 mL
½ tsp	baking soda	2 mL
¼ tsp	salt	1 mL
6 tbsp	butter	90 mL
½ cup	chopped apricots	125 mL
1 cup	buttermilk (see tip, at left)	250 mL
	Milk	

1. In a bowl, combine flour, oats, all but 1 tsp (5 mL) of the sugar, baking powder, orange zest, baking soda and salt. Using a fork or pastry blender, cut in butter until mixture resembles coarse crumbs. Stir in apricots. Add buttermilk; stir until mixture is just combined.

2. On a lightly floured surface, knead dough gently 4 or 5 times. Divide into 3 pieces. Shape each piece into a round about 1 inch (2.5 cm) thick. Transfer to baking sheet.

3. Cut each round into quarters. Brush tops with milk; sprinkle with reserved sugar.

4. Bake in preheated oven for 20 to 25 minutes or until lightly browned.

This recipe courtesy of dietitian Bev Callaghan.

Variation

For a change, substitute ½ cup (125 mL) dates, raisins, currants or dried cranberries for the apricots.

Nutrients per scone	
Calories	212
Fat	7 g
Saturated Fat	4 g
Cholesterol	17 mg
Sodium	121 mg
Carbohydrate	32 g
Fiber	2 g
Sugars	9 g
Protein	5 g
Calcium	149 mg
Iron	2 mg

Triple B Health Muffins

Makes 12 muffins

These healthy muffins are a good choice for breakfast or a mid-morning snack.

- Preheat oven to 400°F (200°C)
- 12-cup muffin tin, lightly greased or lined with paper cups

1 cup	whole wheat flour	250 mL
1 cup	wheat bran or oat bran	250 mL
1 cup	fresh or frozen blueberries	250 mL
1 tsp	baking soda	5 mL
1 tsp	baking powder	5 mL
2	ripe bananas, mashed (about 1 cup/250 mL)	2
1	large egg, lightly beaten	1
½ cup	granulated sugar	125 mL
½ cup	milk	125 mL
¼ cup	vegetable oil	60 mL
1 tsp	vanilla extract	5 mL

1. In a medium bowl, combine flour, wheat bran, blueberries, baking soda and baking powder.

2. In a large bowl, combine bananas, egg, sugar, milk, oil and vanilla. Fold in flour mixture until just combined.

3. Divide batter evenly among prepared muffin cups, filling each two-thirds full.

4. Bake in preheated oven for 20 to 25 minutes or until tops are firm to the touch and a tester inserted in the center of a muffin comes out clean. Let cool in tin for 10 minutes, then remove to a wire rack to cool completely.

This recipe courtesy of Barbara Kajifasz.

Nutrients per muffin	
Calories	154
Fat	6 g
Saturated Fat	1 g
Cholesterol	16 mg
Sodium	140 mg
Carbohydrate	26 g
Fiber	4 g
Sugars	13 g
Protein	3 g
Calcium	42 mg
Iron	1 mg

Cocoa Banana Mini Muffins

**Makes
36 mini muffins**

*Everyone needs a great
breakfast recipe that can
be thrown together in
minutes the night before.
These mini muffins are
just such a recipe.*

Tip

Natural cane confectioners'
(icing) sugar is made
using the same process as
regular confectioners' sugar
(granulated sugar is crushed
to a fine white powder), but
is made with less-processed
natural cane sugar. Regular
confectioners' sugar may
be used in its place.

- Preheat oven to 400°F (200°C)
- Three 12-cup mini muffin pans, sprayed with nonstick cooking spray

1¼ cups	quinoa flour	300 mL
1 cup	quick-cooking rolled oats	250 mL
½ cup	natural cane sugar or packed light brown sugar	125 mL
⅓ cup	unsweetened cocoa powder (not Dutch process)	75 mL
1¼ tsp	baking powder	6 mL
½ tsp	baking soda	2 mL
¼ tsp	fine sea salt	1 mL
2	large eggs	2
⅔ cup	mashed ripe bananas	150 mL
½ cup	milk or plain nondairy milk (such as soy, almond, rice or hemp)	125 mL
¼ cup	virgin coconut oil, warmed, or unsalted butter, melted	60 mL
1 tsp	vanilla extract	5 mL
2 tbsp	natural cane confectioners' (icing) sugar (optional)	30 mL

1. In a large bowl, whisk together quinoa flour, oats, cane sugar, cocoa powder, baking powder, baking soda and salt.

2. In a medium bowl, whisk together eggs, bananas, milk, oil and vanilla until well blended.

3. Add the egg mixture to the flour mixture and stir until just blended.

Nutrients per muffin

Calories	62
Fat	2 g
Saturated Fat	1 g
Cholesterol	11 mg
Sodium	44 mg
Carbohydrate	9 g
Fiber	1 g
Sugars	3 g
Protein	2 g
Calcium	17 mg
Iron	1 mg

Store cooled muffins in an airtight container in the refrigerator for up to 5 days.

4. Divide batter equally among prepared muffin cups.

5. Bake in preheated oven 10 to 12 minutes or until a tester inserted in the center comes out clean. Let cool in pans on a wire rack for 5 minutes, then transfer to the rack to cool. Sprinkle with confectioners' sugar, if desired.

Muffin-Making Tips

- Mix dry and wet ingredients separately before combining them.
- Do not overstir.
- Use an ice cream scoop to transfer the batter to the muffin cups without making a mess.
- Let muffins hot from the oven cool in the pan for 5 minutes before removing them. This will help prevent them from falling apart. But don't leave them in the pan for longer than 5 minutes or they may get soggy.
- Freeze leftover muffins for up to 6 months. Muffins freeze wonderfully.

Artichoke Cheddar Squares

Makes 24 squares

Here, a popular artichoke dip is turned into a casserole, then cut into squares. They're perfect for a buffet or as passed hors d'oeuvres at a party.

- Preheat oven to 325°F (160°C)
- 9-inch (23 cm) glass baking dish, greased

1 tbsp	olive oil	15 mL
1	small onion, minced	1
1	clove garlic, minced	1
2	jars (each 6½ oz/184 mL) marinated artichoke hearts, drained and chopped	2
4	large eggs	4
¼ cup	dry bread crumbs	60 mL
¼ tsp	salt	1 mL
⅛ tsp	freshly ground black pepper	0.5 mL
⅛ tsp	dried oregano	0.5 mL
⅛ tsp	hot pepper sauce	0.5 mL
2 cups	shredded extra-sharp (extra-old) Cheddar cheese	500 mL
2 tbsp	minced fresh parsley	30 mL

1. In a large nonstick skillet, heat oil over medium heat. Sauté onion and garlic for about 5 minutes or until tender. Stir in artichokes. Let cool slightly.

2. In a large bowl, whisk eggs until blended. Stir in bread crumbs, salt, black pepper, oregano and hot pepper sauce. Gently stir in cheese and parsley. Stir in onion mixture. Pour into prepared baking dish.

3. Bake in preheated oven for 30 minutes or until golden. Let cool slightly, then cut into 1-inch (2.5 cm) squares.

Variation

For a different flavor and aroma, substitute smoked mozzarella for the Cheddar.

Nutrients per square	
Calories	71
Fat	6 g
Saturated Fat	2 g
Cholesterol	41 mg
Sodium	144 mg
Carbohydrate	2 g
Fiber	1 g
Sugars	0 g
Protein	4 g
Calcium	76 mg
Iron	0 mg

Whole-Grain Power Bars

Makes 20 bars

Taking their goodness from the homemade power cereal, these high-energy bars are a great snack for active people. Enough said.

- Preheat oven to 375°F (190°C)
- Rimmed baking sheet
- 11- by 7-inch (28 by 18 cm) baking pan

1 cup	coarsely chopped walnuts	250 mL
1/2 cup	sesame seeds	125 mL
2 cups	granola	500 mL
1 1/2 cups	unsweetened crisp brown rice cereal	375 mL
1 cup	dried cherries or cranberries	250 mL
1/4 cup	flax seeds	60 mL
2 tbsp	whole chia seeds	30 mL
1 tbsp	sea salt	15 mL
1/2 cup	brown rice syrup or agave nectar	125 mL
2 tbsp	virgin coconut oil	30 mL
2 tsp	vanilla extract	10 mL

1. On baking sheet, combine walnuts and sesame seeds. Bake in preheated oven for 5 minutes or until lightly browned and toasted.

2. In a large bowl, combine toasted nuts and seeds, granola, rice cereal, cherries, flax seeds, chia seeds and salt.

3. In a saucepan over medium-high heat, heat rice syrup until lightly simmering. Remove from heat and stir in coconut oil and vanilla. Stir until coconut oil is dissolved. Pour over cereal mixture. Press into prepared baking pan and set aside for 15 minutes. Cut into 2-inch (5 cm) squares.

4. Store bars in an airtight container for up to 2 weeks or in the refrigerator for up to 1 month.

Nutrients per bar	
Calories	207
Fat	11 g
Saturated Fat	2 g
Cholesterol	0 mg
Sodium	438 mg
Carbohydrate	23 g
Fiber	5 g
Sugars	10 g
Protein	4 g
Calcium	68 mg
Iron	2 mg

Superpower Breakfast Cookies

The prebiotics and probiotics in these cookies create a synergistic effect in your gut, and that's a great thing!

Tip

Store cooled cookies in an airtight container in the refrigerator for up to 5 days.

- Preheat oven to 350°F (180°C)
- Baking sheets, lined with parchment paper

1/2 cup	quinoa, rinsed	125 mL
1 1/4 cups	quinoa flour	300 mL
3/4 cup	quick-cooking rolled oats	175 mL
1 1/2 tsp	baking powder	7 mL
1 tsp	fine sea salt	5 mL
1/2 tsp	baking soda	2 mL
1	large egg, lightly beaten	1
1/2 cup	liquid honey, pure maple syrup or brown rice syrup	125 mL
1/3 cup	plain yogurt	75 mL
1/4 cup	virgin coconut oil, warmed, or vegetable oil	60 mL
1 tsp	vanilla extract	5 mL
2/3 cup	dried cherries, cranberries or blueberries	150 mL

1. In a pot of boiling salted water, cook quinoa for 9 minutes. Drain and rinse under cold water until cool (quinoa will still be slightly chewy).

2. In a large bowl, whisk together quinoa flour, oats, baking powder, salt and baking soda. Stir in egg, honey, yogurt, oil and vanilla until just blended. Gently fold in quinoa and cherries.

3. Drop batter by 2 tbsp (30 mL) onto prepared baking sheets, spacing cookies 2 inches (5 cm) apart.

4. Bake one sheet at a time in preheated oven for 12 to 15 minutes or until just set in the center. Let cool in pan on a wire rack for 5 minutes, then transfer to the rack to cool.

Nutrients per cookie	
Calories	71
Fat	2 g
Saturated Fat	1 g
Cholesterol	5 mg
Sodium	100 mg
Carbohydrate	12 g
Fiber	2 g
Sugars	5 g
Protein	2 g
Calcium	19 mg
Iron	1 mg

Snacks, Appetizers, Dips and Spreads

Sweet Vanilla Buckwheat Almond Clusters. 188

Crunchy Chocolate Banana Pops 189

Cheese Straws 190

Stuffed Mushroom Caps 191

Vegetable Curry Rolls 192

Buckwheat Blinis. 193

Toasted Tofu with Onion Miso Jam 194

Yogurt Cheese 195

Barbecued Tofu Nuggets. 196

Tofu and Chickpea Garlic Dip 197

Garlic Cheese 197

Quick Zucchini and Jerusalem Artichoke
  on Grilled Crostini 198

Roasted Garlic Sour Cream Dip 199

Cream of Leek and Asparagus on Toast Points 200

French Lentil Dip with Herbed Crostini 201

Caramelized Onion Dip 202

Smoky Eggplant Dip with Yogurt. 203

Cheesy Avocado Dip 204

Artichoke Salsa 205

Gazpacho Salsa. 205

Asparagus Salsa 206

Tomato Garlic Raita. 207

Hummus with Roasted Red Peppers. 208

Artichoke and White Bean Spread 209

Refried Pumpkin 210

Sweet Vanilla Buckwheat Almond Clusters

Makes 7 clusters

These sweet, crunchy and nutrient-dense clusters are the perfect midday pick-me-up.

Tip

Two tablespoons (30 mL) of chia seeds provides about 7 grams of alpha-linolenic acid (ALA), an omega-3 fat that is an essential fatty acid. It is called "essential" because our bodies are unable to make it and must obtain it from food. Good sources of ALA include flax seeds, chia seeds and walnuts.

* Baking sheet lined with parchment

½ cup	raw buckwheat groats	125 mL
2 tbsp	raw almond butter	30 mL
2 tbsp	raw agave nectar	30 mL
1 tbsp	raw chia seeds	15 mL
¼ tsp	raw vanilla extract	1 mL

1. In a bowl, combine buckwheat, almond butter, agave nectar, chia seeds and vanilla extract. Stir together until well incorporated. Using a tablespoon (15 mL), scoop up 7 equal portions and drop onto prepared baking sheet. Freeze for 15 minutes or until firm. Serve immediately or transfer to an airtight container and freeze for up to 2 weeks.

Variations

Chocolate Buckwheat Almond Clusters: Substitute 1 tbsp (15 mL) raw cacao powder for the vanilla and 2 tsp (10 mL) raw cacao nibs for the chia seeds.

Nut-Free Vanilla Buckwheat Clusters: Substitute an equal amount of raw tahini for the almond butter.

Substitute an equal amount of raw cacao nibs, raw shelled hemp seeds or dried shredded coconut for the chia seeds.

Nutrients per cluster	
Calories	95
Fat	3 g
Saturated Fat	0 g
Cholesterol	0 mg
Sodium	10 mg
Carbohydrate	15 g
Fiber	2 g
Sugars	5 g
Protein	3 g
Calcium	28 mg
Iron	0 mg

Crunchy Chocolate Banana Pops

Makes 4 pops

Serve these crunchy sweet treats with a nice tall glass of almond milk for a perfect afternoon snack.

Tip

Coconut oil is solid at room temperature but has a melting point of 76°F (24°C), so it is easy to liquefy. To melt it, place in a shallow glass bowl over a pot of simmering water.

- Blender
- Baking sheet, lined with parchment paper

1/4 cup	melted virgin coconut oil (see tip, at left)	60 mL
1/4 cup	filtered water	60 mL
3 tbsp	raw cacao powder	45 mL
3 tbsp	raw agave nectar	45 mL
4	bananas, peeled	4

1. In blender, combine coconut oil, water, cacao powder and agave nectar. Blend at high speed until smooth. Transfer mixture to a shallow dish large enough to accommodate the bananas.

2. Using your hands, dip each banana in mixture until evenly coated. Place on prepared baking sheet and freeze for 10 minutes or until coating has set and outside is firm enough to handle. Serve immediately or transfer to an airtight container and freeze for up to 5 days.

Nutrients per pop	
Calories	301
Fat	16 g
Saturated Fat	13 g
Cholesterol	0 mg
Sodium	11 mg
Carbohydrate	40 g
Fiber	6 g
Sugars	24 g
Protein	4 g
Calcium	5 mg
Iron	0 mg

Cheese Straws

This recipe deviates slightly from the usual with the addition of fresh whole-grain bread crumbs. To turn this into an easy appetizer, wrap the cooled straws in thin slices of prosciutto or salami.

Tips

If your bread is fresh, it will benefit from being dried out a bit in the oven before processing. Place on a baking sheet in a preheated 325°F (160°C) oven, turning once, for 10 minutes.

Italian-style, whole wheat and sourdough bread all work well in this recipe. Depending on the dimensions of the bread, you may need to increase the number of slices.

Nutrients per 4 straws	
Calories	139
Fat	9 g
Saturated Fat	6 g
Cholesterol	28 mg
Sodium	232 mg
Carbohydrate	8 g
Fiber	0 g
Sugars	0 g
Protein	6 g
Calcium	165 mg
Iron	1 mg

- Preheat oven to 400°F (200°C)
- Food processor
- Baking sheets, lined with parchment paper

3	slices day-old bread, about 1 inch (2.5 cm) thick, crusts removed, broken into chunks (see tips, at left)	3
2 cups	shredded Cheddar cheese, preferably sharp (old)	500 mL
3 tbsp	unsalted butter, softened	45 mL
1 tbsp	chopped fresh dill fronds	15 mL
¾ cup	all-purpose flour	175 mL
¼ cup	milk or buttermilk	60 mL
½ tsp	salt	2 mL
½ tsp	hot or sweet smoked or plain paprika	2 mL

1. In food processor, process bread into fine crumbs. Measure 1½ cups (375 mL) and set aside.

2. In food processor, process cheese, butter and dill until integrated, scraping down sides of the bowl as required. Add bread crumbs, flour, milk, salt and smoked paprika and process until blended and dough comes together when pinched between your fingers. Transfer to a lightly floured surface and knead lightly.

3. On a lightly floured surface, roll out dough to a rectangle about 6 inches (15 cm) wide and ¼ inch (0.5 cm) thick. Cut into strips, each 6 inches (15 cm) long by ½ inch (1 cm) wide. Cut each strip in half crosswise, then fold in half lengthwise. Roll between your hands to make a cylinder, then transfer to work surface and roll until straw is about 4 inches (10 cm) long. Repeat until all dough has been rolled. Place about 2 inches (5 cm) apart on prepared baking sheets.

4. Bake in preheated oven, switching and rotating baking sheets halfway through, until lightly browned, about 15 minutes.

Stuffed Mushroom Caps

Makes 24 caps

Elegant yet easy to make, these tasty tidbits make great finger food.

Tip

If you have a mini-bowl attachment for your food processor, you can use it to mix the ingredients. Combine coarsely chopped artichokes, tomatoes and garlic and pulse until finely chopped, stopping and scraping down sides of the bowl as necessary. Add goat cheese and pulse to blend.

- Preheat oven to 400°F (200°C)

24	large white mushroom caps	24
2 tbsp	olive oil	30 mL
1	jar (6 oz/170 mL) marinated artichokes, drained and finely chopped	1
2	reconstituted sun-dried tomatoes, minced	2
2	cloves garlic, minced	2
4 oz	soft goat cheese	125 g
2 tbsp	pine nuts, finely chopped	30 mL

1. Brush mushroom caps all over with olive oil and place, convex side up, on a baking sheet. Bake in preheated oven for 15 minutes or until nicely softened. Let cool slightly. Leave oven on.

2. Meanwhile, in a bowl, combine artichokes, sun-dried tomatoes and garlic. Mix well. Add goat cheese and mix until blended. Spoon about 1 heaping tsp (7 mL) of mixture into each mushroom cap. Sprinkle with pine nuts. Return to oven and bake until cheese is melted and pine nuts are lightly toasted, about 10 minutes. Serve warm.

Nutrients per cap	
Calories	37
Fat	3 g
Saturated Fat	1 g
Cholesterol	2 mg
Sodium	39 mg
Carbohydrate	1 g
Fiber	0 g
Sugars	1 g
Protein	2 g
Calcium	8 mg
Iron	0 mg

Vegetable Curry Rolls

Makes 30 pastries

An adaptation of traditional Thai curry puffs, with a filling similar to vegetable samosas. Using phyllo pastry makes these easy to assemble, and baking replaces the usual deep-frying. For a vegetarian version, replace the fish sauce with soy sauce.

Tip

Rolls can be baked, cooled, packaged tightly and frozen for up to 3 weeks. To heat, place frozen on a baking sheet lined with parchment paper and bake in a preheated 300°F (150°C) oven for 15 to 18 minutes or until hot throughout.

• Preheat oven to 400°F (200°C)
• Baking sheet, lined with parchment paper

1 tbsp	vegetable oil	15 mL
2	cloves garlic, finely chopped	2
1	onion, chopped	1
1½ cups	diced potato	375 mL
1 cup	diced carrot	250 mL
¼ cup	water	60 mL
½ cup	finely chopped red bell pepper	125 mL
½ cup	green peas	125 mL
2 tbsp	chopped fresh cilantro leaves	30 mL
2 tbsp	fish sauce or soy sauce	30 mL
1 tbsp	packed brown sugar	15 mL
1 tsp	curry powder	5 mL
½ tsp	hot chili sauce	2 mL
10	sheets phyllo pastry	10
¼ cup	vegetable or olive oil	60 mL

1. In a wok or large skillet, heat oil over medium-high heat. Add garlic, onion, potato and carrot. Cook for 2 minutes, stirring.

2. Add water. Cover and cook for 4 to 5 minutes or until vegetables are almost tender.

3. Add red pepper, peas, cilantro, fish sauce, sugar, curry powder and chili sauce. Cook for 4 to 5 minutes, stirring frequently, until vegetables are tender and moisture has evaporated. Transfer to a bowl to cool.

4. To assemble, cut stack of phyllo crosswise into three equal pieces. Working with one or two pieces of pastry at a time (keep remainder covered to prevent drying), place pastry on a flat work surface. Place a full tablespoon of filling about 1 inch (2.5 cm) from bottom narrow edge and sides of pastry. Fold bottom of pastry over filling and fold in long sides. Roll up pastry to form a cigar shape. Place on prepared baking sheet. Brush lightly with oil. Continue with the remaining pastry and filling.

5. Bake pastries in preheated oven for 15 to 18 minutes or until golden and crisp. Serve warm or at room temperature.

Nutrients per pastry	
Calories	53
Fat	3 g
Saturated Fat	0 g
Cholesterol	0 mg
Sodium	129 mg
Carbohydrate	6 g
Fiber	1 g
Sugars	1 g
Protein	1 g
Calcium	6 mg
Iron	0 mg

Buckwheat Blinis

Makes about 50 blinis

These simple traditional Russian pancakes are wonderful topped with caviar, smoked salmon or other smoked fish, gravlax, sour cream and many other hors d'oeuvres toppings.

Tip

Make sure you use regular buckwheat flour (sometimes sold as light buckwheat flour), not the dark variety.

• Blender

1½ tsp	granulated sugar, divided	7 mL
¼ cup	warm water	60 mL
1½ tsp	active dry yeast	7 mL
1	large egg	1
1½ cups	lukewarm milk	375 mL
¼ cup	butter, melted, divided	60 mL
1 cup	all-purpose flour	250 mL
¾ cup	buckwheat flour	175 mL
½ tsp	salt	2 mL

1. In blender, dissolve ½ tsp (2 mL) sugar in warm water. Sprinkle in yeast and let stand until frothy, about 10 minutes. Add egg, milk, 2 tbsp (30 mL) butter and the remaining sugar; blend on low speed until frothy. With motor running, through hole in top, gradually add all-purpose flour, buckwheat flour and salt; blend, scraping down sides as necessary, until thoroughly mixed. Scrape into a bowl, cover and let rise in a warm place until doubled in bulk, about 1 hour.

2. Heat a nonstick skillet over medium heat and brush lightly with some of the remaining butter. Without stirring, spoon in batter by scant 2 tablespoonfuls (30 mL), adding butter as necessary. Cook until bubbles form on top that do not fill in, about 1 minute. Turn and cook until bottom is golden, about 30 seconds. Remove to a warmed platter and repeat with the remaining batter.

Nutrients per blini	
Calories	29
Fat	1 g
Saturated Fat	1 g
Cholesterol	7 mg
Sodium	29 mg
Carbohydrate	4 g
Fiber	0 g
Sugars	1 g
Protein	1 g
Calcium	17 mg
Iron	0 mg

Toasted Tofu with Onion Miso Jam

Makes 4 servings

Delicate toasted tofu is paired with the savory sweetness of the onion miso jam. Miso is another way to sneak in some probiotics.

• Rimmed baking sheet, lightly oiled

Tofu

1 lb	extra-firm tofu	500 g
2 tbsp	olive oil	30 mL
	Salt and freshly ground black pepper	
2 tsp	toasted sesame seeds (optional)	10 mL

Onion Miso Jam

2 tbsp	olive oil	30 mL
2 tbsp	vegan hard margarine	30 mL
2	large sweet onions, such as Vidalia or Walla Walla, thinly sliced	2
1 tsp	granulated sugar	5 mL
2 tbsp	vegan sake	30 mL
2 tbsp	brown rice syrup	30 mL
2 tbsp	rice wine vinegar	30 mL
1 tbsp	white miso	15 mL

1. *Tofu:* Drain tofu well and wrap in a kitchen towel or a few layers of paper towels. Set wrapped tofu on a plate, cover with another plate and place a heavy object (such as a 28-oz/796 mL can of tomatoes) on top. Transfer to the refrigerator and let stand for about 1 hour.

2. Unwrap tofu and cut crosswise into 8 pieces. Place on prepared baking sheet. Brush both sides with oil and lightly season with salt and pepper.

3. *Onion Miso Jam:* Meanwhile, place a large nonstick skillet over medium heat and let pan get hot. Add oil and margarine and tip pan to coat. Add onions, stirring to coat. Cook, stirring frequently, about 6 minutes. Add sugar and cook, stirring occasionally, until onions slowly turn golden, 20 to 30 minutes, reducing heat to medium-low, if necessary.

Nutrients per serving

Calories	369
Fat	25 g
Saturated Fat	4 g
Cholesterol	0 mg
Sodium	231 mg
Carbohydrate	22 g
Fiber	3 g
Sugars	10 g
Protein	13 g
Calcium	110 mg
Iron	2 mg

Tips

Tofu may also be toasted on the stovetop. Heat a cast-iron skillet over medium-high heat until very hot. Carefully add tofu slices and toast until lightly browned, 2 to 3 minutes per side.

If vegan sake is unavailable, substitute mirin or white wine.

4. In a small bowl, combine sake, brown rice syrup, vinegar and miso, mixing well. Stir mixture into onions. Reduce heat to low and simmer, stirring occasionally, until liquid reduces and mixture thickens, about 30 minutes. Set aside.

5. Preheat oven to 450°F (230°C).

6. Bake tofu in preheated oven for 10 minutes. Carefully flip tofu and bake for 8 minutes more. Remove pan from oven and set oven to broil. Carefully spread a thick layer of jam on each piece of tofu, return to oven and broil until jam begins to bubble, 30 seconds to 2 minutes. Sprinkle with sesame seeds (if using) and serve immediately.

Yogurt Cheese

Makes about 1⅓ cups (325 mL)

The longer the yogurt drains, the thicker the resulting "cheese" will be. This is a healthy, low-fat alternative to the mayonnaise and cream cheese in dips and spreads.

| 2 cups | plain yogurt | 500 mL |

1. Spoon yogurt into a sieve lined with cheesecloth and cover with plastic wrap. Set over a bowl to drain. Refrigerate for 2 to 3 hours or until yogurt is thick and reduced to about 1⅓ cups (325 mL).

2. Store cheese, tightly covered, in the refrigerator for up to 2 days.

Nutrients per ⅓ cup (75 mL)

Calories	77
Fat	2 g
Saturated Fat	1 g
Cholesterol	7 mg
Sodium	86 mg
Carbohydrate	9 g
Fiber	0 g
Sugars	9 g
Protein	6 g
Calcium	224 mg
Iron	0 mg

Barbecued Tofu Nuggets

Makes 2 to 4 servings

These tasty nuggets do double duty as finger food for a party or a great main course.

Tip

You can find smoked barbecued tofu in most major supermarkets or natural foods stores. If you can't find it, use the same amount of extra-firm tofu, cubed. Place the cubes on a double layer of paper towels. Let drain for 20 minutes. Pour off water and set tofu aside.

- Preheat oven to 375°F (190°C)
- Rimmed baking sheet, greased

6 oz	smoked barbecued tofu (see tip, at left), cut into 12 cubes	175 g
1/3 cup	barbecue sauce	75 mL
1 1/2 cups	finely crushed plain potato chips or barbecue-flavor potato chips	375 mL

1. Pat tofu dry with paper towels and brush all over with barbecue sauce. Place potato chips in a bowl. One at a time, drop cubes into potato chips, lightly tossing to ensure all sides are coated.

2. Place nuggets on prepared pan, 2 to 3 inches (5 to 7.5 cm) apart. Bake in preheated oven for 12 minutes or until hot and crispy. Let cool on pan for 1 minute. Using a metal spatula, transfer to a serving platter.

Variations

Substitute your favorite flavored potato chips, tortilla chips or wheat crackers for the plain or barbecue-flavored chips.

Substitute 1/3 cup (75 mL) soy mayonnaise for the barbecue sauce.

Nutrients per serving (1 of 4)	
Calories	153
Fat	8 g
Saturated Fat	1 g
Cholesterol	0 mg
Sodium	333 mg
Carbohydrate	15 g
Fiber	1 g
Sugars	6 g
Protein	7 g
Calcium	263 mg
Iron	1 mg

Tofu and Chickpea Garlic Dip

Makes 6 to 8 servings

Nutrients per serving
(1 of 8)

Calories	91
Fat	4 g
Saturated Fat	1 g
Cholesterol	0 mg
Sodium	212 mg
Carbohydrate	10 g
Fiber	2 g
Sugars	1 g
Protein	4 g
Calcium	31 mg
Iron	1 mg

- Food processor

1 cup	rinsed drained canned chickpeas	250 mL
8 oz	silken tofu, drained	250 g
2 tbsp	tahini	30 mL
2 tbsp	freshly squeezed lemon juice	30 mL
1 tsp	minced garlic	5 mL
1/4 cup	chopped fresh dill (or 1 tsp/5 mL dried dillweed)	60 mL
1/4 cup	chopped green onions	60 mL
1/4 cup	chopped green olives	60 mL
1/4 cup	chopped red bell pepper	60 mL
1/4 tsp	freshly ground black pepper	1 mL

1. In food processor, combine chickpeas, tofu, tahini, lemon juice and garlic; purée. Stir in dill, green onions, olives, red pepper and pepper.

2. Chill. Serve with vegetables, crackers or bread.

Garlic Cheese

Makes 4 to 6 servings

Serve with fresh bread or crackers.

Nutrients per serving
(1 of 6)

Calories	136
Fat	13 g
Saturated Fat	7 g
Cholesterol	42 mg
Sodium	122 mg
Carbohydrate	3 g
Fiber	0 g
Sugars	2 g
Protein	2 g
Calcium	43 mg
Iron	0 mg

8 oz	farmer's cheese or cream cheese, softened	250 g
3	cloves garlic, minced	3
1 tbsp	minced lemon zest, bruised	15 mL
1 tsp	granulated sugar	5 mL
1 tsp	coarsely ground black pepper	5 mL
1 tsp	wine vinegar	5 mL

1. In a bowl, combine cheese, garlic, lemon zest, sugar, pepper and vinegar.

2. Transfer to a small plate and shape into a dome.

3. Store in an airtight container in the refrigerator for up to 3 days.

Quick Zucchini and Jerusalem Artichoke on Grilled Crostini

Makes 30 crostini

This quick sauté of vegetables is perfect served on top of crisp crostini, creating a bruschetta-like appetizer.

Tips

Jerusalem artichokes, also known as sunchokes, resemble gingerroot and are sweetest when they are 2 to 3 inches (5 to 7.5 cm) wide by 3 to 4 inches (7.5 to 10 cm) long. They can be peeled using a regular vegetable peeler.

To create Parmesan curls, gently press a vegetable peeler against the cheese and push the peeler away from your body in one long motion.

Nutrients per crostini	
Calories	119
Fat	2 g
Saturated Fat	1 g
Cholesterol	2 mg
Sodium	323 mg
Carbohydrate	20 g
Fiber	1 g
Sugars	1 g
Protein	4 g
Calcium	11 mg
Iron	1 mg

- Preheat oven to 350°F (180°C)
- Ovenproof skillet

1 tbsp	olive oil	15 mL
1/2 cup	diced Jerusalem artichokes (see tip, at left)	125 mL
1 1/4 cups	diced zucchini	300 mL
1/2 cup	minced red onion	125 mL
1 cup	finely chopped roasted red bell peppers (see box, page 225)	250 mL
1/2 cup	sliced cherry tomatoes	125 mL
1 tbsp	thinly sliced garlic	15 mL
1/2 tsp	finely chopped fresh thyme leaves	2 mL
1/2 tsp	finely chopped fresh basil leaves	2 mL
1 tsp	salt	5 mL
1/2 tsp	freshly ground black pepper	2 mL
30	Grilled Herbed Crostini (see recipe, opposite)	30
1/4 cup	Parmesan curls (see tip, at left)	60 mL

1. In ovenproof skillet, heat oil over high heat. Add artichokes and toss to coat. Transfer skillet to a preheated oven and roast until golden brown, about 10 minutes. Add zucchini and red onion and roast in preheated oven until zucchini is tender-crisp, 15 to 20 minutes.

2. Add roasted peppers, tomatoes, garlic, thyme, basil, salt and pepper and toss to combine. Place about 1 tbsp (15 mL) on each crostini and garnish with Parmesan cheese. Serve immediately.

Grilled Herbed Crostini

Makes 24 crostini

Nutrients per crostini

Calories	104
Fat	2 g
Saturated Fat	0 g
Cholesterol	1 mg
Sodium	234 mg
Carbohydrate	19 g
Fiber	1 g
Sugars	0 g
Protein	4 g
Calcium	1 mg
Iron	1 mg

• Preheat barbecue grill to high

24	slices baguette (each about $^1/_2$ inch/1 cm thick)	24
2 tbsp	extra virgin olive oil	30 mL
1 tbsp	unsalted butter, melted	15 mL
$^1/_2$ tsp	freshly ground black pepper	2 mL
$^1/_4$ tsp	salt	1 mL
1 tbsp	finely chopped fresh thyme leaves	15 mL

1. In a bowl, combine bread, olive oil, butter, pepper and salt and toss well to coat. Grill until golden brown, about 1 minute per side. Remove from heat and toss with fresh thyme. Serve immediately.

Roasted Garlic Sour Cream Dip

Makes about 1$^1/_2$ cups (375 mL)

It's amazing how sweet garlic can become when roasted. Delicious and gut-friendly!

Nutrients per $^1/_4$ cup (60 mL)

Calories	105
Fat	8 g
Saturated Fat	3 g
Cholesterol	15 mg
Sodium	119 mg
Carbohydrate	5 g
Fiber	0 g
Sugars	2 g
Protein	2 g
Calcium	65 mg
Iron	0 mg

• Preheat oven to 400°F (200°C)

2	bulbs garlic	2
2 tbsp	extra virgin olive oil	30 mL
$^1/_4$ tsp	salt	1 mL
$^1/_2$ cup	plain yogurt	125 mL
$^1/_2$ cup	sour cream	125 mL
1 tsp	finely chopped fresh chives	5 mL

1. Cut whole garlic bulbs in half along their "equator" and thoroughly coat with olive oil. Combine the two halves and wrap in foil. Roast in preheated oven until bulbs are soft, about 1 hour. Let cool to room temperature. Squeeze garlic out of skins into a bowl to release caramelized cloves. Sprinkle with salt.

2. In a bowl, combine $^1/_2$ cup (125 mL) roasted garlic, yogurt, sour cream and chives. Cover and refrigerate overnight to allow flavors to meld or for up to 3 days.

Cream of Leek and Asparagus on Toast Points

When spring brings wild leeks (ramps) and fresh asparagus, this is one way to combine their fresh tastes. Serve this easy dish as a starter for a light lunch.

Tip

In place of the wild leeks, you can use 1 cup (250 mL) sliced leeks (white and light green parts only).

3 tbsp	olive oil, divided	45 mL
1	bunch wild leeks (about 20), white part and green leaves, sliced	1
2 tbsp	all-purpose flour	30 mL
2 cups	rice milk or soy milk	500 mL
1 lb	fresh asparagus, trimmed and cut into 1-inch (2.5 cm) pieces	500 g
4	slices whole wheat bread, toasted	4
4	wild leek leaves (optional)	4

1. In a saucepan, heat 2 tbsp (30 mL) oil over medium heat. Add leeks and cook, stirring occasionally, for 6 to 8 minutes or until soft. Using a slotted spoon, lift out leeks and set aside.

2. Add the remaining oil to saucepan and stir in flour. Cook, stirring constantly, for 1 minute. Whisk in rice milk and cook, stirring constantly, for 4 minutes or until sauce thickens. Add leeks and asparagus and cook, stirring frequently, for 5 minutes or until asparagus is tender-crisp.

3. Cut each slice of toast into 4 wedges and arrange on plates. Spoon creamed vegetables over toast points and garnish with leek leaves (if using).

Nutrients per serving	
Calories	320
Fat	13 g
Saturated Fat	2 g
Cholesterol	0 mg
Sodium	204 mg
Carbohydrate	46 g
Fiber	7 g
Sugars	14 g
Protein	9 g
Calcium	274 mg
Iron	6 mg

French Lentil Dip with Herbed Crostini

Makes 8 to 10 servings

With a little advance preparation, you can throw this together after work for a quick and easy weeknight get-together. Making the dip in the morning before work gives the flavors time to blend.

Tips

The average 1-lb (500 g) baguette will yield forty to forty-five $\frac{1}{2}$-inch (1 cm) slices.

Crostini can be prepared up to a week in advance. Store in a paper bag at room temperature and crisp on a baking sheet in a 350°F (180°C) oven for 3 to 4 minutes before serving.

Nutrients per serving (1 of 10)	
Calories	287
Fat	8 g
Saturated Fat	1 g
Cholesterol	0 mg
Sodium	535 mg
Carbohydrate	43 g
Fiber	4 g
Sugars	0 g
Protein	12 g
Calcium	15 mg
Iron	3 mg

• Food processor

French Lentil Dip

1 cup	dried French (Puy) lentils, picked through and rinsed	250 mL
1	small onion, finely chopped	1
1	bay leaf	1
2 cups	water	500 mL
1 tbsp	freshly squeezed lemon juice	15 mL
3 tbsp	olive oil, divided	45 mL
1 tbsp	chopped fresh tarragon	15 mL
$\frac{1}{2}$ tsp	fleur de sel or other sea salt	2 mL
$\frac{1}{2}$ tsp	freshly ground black pepper	2 mL
2 tbsp	chopped drained capers	30 mL
2 tbsp	toasted pine nuts	30 mL

Herbed Crostini

1 lb	rustic baguette loaf, sliced into $\frac{1}{2}$-inch (1 cm) pieces (see tip, at left)	500 g
2 tbsp	olive oil	30 mL
2 tsp	dried herbes de Provence, crushed	10 mL

1. *Dip:* In a saucepan, combine lentils, onion and bay leaf and cover with water. Bring to a boil over medium-high heat. Reduce heat and gently simmer until lentils are just tender, 15 to 20 minutes. Let cool. Drain lentils, reserving cooking liquid. Discard bay leaf.

2. In food processor, combine lentils, lemon juice, 2 tbsp (30 mL) oil, tarragon and salt and pulse until rough and creamy but not yet smooth, adding a little reserved cooking liquid if necessary. Taste and adjust seasoning with salt and pepper, if needed, and pulse to combine. If making ahead, cover and refrigerate for up to 5 days. When ready to serve, bring dip to room temperature, transfer to a serving bowl, drizzle with 1 tbsp (15 mL) oil and garnish with capers and pine nuts.

3. Preheat oven to 350°F (180°C).

4. *Crostini:* Arrange baguette slices on a baking sheet. Brush each on both sides lightly with oil and sprinkle with a pinch of herbes de Provence. Bake in preheated oven, turning once, until lightly toasted, 4 to 6 minutes per side (watch closely, as crostini can quickly burn).

5. Place bowl of lentil dip in the center of a large platter and surround with herbed crostini.

Caramelized Onion Dip

**Makes about
1½ cups (375 mL)**

*This dip is one of life's
guilty pleasures. It always
disappears to the very
last drop. Serve with a
nutritious accompaniment
such as spears of Belgian
endive or celery sticks, to
balance the creamy dairy
and complement the range
of nutrients it provides.*

- Small (about 2-quart) slow cooker
- Food processor

2	onions, thinly sliced on the vertical	2
4	cloves garlic, chopped	4
1 tbsp	melted butter	15 mL
4 oz	Neufchâtel cheese, cubed and softened	125 g
½ cup	sour cream	125 mL
1 tbsp	brown rice miso	15 mL
	Sea salt and freshly ground black pepper	
	Finely snipped chives	

1. In slow cooker stoneware, combine onions, garlic and butter. Toss well to ensure onions are thoroughly coated. Place a clean tea towel folded in half (so you will have two layers) over top of stoneware to absorb moisture. Cover and cook on High for 5 hours, stirring two or three times to ensure onions are browning evenly, replacing towel each time, until onions are nicely caramelized.

2. Transfer mixture to food processor. Add cheese, sour cream, miso, and salt and pepper to taste. Process until well blended. Transfer to a serving dish and garnish with chives. Serve immediately.

Variation

For a more herbal flavor, add 2 tbsp (30 mL) fresh thyme leaves along with the Neufchâtel cheese.

Nutrients per ¼ cup (60 mL)	
Calories	110
Fat	8 g
Saturated Fat	5 g
Cholesterol	27 mg
Sodium	204 mg
Carbohydrate	5 g
Fiber	1 g
Sugars	3 g
Protein	3 g
Calcium	84 mg
Iron	0 mg

Smoky Eggplant Dip with Yogurt

Makes about 2¹⁄₂ cups (625 mL)

This dip is delicious with raw vegetables or on pita triangles or crusty French bread. For the most flavor, use a smoker or grill the eggplant on a charcoal barbecue. If you're using a gas barbecue, place dampened wood chips in a smoke box, following the manufacturer's instructions.

Tips

If you are using a smoker, the eggplant will cook in about 1¹⁄₄ hours at 200°F (100°C). The skin will not blister as it will on a barbecue.

Make an effort to get Greek yogurt. It is lusciously thick and adds beautiful depth to this and many other dishes.

- Preheat gas or charcoal barbecue to high
- Food processor

1	eggplant (about 1 lb/500 g)	1
¹⁄₃ cup	full-fat plain yogurt (preferably Greek)	75 mL
6	cherry tomatoes	6
1	green onion, cut into chunks	1
1	clove garlic, coarsely chopped	1
1 tsp	freshly squeezed lemon juice	5 mL
¹⁄₂ tsp	salt	2 mL
	Freshly ground black pepper	
1 tbsp	finely chopped dill fronds	15 mL
	Finely chopped black olives (optional)	

1. Prick eggplant in several places with a fork. Place eggplant on preheated grill. Cook, turning several times, until skin is blackened and blistered, about 30 minutes. Set aside until cool enough to handle.

2. Scoop out eggplant flesh and place in food processor. Discard skin and stem. Add yogurt, tomatoes, green onion, garlic, lemon juice, salt, and pepper to taste. Process until smooth.

3. Transfer to a serving bowl and cover and refrigerate for at least 3 hours, until thoroughly chilled, or for up to 2 days. To serve, garnish with dill and olives (if using).

Nutrients per ¹⁄₄ cup (60 mL)	
Calories	18
Fat	0 g
Saturated Fat	0 g
Cholesterol	1 mg
Sodium	122 mg
Carbohydrate	4 g
Fiber	2 g
Sugars	2 g
Protein	1 g
Calcium	16 mg
Iron	0 mg

Cheesy Avocado Dip

Makes about 3 cups (750 mL)

If you're looking for an avocado-based dip that differs from guacamole, the addition of feta cheese, parsley and dill turns this relative into a deliciously different treat. Serve it on warm pita bread or, if you don't want to stray too far from the original, with tostadas or tortilla chips.

- Food processor

1 cup	cherry or grape tomatoes	250 mL
4	green onions (white parts with a bit of green), cut into chunks	4
1/4 cup	fresh flat-leaf (Italian) parsley leaves	60 mL
1/4 cup	fresh dill fronds	60 mL
1	clove garlic	1
2	avocados, cut into chunks	2
4 oz	feta cheese	125 g
1 tbsp	freshly squeezed lemon juice	15 mL
	Salt and freshly ground black pepper	

1. In food processor, pulse tomatoes, green onions, parsley, dill and garlic until chopped, about 10 times. Add avocados, feta and lemon juice and process until smooth, about 30 seconds. Season to taste with salt and pepper.

2. Transfer to a serving bowl. Serve immediately or cover with plastic wrap, pressing down onto surface of dip, and refrigerate for up to 4 hours.

Nutrients per 1/4 cup (60 mL)

Calories	83
Fat	7 g
Saturated Fat	2 g
Cholesterol	8 mg
Sodium	110 mg
Carbohydrate	4 g
Fiber	2 g
Sugars	1 g
Protein	2 g
Calcium	56 mg
Iron	0 mg

Artichoke Salsa

Makes about 1½ cups (375 mL)

This yummy salsa offers another easy way to be kind to your gut!

Nutrients per ¼ cup (60 mL)	
Calories	68
Fat	7 g
Saturated Fat	0 g
Cholesterol	0 mg
Sodium	68 mg
Carbohydrate	3 g
Fiber	1 g
Sugars	0 g
Protein	1 g
Calcium	2 mg
Iron	0 mg

- Food processor

1	jar (6 oz/170 mL) marinated artichoke hearts, drained	1
1	small clove garlic	1
⅓ cup	pine nuts	75 mL
	Juice of ½ large lemon	

1. In food processor, combine artichokes, garlic, pine nuts and lemon juice; process until finely chopped.

Gazpacho Salsa

Makes about 3 cups (750 mL)

Inulin, a type of fructo-oligosaccaride, is naturally found in tomatoes.

Nutrients per ¼ cup (60 mL)	
Calories	27
Fat	2 g
Saturated Fat	0 g
Cholesterol	0 mg
Sodium	4 mg
Carbohydrate	1 g
Fiber	0 g
Sugars	1 g
Protein	0 g
Calcium	4 mg
Iron	0 mg

- Food processor

2	large tomatoes, quartered	2
1	small clove garlic	1
¼	small cucumber, peeled and cut into chunks	¼
¼	jalapeño pepper, halved and seeded	¼
1 tbsp	chopped onion	15 mL
2 tbsp	extra virgin olive oil	30 mL
1 tbsp	red wine vinegar	15 mL

1. In food processor, combine tomatoes, garlic, cucumber, jalapeño, onion, olive oil and vinegar; process until finely chopped.

2. Store in an airtight container in the refrigerator for up to 2 days.

Asparagus Salsa

Asparagus is key to gut health! Enjoy this salsa as an appetizer or a snack.

Tips

When blanching green vegetables, salt is very useful for adding flavor. It is also quite instrumental in bringing the vibrant green color out long before the vegetable is overcooked. For maximum effect, use 1 tbsp (15 mL) salt for every 6 cups (1.5 L) water.

To grill corn, preheat barbecue grill to high. Grill ears of corn, husks on, rotating often until dark brown all over, about 20 minutes. Transfer to a plate and let cool for 5 minutes or until cool enough to handle. Remove husk and silks and, using a serrated knife, cut kernels from cob.

1¹/₄ cups	finely chopped asparagus	300 mL
	Ice water	
¹/₃ cup	finely diced cherry tomatoes	75 mL
¹/₃ cup	grilled corn kernels (see tip, at left)	75 mL
2 tbsp	minced red onion	30 mL
1 tbsp	coarsely chopped dried cranberries	15 mL
1 tbsp	coarsely chopped toasted almonds	15 mL
1 tsp	malt vinegar	5 mL
1 tsp	extra virgin olive oil	5 mL
¹/₂ tsp	chopped fresh basil leaves	2 mL
¹/₄ tsp	salt	1 mL
¹/₄ tsp	freshly ground black pepper	1 mL
¹/₈ tsp	hot pepper flakes	0.5 mL

1. In a pot of boiling salted water, blanch asparagus until vibrant green and al dente, about 2 minutes. Drain and immediately plunge into a bowl of ice water to stop the cooking process. Let stand until well chilled. Drain well.

2. In a bowl, combine asparagus, tomatoes, corn, red onion, cranberries, almonds, vinegar, olive oil, basil, salt, pepper and hot pepper flakes. Let stand at room temperature for at least 1 hour to allow flavors to meld, or cover and refrigerate for up to 8 hours before serving.

Nutrients per ¹/₄ cup (60 mL)	
Calories	33
Fat	2 g
Saturated Fat	0 g
Cholesterol	0 mg
Sodium	99 mg
Carbohydrate	5 g
Fiber	1 g
Sugars	2 g
Protein	1 g
Calcium	12 mg
Iron	1 mg

Tomato Garlic Raita

Makes about 1½ cups (375 mL)

Gently spiced and tomato-tart, this yogurt sauce makes a pleasant side sauce and also works well as a dip for chips or raw vegetables.

Tip

Use full-fat Greek-style or Balkan-style yogurt for the best texture. To use a lower-fat yogurt, place about 1½ cups (375 mL) into a sieve lined with a coffee filter or cheesecloth and placed over a bowl. Refrigerate and let drain until thickened but not dry, about 4 hours.

1 cup	thick plain yogurt (see tip, at left)	250 mL
¼ tsp	salt	1 mL
1 cup	finely diced seeded tomato	250 mL
1 tbsp	vegetable oil	15 mL
¼ tsp	cumin seeds	1 mL
2 tbsp	minced garlic	30 mL
	Chopped fresh cilantro	

1. In a bowl, stir together yogurt and salt until smooth and blended. Fold in tomato until well mixed. Set aside.

2. In a small skillet, heat oil over medium heat until hot but not smoking. Add cumin seeds and cook, stirring, until the seeds start to pop, about 1 minute. Add garlic and cook, stirring, just until garlic is fragrant, about 30 seconds. Remove from heat and stir gently into the yogurt mixture. Transfer to a serving bowl, if desired, and sprinkle with cilantro. Serve at room temperature.

Nutrients per ¼ cup (60 mL)

Calories	67
Fat	4 g
Saturated Fat	1 g
Cholesterol	2 mg
Sodium	127 mg
Carbohydrate	5 g
Fiber	0 g
Sugars	4 g
Protein	2 g
Calcium	79 mg
Iron	0 mg

Hummus with Roasted Red Peppers

**Makes about
1¼ cups (300 mL)**

*This versatile spread has
many applications. Serve
it as an appetizer with
sliced vegetables, as a dip
for crackers or in a pita.*

Tips

If you're using a 19-oz
(540 mL) can of beans,
you may want to adjust
the seasoning by adding a
pinch of cumin and salt.

You can use bottled roasted
red bell peppers in this
hummus or roast your own
(see box, page 225).

Store, tightly covered, in
the refrigerator for 3 or
4 days.

- Food processor or blender

1	can (14 to 19 oz/398 to 540 mL) chickpeas, drained and rinsed	1
¼ cup	tahini	60 mL
¼ cup	freshly squeezed lemon juice	60 mL
2	cloves garlic, minced	2
½	roasted red bell pepper, thinly sliced (see tip, at left)	½
1 tsp	ground cumin	5 mL
¼ tsp	salt (or to taste)	1 mL
	Water (optional)	

1. In food processor, combine chickpeas, tahini, lemon juice and garlic; process until smooth.

2. Add roasted pepper, ground cumin and salt and process until smooth. If you prefer a creamier consistency, add water, 1 tbsp (15 mL) at a time, processing until the desired texture is achieved.

3. Transfer to an airtight container and refrigerate for at least 2 hours or overnight.

Variations

Hummus with Black Olives: Substitute ½ cup
(125 mL) chopped pitted kalamata olives for the
roasted pepper.

Lemony Hummus: Substitute 1 tbsp (15 mL) grated
lemon zest for the roasted pepper.

Nutrients per ¼ cup (60 mL)	
Calories	146
Fat	6 g
Saturated Fat	1 g
Cholesterol	0 mg
Sodium	300 mg
Carbohydrate	19 g
Fiber	4 g
Sugars	1 g
Protein	5 g
Calcium	41 mg
Iron	2 mg

Artichoke and White Bean Spread

**Makes about
3 cups (750 mL)**

*The flavor combination
in this spread — onion,
garlic, cannellini beans,
artichokes, Parmesan
and parsley — is simple,
elegant and synergistically
delicious. Serve on
crackers or crudités.*

Tips

For this quantity of beans,
soak, cook and drain 1 cup
(250 mL) dried cannellini
beans, or drain and rinse
1 can (14 to 19 oz/398 to
540 mL) no-salt-added
cannellini beans.

If you prefer, use frozen
artichokes, thawed, to
make this recipe. You will
need 6 artichoke hearts.

- Small (about 2-quart) slow cooker
- Food processor

1/2	red onion, finely chopped	1/2
2	cloves garlic, minced	2
1/4 cup	extra virgin olive oil, divided	60 mL
2 cups	cooked cannellini (white kidney) beans (see tip, at left)	500 mL
1	can (14 oz/398 mL) artichoke hearts, drained and coarsely chopped (see tip, at left)	1
1/2 cup	freshly grated Parmesan cheese or vegan alternative	125 mL
1 tsp	sweet paprika	5 mL
1/2 tsp	sea salt	2 mL
1/4 tsp	freshly ground black pepper	1 mL
1/2 cup	finely chopped fresh parsley leaves	125 mL

1. In slow cooker stoneware, combine onion, garlic and 2 tbsp (30 mL) oil. Place a clean tea towel folded in half (so you will have two layers) over top of stoneware to absorb moisture. Cover and cook on High for 30 minutes, until onion is softened.

2. Meanwhile, in food processor, in batches if necessary, pulse beans and artichokes until desired consistency is achieved. After onions have softened, add bean mixture to stoneware along with Parmesan, paprika, salt, pepper and the remaining oil. Replace tea towel. Cover and cook on Low for 4 hours or on High for 2 hours, until hot and bubbly. Add parsley and stir well.

Nutrients per 1/4 cup (60 mL)	
Calories	113
Fat	6 g
Saturated Fat	1 g
Cholesterol	3 mg
Sodium	170 mg
Carbohydrate	12 g
Fiber	5 g
Sugars	1 g
Protein	5 g
Calcium	60 mg
Iron	1 mg

Refried Pumpkin

Makes 4 servings

Spread this sweet and savory dip on any whole wheat bread, crackers or pitas.

- Food processor

2 tbsp	vegetable oil, divided	30 mL
3	garlic cloves	3
1/2 cup	fresh bread cubes	125 mL
1/3 cup	green pumpkin seeds (pepitas)	75 mL
1	jalapeño pepper, minced	1
1/3 cup	finely chopped onion	75 mL
1/2 tsp	ground cumin	2 mL
1/2 tsp	ground cinnamon	2 mL
2 tbsp	packed light brown sugar	30 mL
1 tbsp	red wine vinegar	15 mL
1	can (28 oz/796 mL) pumpkin purée (not pie filling)	1
	Salt and freshly ground black pepper	

1. In a large skillet, heat half the oil over medium-high heat. Sauté garlic, bread cubes and pumpkin seeds until toasted. Add jalapeño, onion, cumin and cinnamon; sauté for 30 seconds.

2. Transfer to food processor, add brown sugar and vinegar, and process to a paste.

3. Wipe out skillet and heat the remaining oil over medium-high heat. Add spice paste, pumpkin purée, and salt and pepper to taste; cook, stirring occasionally, until mixture bubbles vigorously and starts to brown at the edges.

Nutrients per serving	
Calories	240
Fat	13 g
Saturated Fat	2 g
Cholesterol	0 mg
Sodium	37 mg
Carbohydrate	29 g
Fiber	7 g
Sugars	14 g
Protein	6 g
Calcium	82 mg
Iron	4 mg

Soups

Vegetable Stock 212

Jerusalem Artichoke Soup 214

Cauliflower and Cheese Soup 215

Garlic Soup 216

Classic French Onion Soup 217

Roasted Tomato and Pesto Soup 218

Roasted Summer Vegetable Soup 219

Turkish-Style Barley Soup 220

Mushroom Barley Soup with Miso 221

Lentil Soup Italian-Style 222

Black Bean Coconut Soup 223

Chilled Curried Banana Coconut Soup 224

Chilled Yogurt Soup with Roasted Red Pepper
    and Pesto Swirls 225

Chilled Fruited Gazpacho 226

Vegetable Stock

The backbone of whole, fresh cooking is often a good vegetable stock. One way to ensure a supply of vegetables for the stockpot is to freeze trimmings — the tougher asparagus or broccoli stalks, peelings and leafy tops of celery — and drop them directly into the simmering stock. Similarly, freezing homemade stock makes it easy to thaw and use in recipes.

Tip

Roasting the onion, garlic and leek lends a more complex taste and rich color to the stock. If time does not permit roasting, simply sauté them with oil in the stockpot first, then add all the other items. Or, for an extremely easy and fat-free stock, omit the oil and toss all the ingredients into the pot, simmer for 1 hour and strain.

Nutrients per ½ cup (125 mL)	
Calories	39
Fat	2 g
Saturated Fat	0 g
Cholesterol	0 mg
Sodium	17 mg
Carbohydrate	6 g
Fiber	1 g
Sugars	2 g
Protein	1 g
Calcium	30 mg
Iron	0 mg

- Preheat oven to 400°F (200°C)
- Baking sheet
- Large stockpot

1	onion, peeled and quartered	1
4	cloves garlic, peeled	4
1	leek, trimmed and cut into large chunks	1
2 tbsp	olive oil	30 mL
8 cups	water	2 L
½	green cabbage, quartered	½
1 cup	coarsely chopped broccoli or asparagus stems (optional)	250 mL
1	stalk celery, cut into chunks	1
1	carrot, cut into chunks	1
1	apple, cut into chunks	1
1	whole dried cayenne pepper	1
6	sprigs fresh parsley	6
5	allspice berries	5
5	whole cloves	5
5	whole black peppercorns	5
1	bay leaf	1
	A few sprigs fresh thyme and sage	
3	dried astragalus root wafers	3
1	1-inch (2.5 cm) piece gingerroot	1
1	1-inch (2.5 cm) piece burdock root	1
1	1-inch (2.5 cm) piece dandelion root	1

1. On baking sheet, toss onion, garlic and leek with olive oil. Roast in preheated oven, stirring once, for 30 to 40 minutes or until vegetables are soft and brown (some edges may be charred).

Tips

Be sure to include the asparagus, burdock root and dandelion root for their prebiotic benefits.

Other vegetables to use: parsnips, mushrooms, rutabaga, fennel bulb, zucchini, tomatoes, kale, bok choy and Swiss chard.

Store stock in clean jars with lids in the refrigerator for up to 2 days, or freeze in 2- or 4-cup (500 mL or 1 L) portions in freezer containers for up to 2 months.

2. In stockpot, bring water to a boil over high heat. Add cabbage, broccoli (if using), celery, carrot, apple, cayenne, parsley, allspice, cloves, peppercorns, bay leaf, thyme, sage, astragalus, ginger, burdock, dandelion root and roasted vegetables. Cover, reduce heat and simmer for 1 hour. Remove from heat and let cool slightly. Strain off and discard solids. Let stock cool completely and store.

Double-Strength Stock

For the enhanced flavor requirements of sauces (as opposed to soups), prepare a concentrated version of stock by boiling it down to reduce its volume by half.

Jerusalem Artichoke Soup

Makes 4 servings

Jerusalem artichokes, or sunchokes, are a delicious root vegetable native to North America. Because of their rich artichoke-like flavor, they need few additions to make a wonderful soup. They pair naturally with butter and cream. This soup is well worth the trouble of peeling the gnarled roots.

Tips

You can also serve the soup chilled: just replace the butter with an equal amount of olive oil. Add lemon juice to blender. Refrigerate puréed soup until chilled and stir in chilled cream just before serving.

Garnish with chopped chives or chopped fresh parsley, if desired.

Using reduced-sodium broth will lower the sodium content of each serving to 347 mg.

Nutrients per serving	
Calories	265
Fat	18 g
Saturated Fat	11 g
Cholesterol	61 mg
Sodium	1081 mg
Carbohydrate	24 g
Fiber	2 g
Sugars	13 g
Protein	4 g
Calcium	44 mg
Iron	4 mg

- **Blender**

2 tbsp	butter	30 mL
1	white onion, chopped	1
1 lb	Jerusalem artichokes, peeled and sliced	500 g
2 cups	ready-to-use chicken broth	500 mL
1 cup	water	250 mL
1/2 tsp	salt	2 mL
1/4 tsp	freshly ground black pepper	1 mL
Pinch	ground mace or nutmeg	Pinch
2 tsp	freshly squeezed lemon juice	10 mL
1/2 cup	heavy or whipping (35%) cream	125 mL

1. In a large saucepan, melt butter over medium-high heat. Add onion and cook, stirring, for 3 to 4 minutes or until soft. Add Jerusalem artichokes and cook, stirring, until very lightly browned, about 2 minutes. Add broth, water, salt, pepper and mace; bring to a boil. Cover, reduce heat to low and simmer until artichokes are very tender, about 30 minutes.

2. Transfer to blender in batches and purée on high speed.

3. Return purée to saucepan, add lemon juice and bring back to a simmer over medium heat. Add cream and simmer until heated through. Ladle into bowls.

Cauliflower and Cheese Soup

Cauliflower and cheese are a match made in heaven.

Tips

If you have homemade Vegetable Stock (page 212) on hand, use it in this recipe in place of store-bought broth.

Using reduced-sodium broth will lower the sodium content of each serving to 170 mg.

• Blender

1	head cauliflower, coarsely chopped	1
1	white onion, quartered	1
²/₃ cup	cubed Gruyère, aged Gouda or extra-sharp (extra-old) Cheddar cheese	150 mL
2 tbsp	butter	30 mL
¼ cup	heavy or whipping (35%) cream or sour cream	60 mL
Pinch	ground nutmeg	Pinch
Pinch	cayenne pepper	Pinch
Pinch	freshly ground white pepper	Pinch
2½ cups	ready-to-use chicken or vegetable broth	625 mL
2 tbsp	chopped fresh chives or parsley	30 mL

1. In a large saucepan of boiling salted water, cook cauliflower and onion until very tender, about 10 minutes. Drain, reserving ½ cup (125 mL) cooking water.

2. Transfer cauliflower, onion and reserved cooking water to blender and add Gruyère, butter, cream, nutmeg, cayenne and white pepper. Purée on high speed.

3. Return purée to saucepan, stir in broth and bring to a boil over medium-high heat. Reduce heat and simmer, stirring, for 2 minutes.

4. Ladle into bowls and garnish with chives.

Nutrients per serving	
Calories	263
Fat	20 g
Saturated Fat	11 g
Cholesterol	66 mg
Sodium	1088 mg
Carbohydrate	11 g
Fiber	3 g
Sugars	5 g
Protein	11 g
Calcium	272 mg
Iron	1 mg

Garlic Soup

Makes 4 to 6 servings

Garlic has been used as food and medicine in various cultures for thousands of years.

Tips

If you prefer a less peppery soup, halve the amount of black pepper.

Serve this soup with freshly baked croutons. To bake croutons, toss together 1¼ cups (300 mL) cubed fresh bread, 1 tbsp (15 ml) melted butter or extra virgin olive oil, and a generous pinch each of salt and pepper. Spread on a baking sheet and toast in a 400°F (200°C) oven or toaster oven for 8 to 10 minutes or until crisp and golden.

Using reduced-sodium broth will lower the sodium content of each serving to 420 mg.

Nutrients per serving (1 of 6)	
Calories	95
Fat	5 g
Saturated Fat	1 g
Cholesterol	3 mg
Sodium	909 mg
Carbohydrate	10 g
Fiber	1 g
Sugars	2 g
Protein	2 g
Calcium	26 mg
Iron	1 mg

- Blender

2 tbsp	extra virgin olive oil or butter	30 mL
16	cloves garlic (about 2 large heads)	16
1	white onion, chopped	1
½ tsp	freshly ground black pepper	2 mL
1	potato, peeled and diced	1
2 cups	ready-to-use chicken broth	500 mL
2 cups	water	500 mL
1 tsp	salt	5 mL
¼ cup	chopped fresh parsley	60 mL

1. In a large saucepan, heat oil over medium heat. Add garlic, onion and pepper; cook, stirring often, until onion is soft and garlic is lightly browned, about 6 minutes. Add potato, broth, water and salt; bring to a boil. Cover, reduce heat to low and simmer until potato is soft, about 20 minutes.

2. Transfer to blender in batches and purée on high speed.

3. Return purée to saucepan and simmer until heated through. Stir in parsley. Ladle into bowls.

Classic French Onion Soup

Makes 6 servings

On a chilly day, there's nothing more appetizing than a bowl of steaming onion soup, bubbling away under a blanket of browned cheese.

Tips

If you are pressed for time, skip step 1 and soften the onions on the stovetop. Heat the butter in a large skillet over medium heat. Add the onions and cook, stirring, until they soften, about 10 minutes. Transfer to stoneware and continue with step 2.

To make ahead, complete steps 1 and 2. Cover and refrigerate onions for up to 2 days. When you're ready to cook, complete the recipe, adding 1 hour to the cooking time in step 3.

Using reduced-sodium broth will lower the sodium content of each serving to 1069 mg.

Nutrients per serving	
Calories	433
Fat	14 g
Saturated Fat	9 g
Cholesterol	43 mg
Sodium	2135 mg
Carbohydrate	57 g
Fiber	4 g
Sugars	10 g
Protein	19 g
Calcium	315 mg
Iron	3 mg

* Medium to large (3½- to 5-quart) slow cooker
* 6 ovenproof soup bowls

10	onions, thinly sliced on the vertical	10
2 tbsp	melted butter	30 mL
1 tbsp	granulated sugar	15 mL
8 cups	enhanced ready-to-use vegetable broth (see box, below)	2 L
2 tbsp	brandy or cognac	30 mL
1 tsp	salt	5 mL
1 tsp	cracked black peppercorns	5 mL
12	slices baguette, about ½ inch (1 cm) thick	12
2 cups	shredded Swiss or Gruyère cheese	500 mL

1. In slow cooker stoneware, combine onions and butter. Toss well to ensure onions are thoroughly coated. Cover and cook on High for 1 hour, until onions are softened.

2. Add sugar and stir well. Place a clean tea towel, folded in half (so you will have two layers), over top of stoneware to absorb moisture. Cover and cook on High for 4 hours, stirring two or three times to ensure that onions are browning evenly, replacing towel each time.

3. Add broth, brandy, salt and peppercorns and stir well. Remove towel, cover and cook on High for 2 hours.

4. Preheat broiler. Ladle soup into ovenproof bowls. Place 2 baguette slices in each bowl. Sprinkle liberally with cheese and broil until top is bubbly and brown, 2 to 3 minutes. Serve immediately.

Enhanced Broth

To enhance 8 cups (2 L) ready-to-use vegetable broth, add it to a large saucepan over medium heat with 2 carrots, peeled and coarsely chopped, 1 tbsp (15 mL) tomato paste, 1 tsp (5 mL) celery seed, 1 tsp (5 mL) cracked black peppercorns, ½ tsp (2 mL) dried thyme, 4 parsley sprigs, 1 bay leaf and 1 cup (250 mL) white wine. Bring to a boil. Reduce heat to low and simmer, covered, for 30 minutes, then strain and discard solids.

Roasted Tomato and Pesto Soup

You'll be surprised at the difference roasting the cherry tomatoes makes. This easy step gives the soup a slightly sweet, deep tomato flavor that still manages to retain all of its freshness.

Tips

If you're using a blender or food processor to purée hot soup, make sure not to fill the container more than one-third full. The buildup of pressure from the steam can sometimes blow the cover off, sending hot liquid flying.

If you're watching your sodium intake, use a reduced-sodium broth. This will lower the sodium content of each serving to 745 mg.

- Preheat oven to 400°F (200°C)
- Rimmed baking sheet
- Immersion blender, food processor or blender

6 cups	cherry tomatoes	1.5 L
3 tbsp	olive oil, divided	45 mL
1 tsp	salt	5 mL
½ tsp	freshly ground black pepper	2 mL
2 tbsp	unsalted butter	30 mL
6	cloves garlic, minced	6
1 cup	chopped onion	250 mL
¼ tsp	hot pepper flakes	1 mL
1	can (28 oz/796 mL) diced tomatoes, with juice	1
4 cups	ready-to-use chicken broth	1 L
½ tsp	dried thyme	2 mL
	Pesto	

1. On baking sheet, combine cherry tomatoes, 2 tbsp (30 mL) oil, salt and black pepper; toss to coat evenly and spread in a single layer. Roast in preheated oven until tomatoes are shriveled and have brown spots, 35 to 45 minutes.

2. In a large pot, heat butter and the remaining oil over medium heat. Add garlic, onion and hot pepper flakes; sauté until onion starts to brown, about 10 minutes. Add canned tomatoes, broth, thyme and roasted tomatoes, including liquid on baking sheet; bring to a boil. Reduce heat and simmer for 40 minutes.

3. Using an immersion blender, or in batches in a food processor or blender, purée soup until smooth. Return to the pot, if necessary. Taste and adjust seasoning with salt and black pepper, if necessary.

4. Ladle into heated bowls and swirl a dollop of pesto into each.

Nutrients per serving	
Calories	172
Fat	12 g
Saturated Fat	4 g
Cholesterol	17 mg
Sodium	1724 mg
Carbohydrate	12 g
Fiber	3 g
Sugars	6 g
Protein	3 g
Calcium	61 mg
Iron	0 mg

Roasted Summer Vegetable Soup

Makes 6 servings

This mouthwatering soup features eggplant, zucchini, tomatoes, corn, garlic and onions — a team that never fails to win.

Tips

When purchasing eggplants, look for those with shiny, smooth skin.

Using reduced-sodium broth will lower the sodium content of each serving to 483 mg.

- Preheat oven to 425°F (220°C)
- 2 large rimmed baking sheets

10	cloves garlic (unpeeled)	10
2	eggplants, cut into $\frac{1}{2}$-inch (1 cm) dice	2
2	zucchini, cut into $\frac{1}{2}$-inch (1 cm) dice	2
1	large onion, cut into 8 wedges	1
4 cups	cherry tomatoes	1 L
$\frac{1}{4}$ cup	olive oil	60 mL
1 tsp	salt	5 mL
$\frac{1}{2}$ tsp	freshly ground black pepper	2 mL
6 cups	ready-to-use chicken broth, divided	1.5 L
2 cups	fresh or frozen corn kernels	500 mL
3	sprigs fresh thyme	3
	Pesto	

1. On baking sheets, combine garlic, eggplants, zucchini, onion, tomatoes, oil, salt and pepper; toss to coat evenly and spread in a single layer. Roast in preheated oven, stirring occasionally, until vegetables are browned and tender, 35 to 45 minutes. Remove garlic cloves from pan, squeeze garlic from skins, mash into a paste and set aside. Discard skins.

2. Pour $\frac{1}{4}$ cup (60 mL) broth onto each baking sheet and scrape up any brown bits. Transfer broth and vegetables to a large pot and add the remaining broth, corn, thyme and roasted garlic; bring to a boil over medium heat. Reduce heat and simmer for 20 minutes to blend the flavors.

3. Ladle into heated bowls and swirl a dollop of pesto into each.

Nutrients per serving	
Calories	252
Fat	12 g
Saturated Fat	2 g
Cholesterol	10 mg
Sodium	1951 mg
Carbohydrate	32 g
Fiber	10 g
Sugars	14 g
Protein	8 g
Calcium	56 mg
Iron	2 mg

Turkish-Style Barley Soup

Makes 8 servings

This simple soup is an exquisite combination of textures and flavors. Serve it as a light main course or in small quantities as a prelude to dinner.

Tips

After adding the probiotic-rich yogurt, cooking on Low ensures that the soup doesn't boil, in which case the yogurt would curdle.

To make ahead, complete step 1. Cover and refrigerate for up to 2 days. When you're ready to cook, complete the recipe. Because the barley soaks up liquid on sitting, add an extra ½ cup (125 mL) broth or water before cooking.

- Medium to large (3½ to 5-quart) slow cooker

1 tbsp	olive oil	15 mL
1	onion, finely chopped	1
3	leeks (white part with just a bit of green), cleaned (see tip, page 268) and thinly sliced	3
4	cloves garlic, peeled	4
1 tsp	salt	5 mL
½ tsp	cracked black peppercorns	2 mL
1	2-inch (5 cm) cinnamon stick	1
2 tbsp	all-purpose flour	30 mL
½ cup	barley (see tips, page 221)	125 mL
6 cups	Vegetable Stock (page 212) or ready-to-use vegetable broth, divided	1.5 L
2 tsp	sweet paprika, dissolved in 2 tbsp (30 mL) freshly squeezed lemon juice	10 mL
2	long green or red chile peppers, minced	2
¾ cup	full-fat yogurt or vegan alternative	175 mL
2 tbsp	finely chopped fresh mint	30 mL

1. In a skillet, heat oil over medium heat. Add onion and leeks and cook, stirring, until softened, about 4 minutes. Add garlic, salt, peppercorns, cinnamon stick and flour and cook, stirring, for 1 minute. Add barley and toss to coat. Add 2 cups (500 mL) broth and bring to a boil. Boil for 2 minutes. Transfer to slow cooker stoneware.

2. Stir in the remaining broth. Cover and cook on Low for 6 to 8 hours or on High for 3 to 4 hours, until barley is tender. Discard cinnamon stick.

3. Add paprika solution to slow cooker along with chiles, yogurt and mint. Cover and cook on Low for 15 minutes to meld flavors.

Nutrients per serving	
Calories	170
Fat	6 g
Saturated Fat	1 g
Cholesterol	3 mg
Sodium	337 mg
Carbohydrate	28 g
Fiber	6 g
Sugars	7 g
Protein	5 g
Calcium	114 mg
Iron	2 mg

Mushroom Barley Soup with Miso

Miso is a traditional Japanese seasoning made by fermenting soybeans with salt, koji and sometimes whole-grain barley, rice and other ingredients.

Tips

Use the type of barley you prefer — pearled, pot or whole. Whole (also known as hulled) barley is the most nutritious form of the grain.

Barley, like all whole grains, really soaks up liquid. If you've refrigerated this soup and are reheating it, you'll need to add water to ensure an appropriate consistency.

To make ahead, complete step 1. Cover and refrigerate for up to 2 days. When you're ready to cook, complete the recipe. Because the barley soaks up liquid on sitting, add an extra ½ cup (125 mL) broth or water before cooking.

Nutrients per serving

Calories	249
Fat	11 g
Saturated Fat	1 g
Cholesterol	0 mg
Sodium	1795 mg
Carbohydrate	33 g
Fiber	7 g
Sugars	10 g
Protein	8 g
Calcium	60 mg
Iron	2 mg

- Medium (about 4-quart) slow cooker

2 tbsp	vegetable oil or butter	30 mL
2	onions, finely chopped	2
4	stalks celery, diced	4
4	cloves garlic, minced	4
1 tsp	dried thyme	5 mL
1 tsp	salt	5 mL
½ tsp	cracked black peppercorns	2 mL
1	bay leaf	1
½ cup	barley (see tips, at left)	125 mL
6 cups	ready-to-use mushroom broth	1.5 L
1 lb	cremini mushrooms, trimmed and quartered	500 g
¼ cup	white miso	60 mL
	Finely chopped green onions or fresh parsley	

1. In a skillet, heat oil over medium heat. Add onions and celery and cook, stirring, until softened, about 5 minutes. Add garlic, thyme, salt, peppercorns and bay leaf and cook, stirring, for 1 minute. Add barley and toss until coated. Transfer to slow cooker stoneware. Add mushroom broth.

2. Stir in mushrooms. Cover and cook on Low for 6 hours or on High for 3 hours. Stir in miso. Cover and cook on High for 15 minutes to meld flavors. Discard bay leaf. Ladle soup into bowls and garnish with green onions.

Lentil Soup Italian-Style

*Lentils are nutritious,
delicious and adaptable.
You'll find this recipe
fuss-free, since all the
ingredients are cooked
together instead of being
sautéed separately.*

Tip

Fennel bulb comes
attached to woody branches
and thin leaves that look
like dill. Cut off and
discard the woody branches
and thin leaves. Quarter
the bulb vertically, then cut
out and discard the hard
triangular sections of core.
What remains is the usable
part of the fennel.

2¹/₂ cups	dried green lentils, rinsed and drained	625 mL
12 cups	water	3 L
1 tsp	salt	5 mL
2 cups	chopped onions	500 mL
1	large carrot, diced	1
1	fennel bulb, thinly sliced (see tip, at left)	1
6	cloves garlic, chopped	6
1	can (28 oz/796 mL) crushed tomatoes	1
3	bay leaves	3
¹/₂ cup	packed chopped fresh parsley	125 mL
1¹/₂ tbsp	balsamic vinegar	22 mL
¹/₄ cup	olive oil	60 mL
1 tsp	fennel seeds	5 mL
¹/₂ tsp	hot pepper flakes	2 mL
¹/₂ tsp	freshly ground black pepper	2 mL
	Freshly grated pecorino or Parmesan cheese	
	Extra virgin olive oil	

1. In a large saucepan or soup pot, cover lentils with the
   water; add salt and let lentils soak for about 20 minutes.

2. Add onions, carrot, fennel, garlic, tomatoes, bay leaves,
   parsley and balsamic vinegar. Bring to a boil, stirring
   occasionally.

3. Meanwhile, in a small frying pan, heat oil over high
   heat for 30 seconds. Add fennel seeds, hot pepper
   flakes and black pepper. Stir-fry for just under 1 minute
   and remove from heat. Set aside.

4. When the soup has come to a boil, add the oil and
   spices; mix well. Reduce heat to medium-low and let
   bubble slowly for 1 hour, stirring occasionally, until all
   the ingredients are soft. If the soup is too thick, add
   1 to 2 cups (250 to 500 mL) water and, raising heat,
   bring back to a quick bubble. Take off heat, cover and
   let rest for 10 to 15 minutes. Serve accompanied by
   grated cheese and a beaker of olive oil.

Nutrients per serving
(1 of 10)

Calories	269
Fat	7 g
Saturated Fat	1 g
Cholesterol	0 mg
Sodium	373 mg
Carbohydrate	41 g
Fiber	8 g
Sugars	2 g
Protein	14 g
Calcium	88 mg
Iron	5 mg

Black Bean Coconut Soup

Don't be fooled by the short ingredients list; this spicy soup has a surprisingly complex flavor.

Tips

If you only have sweet smoked paprika, add $\frac{1}{8}$ tsp (0.5 mL) cayenne pepper.

Store the cooled soup in an airtight container in the refrigerator for up to 2 days or in the freezer for up to 6 months. Thaw overnight in the refrigerator or in the microwave using the Defrost function. Warm soup in a medium saucepan over medium-low heat.

2	cans (each 14 to 19 oz/398 to 540 mL) black beans, drained and rinsed	2
1	can (10 oz/284 mL) diced tomatoes with chiles, with juice	1
1 tbsp	ground cumin	15 mL
1 tsp	chipotle chile powder or hot smoked paprika	5 mL
	Fine sea salt	
2 cups	coconut water	500 mL
2 tbsp	freshly squeezed lime juice, divided	30 mL
	Freshly ground black pepper	
$\frac{1}{2}$ cup	well-stirred coconut milk (full-fat)	125 mL

Suggested Accompaniments

Chopped green onions

Toasted unsweetened flaked or shredded coconut

1. In a medium saucepan, mash one can of beans. Add the remaining beans, tomatoes, cumin, chile powder, $\frac{3}{4}$ tsp (3 mL) salt and coconut water. Bring to a boil over medium-high heat. Reduce heat and simmer, stirring occasionally, for 25 to 30 minutes or until thickened. Stir in 1 tbsp (15 mL) lime juice and season to taste with salt and pepper.

2. In a small bowl, whisk together coconut milk and the remaining lime juice until blended. Season to taste with salt.

3. Ladle soup into bowls and drizzle with coconut milk mixture. Serve with any of the suggested accompaniments, as desired.

Nutrients per serving	
Calories	269
Fat	9 g
Saturated Fat	7 g
Cholesterol	0 mg
Sodium	806 mg
Carbohydrate	37 g
Fiber	10 g
Sugars	6 g
Protein	12 g
Calcium	122 mg
Iron	4 mg

Chilled Curried Banana Coconut Soup

*Farmers from Southeast
Asia and New Guinea
first domesticated
bananas. Eating them raw
maximizes their prebiotics.*

Tips

If lime leaves aren't
available, substitute ¹/₂ tsp
(2 mL) grated lime zest and
add with the lime juice.

For the best flavor and
creamiest texture, be sure
bananas are very ripe
(speckled with brown spots).

• Blender

³/₄ cup	coconut milk, divided	175 mL
2	wild lime leaves (see tip, at left)	2
1 tbsp	minced gingerroot	15 mL
	Salt	
¹/₂ tsp	ground coriander	2 mL
¹/₄ tsp	ground cumin	1 mL
1 tsp	mild Indian yellow curry paste or masala blend	5 mL
2 tbsp	freshly squeezed lime juice	30 mL
4	very ripe bananas	4
³/₄ cup	plain yogurt	175 mL
³/₄ cup	cold water	175 mL
1 tsp	granulated sugar (or to taste)	5 mL
	Chopped fresh mint	

1. In a small skillet, heat 2 tbsp (30 mL) coconut milk over medium-low heat until bubbling. Add lime leaves and cook, stirring, until fragrant, about 2 minutes. Reduce heat to low. Add ginger, ¹/₂ tsp (2 mL) salt, coriander, cumin and curry paste; cook, stirring often, until ginger is softened and spices are fragrant, about 5 minutes. Remove from heat and stir in lime juice, scraping up any bits stuck to pan.

2. Discard lime leaves and transfer spice mixture to blender. Add the remaining coconut milk and bananas; purée until smooth.

3. Transfer to a bowl and whisk in yogurt and cold water. Cover and refrigerate until chilled, about 2 hours, or for up to 8 hours.

4. If soup is very thick, let stand at room temperature for 15 minutes to allow coconut milk to warm slightly. Whisk to blend and season to taste with sugar and salt. Ladle into chilled bowls and serve sprinkled with mint.

Nutrients per serving (1 of 8)

Calories	123
Fat	6 g
Saturated Fat	5 g
Cholesterol	1 mg
Sodium	21 mg
Carbohydrate	17 g
Fiber	2 g
Sugars	10 g
Protein	2 g
Calcium	51 mg
Iron	1 mg

Chilled Yogurt Soup with Roasted Red Pepper and Pesto Swirls

Makes 6 servings

The yogurt in this recipe carries the flavors of the onion, garlic, roasted peppers and pesto even further, making this one delicious soup. As a bonus, yogurt is an excellent source of probiotics.

Tips

If you have homemade Vegetable Stock (page 212) on hand, use it in this recipe in place of store-bought broth.

Choose a reduced-sodium broth to lower the amount of sodium to 410 mg per serving.

- Immersion blender (optional)
* Food processor or blender

2 tbsp	olive oil	30 mL
1/2 cup	minced onion	125 mL
1	clove garlic, minced	1
4 cups	ready-to-use chicken or vegetable broth	1 L
3 cups	plain yogurt	750 mL
1/2 tsp	salt	2 mL
1/4 tsp	freshly ground black pepper	1 mL
2	roasted red bell peppers (see box, below)	2
1 tbsp	balsamic vinegar	15 mL
1/4 cup	pesto	60 mL

1. In a skillet, heat oil over medium heat. Add onion and sauté until lightly browned, about 10 minutes. Add garlic and sauté for 1 minute. Add broth and bring to a boil. Reduce heat and simmer for about 5 minutes to blend the flavors. Let cool to room temperature.

2. Using an immersion blender, or in batches in a food processor or blender, purée soup until smooth. Add yogurt, salt and pepper; pulse until just blended. Transfer to a bowl, cover and refrigerate until cold, about 3 hours. Taste and adjust seasoning with salt and pepper, if necessary.

3. In food processor or blender, pulse roasted peppers and vinegar until smooth.

4. Ladle soup into chilled bowls and top each with a dollop of pesto and a dollop of roasted pepper purée. Swirl a knife around the bowl to create a marbled effect.

Nutrients per serving

Calories	216
Fat	13 g
Saturated Fat	3 g
Cholesterol	17 mg
Sodium	1389 mg
Carbohydrate	15 g
Fiber	1 g
Sugars	13 g
Protein	10 g
Calcium	306 mg
Iron	1 mg

Roasting Peppers

To roast peppers, lay seeded halved peppers on a baking sheet and broil until skins char and blacken. Transfer to a heatproof bowl and cover with plastic wrap. When cool enough to handle, scrape off the blackened skins with the back of a knife. Don't worry about a little bit of black remaining on the peppers.

Chilled Fruited Gazpacho

Makes 4 to 6 servings

Tomatoes are a natural source of inulin, which helps maintain a healthy gut.

Tips

If raspberry vinegar is not available, combine 1 tbsp (15 mL) each wine vinegar and raspberry jam.

If you have homemade Vegetable Stock (page 212) on hand, use it in this recipe in place of store-bought broth.

- Food processor or blender

4 cups	sliced fresh strawberries	1 L
2 cups	chopped seeded peeled tomatoes	500 mL
³/₄ cup	diced seeded peeled cucumber	175 mL
3 tbsp	chopped fresh chives	45 mL
1 cup	apple juice	250 mL
3 tbsp	freshly squeezed lemon juice	45 mL
2 tbsp	raspberry vinegar (see tip, at left)	30 mL
2 tbsp	pesto	30 mL
¹/₂ tsp	salt	2 mL
¹/₂ to 1 cup	ready-to-use vegetable broth	125 to 250 mL
4 to 6	whole strawberries (optional)	4 to 6

1. In a large bowl, combine strawberries, tomatoes, cucumber, chives, apple juice, lemon juice, vinegar, pesto and salt, stirring to mix well. Using a slotted spoon, lift out about 3 cups (750 mL) solids and transfer to food processor. Process for 30 seconds or until smooth. Return to remaining mixture in bowl. Mix well. Stir broth into soup in ¹/₄-cup (60 mL) portions until desired consistency is achieved.

2. Cover and refrigerate for a minimum of 2 hours or for up to 24 hours. Taste and add more salt, lemon juice or vinegar, if required. Serve well chilled and garnish with a whole strawberry (if using).

Nutrients per serving (1 of 6)	
Calories	105
Fat	3 g
Saturated Fat	1 g
Cholesterol	2 mg
Sodium	318 mg
Carbohydrate	19 g
Fiber	3 g
Sugars	14 g
Protein	2 g
Calcium	68 mg
Iron	1 mg

Salads and Dressings

Mexican Jicama Slaw. 228

Arugula, Apricot and Crispy Chickpea Salad. 229

Warm Pear and Snow Pea Salad with Miso Dressing. 230

Summer Artichoke Salad. 231

Dandelion Salad with Citrus Dressing. 232

Tomato Mozzarella Salad. 233

Sautéed Eggplant Salad. 234

Tabbouleh. 236

Bulgur Asparagus Salad. 237

Roasted Red Peppers with Moroccan Couscous 238

North African Carrot Quinoa Salad 239

Pasta Salad with Yellow Tomato Sauce. 240

Lentil Salad with Tomatoes and Tarragon 241

Greek Bean Salad 242

"Roasted" Garlic, Hemp and Parsley Dressing 243

Tomato Basil Dressing 244

Creamy Miso Dressing. 244

Mexican Jicama Slaw

*Jicama is a refreshing
vegetable that tastes like
a blend of apple, celery
and potato. In this salad
it is mixed with cumin
and chili powder for
an authentic Mexican
experience.*

Tips

To peel the jicama, use a
sharp chef's knife to cut
a small slice from each
end, exposing the flesh.
Starting from the top,
in a downward motion,
cut away the dark brown
skin around the flesh
and discard.

Use a mandoline to slice
the jicama approximately
1/4 inch (0.5 cm) thick.
Then stack the slices on a
cutting board and, using
a sharp chef's knife, cut
into thin, even strips.

Nutrients per side salad	
Calories	296
Fat	27 g
Saturated Fat	4 g
Cholesterol	0 mg
Sodium	379 mg
Carbohydrate	13 g
Fiber	7 g
Sugars	3 g
Protein	1 g
Calcium	27 mg
Iron	1 mg

- Food processor

1/4 cup	cold-pressed extra virgin olive oil	60 mL
3 tbsp	freshly squeezed lime juice	45 mL
1 tsp	chili powder	5 mL
1/2 tsp	ground cumin	2 mL
1/4 tsp	fine sea salt	1 mL
2 cups	finely sliced peeled jicama (see tips, at left)	500 mL

1. In food processor, process olive oil, lime juice, chili powder, cumin and salt. Transfer to a bowl.

2. Add jicama to dressing and toss until well coated. Cover and set aside for 10 minutes, until softened. Serve immediately or cover and refrigerate for up to 2 days.

Arugula, Apricot and Crispy Chickpea Salad

Makes 6 servings

Garam masala, fresh lemon and sweet chunks of dried apricot give bitter arugula multidimensional flavor, while crispy chickpeas give croutons a run for their money.

Tips

An equal amount of tender watercress sprigs, baby spinach leaves or mesclun can be used in place of the arugula.

For even more crunch, replace the toasted coconut with an equal amount of toasted green pumpkin seeds (pepitas) or sunflower seeds.

- Preheat oven to 450°F (230°C)
- Large rimmed baking sheet, greased with virgin coconut oil

1	can (14 to 19 oz/398 to 540 mL) chickpeas, drained, rinsed and patted dry	1
1½ tsp	garam masala	7 mL
¼ tsp	fine sea salt, divided	1 mL
3 tbsp	virgin coconut oil, divided	45 mL
2 tsp	finely grated lemon zest	10 mL
2 tbsp	freshly squeezed lemon juice	30 mL
6 cups	packed arugula leaves	1.5 L
½ cup	chopped dried apricots or golden raisins	125 mL
¼ cup	unsweetened flaked or shredded coconut, toasted	60 mL

1. In a medium bowl, combine chickpeas, garam masala, half the salt and 1 tbsp (15 mL) coconut oil. Spread in a single layer on prepared baking sheet. Roast in preheated oven for 10 to 15 minutes or until chickpeas are golden brown and crisp. Let cool completely in pan.

2. In a small bowl, whisk together the remaining salt, lemon zest, lemon juice and the remaining oil.

3. In a large bowl, combine chickpeas, arugula and apricots. Add dressing and gently toss to coat. Sprinkle with coconut.

Variation

Island Chickpea Salad: Replace the garam masala with an equal amount of salt-free jerk seasoning and replace the lemon zest and lemon juice with equal amounts of lime zest and lime juice.

Nutrients per serving	
Calories	197
Fat	10 g
Saturated Fat	8 g
Cholesterol	0 mg
Sodium	322 mg
Carbohydrate	24 g
Fiber	5 g
Sugars	7 g
Protein	4 g
Calcium	60 mg
Iron	2 mg

Warm Pear and Snow Pea Salad with Miso Dressing

In winter, the warmed pears make a cozy starter, but this salad is just as nice without warming the pears — simply slice and pile on top of the other salad ingredients.

- Preheat oven to 400°F (200°C)
- Rimmed baking sheet, lightly oiled

2	ripe pears, halved lengthwise and cored, stem intact	2
1/4 cup	agave nectar	60 mL
1 tbsp	freshly squeezed lemon juice	15 mL
1 tbsp	fresh thyme leaves	15 mL
1 1/2 cups	bean sprouts	375 mL
2 oz	snow peas, cut lengthwise into matchsticks	60 g
2	green onions, halved lengthwise and sliced crosswise on the diagonal	2
1	carrot, shredded	1
3 tbsp	sesame seeds	45 mL

Miso Dressing

2 tbsp	tamari or soy sauce	30 mL
2 tbsp	agave nectar	30 mL
2 tbsp	grapeseed oil	30 mL
1 tbsp	rice vinegar	15 mL
2 tsp	toasted sesame oil	10 mL
2 tsp	miso	10 mL

1. Place a pear half on working surface, cut side down. Starting 1/2 inch (1 cm) down from stem, cut lengthwise to bottom of pear in scant 1/2-inch (1 cm) slices, keeping pear intact at stem. Arrange on prepared baking sheet and press to fan slices.

2. In a bowl, combine agave nectar, lemon juice and thyme. Drizzle over pears. Bake in preheated oven for 10 to 15 minutes or until tender. Let cool slightly.

3. In a salad bowl, combine bean sprouts, snow peas, green onions and carrot.

4. *Dressing:* In a jar with a tight-fitting lid, combine tamari, agave nectar, grapeseed oil, vinegar, sesame oil and miso. Place lid on jar and shake well.

5. Arrange bean sprout mixture on a salad plate. Lift pear halves onto salad, drizzle with dressing and sprinkle sesame seeds over salad.

Nutrients per serving	
Calories	321
Fat	15 g
Saturated Fat	2 g
Cholesterol	0 mg
Sodium	626 mg
Carbohydrate	47 g
Fiber	5 g
Sugars	35 g
Protein	7 g
Calcium	110 mg
Iron	2 mg

Summer Artichoke Salad

Baby artichokes are a gift of nature — all the glory of grown-up artichokes, but with an edible choke (the fuzz that grows out and protects the heart), which means zero work and all pleasure.

Tip

Baby artichokes are available bottled in oil or canned in water. If using fresh, remove the outer leaves, cut $\frac{1}{2}$ inch (1 cm) off the top, trim the stalk and boil over medium heat for 15 minutes until the hearts (bottoms) are easily pierced.

6	baby artichokes, cooked (or 14-oz/ 398 mL can artichoke hearts, drained and rinsed)	6
$\frac{1}{2}$	red bell pepper, cut into thin strips	$\frac{1}{2}$
$\frac{1}{4}$ cup	thinly sliced red onion	60 mL
1	1-inch (2.5 cm) piece English cucumber, thinly sliced	1
5	black olives, pitted and halved	5
1	ripe large tomato, cut into $\frac{1}{2}$-inch (1 cm) wedges	1
12	seedless grapes, halved	12
1 tsp	drained capers	5 mL
1	clove garlic, pressed	1
2 tbsp	extra virgin olive oil	30 mL
1 tbsp	white wine vinegar	15 mL
1 tbsp	freshly squeezed lemon juice	15 mL
$\frac{1}{4}$ tsp	salt	1 mL
$\frac{1}{8}$ tsp	freshly ground black pepper	0.5 mL
	A few sprigs fresh parsley, chopped	

1. Cut artichokes in half and put in a salad bowl. Add red pepper, onion, cucumber, olives, tomato, grapes and capers. Toss gently to mix.

2. In a small bowl, whisk together garlic, olive oil, vinegar, lemon juice, salt and pepper until slightly emulsified. Drizzle over the salad and toss gently to dress all the pieces, but without breaking up the artichokes too much. Garnish with parsley, and serve within 1 hour (cover if it has to wait, but do not refrigerate).

Nutrients per serving	
Calories	130
Fat	7 g
Saturated Fat	1 g
Cholesterol	0 mg
Sodium	413 mg
Carbohydrate	13 g
Fiber	2 g
Sugars	5 g
Protein	3 g
Calcium	22 mg
Iron	2 mg

Dandelion Salad with Citrus Dressing

Makes 4 servings

Dandelion greens contain inulin, a prebiotic fiber that feeds "friendly" gut bacteria.

2 cups	fresh dandelion leaves or other greens (see variations, below)	500 mL
2 cups	fresh spinach, trimmed and patted dry	500 mL
1/2 cup	bean sprouts	125 mL
1/4 cup	sliced green onions	60 mL
1/4 cup	chopped fresh parsley	60 mL
1/4 cup	fresh dandelion petals (optional)	60 mL
1/4 cup	Citrus Dressing (see recipe, below)	60 mL

1. In a large salad bowl, combine dandelion leaves, spinach, sprouts, green onions, parsley and dandelion petals (if using). Drizzle Citrus Dressing over top and toss well. Serve immediately.

Variation

Use radicchio, endive, chicory, watercress or sorrel for greens with the same bitter qualities as dandelion.

Nutrients per serving

Calories	114
Fat	10 g
Saturated Fat	1 g
Cholesterol	0 mg
Sodium	37 mg
Carbohydrate	6 g
Fiber	2 g
Sugars	1 g
Protein	3 g
Calcium	85 mg
Iron	2 mg

Citrus Dressing

Makes about 1/2 cup (125 mL)

1/3 cup	olive oil	75 mL
1/4 cup	freshly squeezed orange juice	60 mL
1 tsp	grated lemon zest	5 mL
1 tbsp	freshly squeezed lemon juice	15 mL
1 tbsp	fresh lemon thyme leaves	15 mL
1 tbsp	chopped fresh lemon balm	15 mL
	Salt	

1. In a jar with a lid or a small bowl, combine oil, orange juice, lemon zest, lemon juice, thyme and lemon balm. Shake or whisk to mix well. Taste and add salt or extra lemon juice, if required.

Nutrients per 1 tbsp (15 mL)

Calories	84
Fat	9 g
Saturated Fat	1 g
Cholesterol	0 mg
Sodium	0 mg
Carbohydrate	1 g
Fiber	0 g
Sugars	1 g
Protein	0 g
Calcium	3 mg
Iron	0 mg

Tomato Mozzarella Salad

Makes 4 servings

Did you know that the tomato is actually a fruit and not a vegetable?

Tips

When tomatoes are in season, there's no better way to enjoy them than in this simple but delicious salad with an Italian flair. If desired, substitute fresh or buffalo mozzarella for the part-skim version, but be aware that the fat content will go up.

To ripen tomatoes, place them in a brown paper bag with an apple or a pear. These fruits give off ethylene dioxide, which causes the tomatoes to ripen.

Vinaigrette

1/4 cup	vegetable or olive oil	60 mL
2 tbsp	white vinegar	30 mL
1 tbsp	chopped fresh parsley	15 mL
2 tsp	Dijon mustard	10 mL
1 tsp	granulated sugar	5 mL
2	cloves garlic, minced	2
1/2 tsp	dried basil	2 mL
1/2 tsp	freshly ground black pepper	2 mL
1/4 tsp	salt	1 mL
2 tbsp	water	30 mL

Salad

3	large tomatoes (preferably beefsteak)	3
16	romaine or Boston lettuce leaves	16
1/2 cup	cubed part-skim mozzarella cheese	125 mL
6	green onions, sliced	6

1. *Vinaigrette:* In a jar with tight-fitting lid, whisk together oil, vinegar, parsley, mustard, sugar, garlic, basil, pepper, salt and water; chill. Shake before using.

2. *Salad:* Cut tomatoes in half; cut each half crosswise into slices. Arrange 4 lettuce leaves on each of 4 salad plates. Arrange tomato slices on lettuce; sprinkle with cheese and green onions.

3. At serving time, pour vinaigrette over each salad.

This recipe courtesy of chef Yvonne C. Levert and dietitian Nanette Porter-MacDonald.

Nutrients per serving

Calories	215
Fat	18 g
Saturated Fat	3 g
Cholesterol	9 mg
Sodium	324 mg
Carbohydrate	10 g
Fiber	3 g
Sugars	5 g
Protein	6 g
Calcium	155 mg
Iron	1 mg

Sautéed Eggplant Salad

A huge favorite in southern Europe and all over the sunbelt, eggplant appears in countless recipes. This adaptation uses ratatouille as a base and touches on the various stewed and sautéed eggplant salads of the Middle East.

4 cups	eggplant, cut into $\frac{1}{2}$-inch (1 cm) cubes	1 L
	Salted water	
3 tbsp	vegetable oil	45 mL
3 tbsp	olive oil	45 mL
$\frac{1}{2}$ tsp	salt	2 mL
$\frac{1}{4}$ tsp	freshly ground black pepper	1 mL
$\frac{1}{4}$ tsp	hot pepper flakes	1 mL
1	onion, cut into $\frac{1}{4}$-inch (0.5 cm) slices	1
$\frac{1}{2}$	green bell pepper, cut into $\frac{1}{2}$-inch (1 cm) squares	$\frac{1}{2}$
$\frac{1}{2}$	red bell pepper, cut into $\frac{1}{2}$-inch (1 cm) squares	$\frac{1}{2}$
4	cloves garlic, thinly sliced	4
4	sun-dried tomatoes, thinly sliced	4
1	tomato, cut into $\frac{1}{2}$-inch (1 cm) wedges	1
1 tsp	red wine vinegar	5 mL
$\frac{1}{2}$ tsp	dried basil	2 mL
$\frac{1}{2}$ tsp	dried oregano	2 mL
$\frac{1}{4}$ cup	water	60 mL
	A few sprigs chopped fresh basil and/or parsley	

1. Immerse cubed eggplant in cold salted water as soon as possible after cutting it (eggplant turns brown soon after it is cut); let soak 5 to 10 minutes.

2. In a large nonstick frying pan, heat vegetable oil over medium-high heat for 1 minute. Drain eggplant and add to the pan (watch for splutters). It will absorb all the oil almost immediately. Cook, stirring actively, for 6 to 7 minutes or until the eggplant is soft and browned all over. Transfer the cooked eggplant to a dish; set aside.

Nutrients per serving	
Calories	237
Fat	21 g
Saturated Fat	2 g
Cholesterol	0 mg
Sodium	339 mg
Carbohydrate	12 g
Fiber	5 g
Sugars	6 g
Protein	2 g
Calcium	33 mg
Iron	1 mg

If you like things less spicy, just omit the hot pepper flakes.

3. Using the same frying pan, heat olive oil over medium-high heat for 30 seconds. Add salt, black pepper and hot pepper flakes; stir-fry for 30 seconds. Add onion, green pepper and red pepper; stir-fry for 2 to 3 minutes or until wilted and beginning to char. Add garlic and sun-dried tomatoes; stir-fry for 1 minute. Add tomato, vinegar, basil and oregano; stir-fry for 2 minutes or until tomato has broken down and a sauce is forming. Add water and immediately reduce heat to medium. Stir in eggplant. Gently mix and fold all ingredients together; cook for 2 minutes or until heated through.

4. Transfer to a flat dish and let rest for about 10 minutes. Garnish with fresh herbs. Serve lukewarm.

Tabbouleh

Makes 8 servings

Mint and lemon are the traditional flavors found in this classic Middle Eastern salad.

Tips

To keep parsley and mint fresh, store in a tightly covered container in refrigerator.

Tomatoes, green onions, parsley and mint help to create a salad that is rich in vitamin C. For a quick lunch and added vitamins and fiber, tuck the tabbouleh into a whole wheat pita and serve with raw vegetables.

• Food processor

1 cup	medium-grain bulgur	250 mL
1 cup	boiling water	250 mL
5 to 6	green onions	5 to 6
1 1/2 cups	lightly packed sprigs fresh parsley	375 mL
1/3 cup	lightly packed fresh mint leaves	75 mL
2	tomatoes, chopped	2

Dressing

1/4 cup	freshly squeezed lemon juice	60 mL
3 tbsp	olive oil	45 mL
1	small clove garlic, minced	1
1/2 tsp	grated lemon zest	2 mL
1/2 tsp	granulated sugar	2 mL
1/2 tsp	dry mustard	2 mL
1/4 tsp	paprika	1 mL
1/4 tsp	salt	1 mL
	Freshly ground black pepper	

1. In a covered saucepan, cook bulgur in boiling water for about 5 minutes or until liquid is absorbed (bulgur should still be crunchy). Spoon into a large bowl; cool.

2. In food processor, coarsely chop onions, parsley and mint leaves; add to bulgur. Stir in tomatoes.

3. *Dressing:* Whisk together lemon juice, olive oil, garlic, lemon zest, sugar, mustard, paprika, salt, and pepper to taste. Pour dressing over bulgur mixture; mix together lightly. Cover and refrigerate for several hours or overnight.

This recipe courtesy of dietitian Johanne Trudeau.

Nutrients per serving

Calories	123
Fat	6 g
Saturated Fat	1 g
Cholesterol	0 mg
Sodium	87 mg
Carbohydrate	17 g
Fiber	4 g
Sugars	2 g
Protein	3 g
Calcium	34 mg
Iron	1 mg

Bulgur Asparagus Salad

Makes 4 servings

In this salad, the bulgur and asparagus are made pleasantly pungent with lemon juice and almonds.

Tips

When whole wheat berries are steamed, hulled, dried and cracked, the resulting product is called bulgur. It is often confused with couscous, a totally different wheat product.

If you have homemade Vegetable Stock (page 212) on hand, use it in this recipe in place of store-bought broth.

- Preheat oven to 400°F (200°C)
- Rimmed baking sheet, lightly oiled

1 lb	asparagus, trimmed	500 g
5 tbsp	olive oil, divided	75 mL
3 tbsp	freshly squeezed lemon juice	45 mL
1/2 cup	finely chopped onion	125 mL
1	clove garlic, minced	1
2 tbsp	finely chopped fresh parsley	30 mL
1 cup	fine or coarse bulgur	250 mL
1 1/4 cups	boiling water or ready-to-use vegetable broth	300 mL
1/2 cup	finely chopped almonds	125 mL

1. Arrange asparagus on prepared baking sheet in a single layer. Drizzle or brush 2 tbsp (30 mL) oil and the lemon juice over. Bake in preheated oven for 20 minutes or until tender when pierced with the tip of a knife.

2. Meanwhile, in a skillet, heat 2 tbsp (30 mL) oil over medium heat. Add onion and garlic and cook, stirring occasionally, for 6 to 8 minutes or until soft. Add parsley, bulgur and water. Cover, reduce heat to medium-low and simmer for 15 to 20 minutes or until the liquid has been absorbed. Fluff with a fork and transfer to a bowl.

3. Add the remaining oil to skillet and return to medium heat. Stir in almonds and toast, stirring frequently, for 2 minutes or until lightly browned.

4. Divide bulgur evenly among 4 salad plates. Top each plate with 4 or 5 asparagus spears and sprinkle with toasted almonds. Serve warm or at room temperature.

Nutrients per serving	
Calories	382
Fat	24 g
Saturated Fat	3 g
Cholesterol	0 mg
Sodium	14 mg
Carbohydrate	37 g
Fiber	11 g
Sugars	4 g
Protein	10 g
Calcium	87 mg
Iron	4 mg

Roasted Red Peppers with Moroccan Couscous

Makes 6 servings

Serve this dish on its own as a colorful, self-contained side salad, or add rice or a green salad to serve it as an entrée.

Tip

If you have homemade Vegetable Stock (page 212) on hand, use it in this recipe in place of store-bought broth.

- Preheat oven to 375°F (190°C)
- Baking sheet, lightly oiled

3	red bell peppers, halved crosswise	3
2 tbsp	olive oil	30 mL

Moroccan Couscous

1 tbsp	olive oil	15 mL
1/2 cup	chopped onion	125 mL
1	clove garlic, minced	1
1 1/2 cups	couscous	375 mL
1 cup	ready-to-use vegetable broth or water	250 mL
1/4 cup	raisins	60 mL
1/4 cup	orange marmalade	60 mL
1/4 tsp	ground cinnamon	1 mL
1/4 tsp	ground cumin	1 mL
	Sea salt and freshly ground black pepper	

1. Arrange pepper halves, cut side down, on prepared baking sheet. Brush or drizzle with oil. Bake in preheated oven for 40 minutes or until the skin bubbles and blackens in places. Transfer to a bowl and let cool. Slip the skins off and arrange, cut sides up, on a serving platter.

2. *Couscous:* Meanwhile, in a skillet, heat oil over medium heat. Add onion and cook, stirring occasionally, for 6 to 8 minutes or until onion is soft. Add garlic and cook, stirring, for 1 minute.

3. Add couscous and cook, stirring constantly, for 1 minute to lightly toast the grains. Add broth, raisins, marmalade, cinnamon and cumin. Increase heat to high and bring to a boil. Turn off heat, leaving the pan on the burner or element, and cover pan. Let stand for 10 minutes or until liquid is absorbed. Fluff with a fork and season to taste with salt and pepper. Divide couscous into 6 portions and stuff each portion into a pepper half. Serve warm or cold.

Nutrients per serving	
Calories	300
Fat	7 g
Saturated Fat	1 g
Cholesterol	0 mg
Sodium	172 mg
Carbohydrate	53 g
Fiber	4 g
Sugars	15 g
Protein	7 g
Calcium	29 mg
Iron	1 mg

North African Carrot Quinoa Salad

A Moroccan-inspired carrot and quinoa salad is versatile enough to accompany almost any meal.

Tip

To mash garlic, working with one clove at a time, place the side of a chef's knife flat against the clove. Place the heel of your hand on the side of the knife and apply pressure so that the clove flattens slightly (this will loosen the peel). Remove and discard the peel, then roughly chop the garlic. Sprinkle a pinch of coarse salt over the garlic. Use the flat part of the knife as before to press the garlic against the cutting board. Repeat until the garlic turns into a fine paste. The mashed garlic is now ready for use in your favorite recipe.

2 cups	cooked black or white quinoa, cooled	500 mL
3 cups	coarsely shredded carrots (about 12 oz/375 g)	750 mL
3/4 cup	packed fresh cilantro or flat-leaf (Italian) parsley leaves, chopped	175 mL
1/3 cup	golden raisins	75 mL
3	cloves garlic, mashed (see tip, at left) or minced	3
1 1/2 tsp	ground cumin	7 mL
3/4 tsp	hot smoked paprika	3 mL
1/2 tsp	ground cinnamon	2 mL
2 tbsp	extra virgin olive oil	30 mL
2 tbsp	freshly squeezed lemon juice	30 mL
	Fine sea salt and cracked black peppercorns	

1. In a large bowl, combine quinoa, carrots, cilantro and raisins.

2. In a small bowl, whisk together garlic, cumin, paprika, cinnamon, oil and lemon juice. Add to quinoa mixture and gently toss to coat. Season to taste with salt and peppercorns. Cover and refrigerate for at least 1 hour, until chilled, or for up to 4 hours.

Nutrients per serving	
Calories	126
Fat	5 g
Saturated Fat	1 g
Cholesterol	0 mg
Sodium	34 mg
Carbohydrate	20 g
Fiber	3 g
Sugars	6 g
Protein	3 g
Calcium	32 mg
Iron	1 mg

Pasta Salad with Yellow Tomato Sauce

Makes 6 to 8 servings

Sweet yellow tomatoes make an attractive and delicious sauce for pasta salad.

Tips

You can also make the sauce with sweet green tomatoes, such as green zebras.

To peel and seed tomatoes, blanch in boiling water until skins begin to peel away, about 15 seconds. With a slotted spoon, remove tomatoes and place in ice water. With a paring knife, peel off skin, then scrape out seeds with a spoon.

- Blender

Yellow Tomato Sauce

5	ripe yellow or green tomatoes (about 1¼ lbs/625 g), peeled and seeded (see tips, at left)	5
2	cloves garlic, chopped	2
¾ cup	loosely packed basil leaves	175 mL
3 tbsp	extra virgin olive oil	45 mL
1 tsp	grated lemon zest	5 mL
¾ tsp	salt	3 mL
¼ tsp	freshly ground white or black pepper	1 mL

Pasta Salad

2	stalks celery	2
1 lb	short pasta	500 g
1	yellow bell pepper	1
1 cup	cubed bocconcini or mozzarella cheese	250 mL
½ cup	chopped toasted walnuts	125 mL

1. *Tomato Sauce:* In blender, on low speed, blend tomatoes, garlic, basil, oil, lemon zest, salt and pepper until slightly chunky. Set aside.

2. *Pasta Salad:* In a large pot of boiling salted water, blanch celery for 20 seconds. Remove with tongs and chill under cold water. Drain, chop and set aside.

3. Add pasta to water in pot and cook according to package directions until al dente (tender to the bite). Drain, rinse under cold water and drain well.

4. Meanwhile, preheat broiler. Cut yellow pepper in half and place on a baking sheet. Broil, skin side up, until skin is charred. Let cool, peel and cut into strips.

5. In a large bowl, combine pasta, celery, yellow pepper, cheese, walnuts and tomato sauce until well mixed.

Nutrients per serving (1 of 8)	
Calories	383
Fat	14 g
Saturated Fat	3 g
Cholesterol	9 mg
Sodium	369 mg
Carbohydrate	50 g
Fiber	4 g
Sugars	2 g
Protein	15 g
Calcium	170 mg
Iron	3 mg

Lentil Salad with Tomatoes and Tarragon

Makes 4 to 6 servings

This salad, which combines the refreshing flavors of tarragon, lemon and garlic, may even be better the day after it is made.

Tips

Unlike dried beans, lentils don't need to be soaked before cooking. You should, however, submerge them in water and remove any impurities that float to the top. Drain in a colander, remove any remaining impurities or blackened lentils and rinse thoroughly under cold running water before using in a recipe.

Cooking times will vary depending on the kind of lentils you use and how long they have been in storage. Generally, the longer they are stored, the longer they take to cook.

Nutrients per serving (1 of 6)	
Calories	202
Fat	10 g
Saturated Fat	1 g
Cholesterol	0 mg
Sodium	1197 mg
Carbohydrate	22 g
Fiber	4 g
Sugars	1 g
Protein	8 g
Calcium	30 mg
Iron	3 mg

6 cups	water	1.5 L
1 tbsp	salt	15 mL
1 cup	dried brown or green lentils, washed, rinsed and drained (see tips, at left)	250 mL
1/2 cup	finely chopped red bell pepper	125 mL
1/4 cup	olive oil	60 mL
1/2 tsp	grated lemon zest	2 mL
2 tbsp	freshly squeezed lemon juice	30 mL
1	clove garlic, minced	1
1 tbsp	chopped fresh tarragon, divided (or 1 tsp/5 mL dried, divided)	15 mL
1 tsp	Dijon mustard	5 mL
1/4 tsp	freshly ground black pepper	1 mL
1 cup	quartered cherry tomatoes	250 mL
1 tsp	red wine vinegar	5 mL
	Salt (optional)	

1. In a large pot, bring water and salt to a boil over high heat. Add lentils and return to a boil. Reduce heat and simmer, uncovered, for 20 to 30 minutes or until lentils are tender but firm. Drain, shaking strainer well to remove excess moisture.

2. In a bowl, whisk together red pepper, olive oil, lemon zest and juice, garlic, 2 tsp (10 mL) tarragon, mustard and black pepper until well blended. Add lentils and toss until evenly coated. Transfer to a serving bowl.

3. In a small bowl, combine tomatoes, the remaining tarragon, vinegar and salt to taste (if using). Arrange tomato mixture over lentil mixture or around the edge of the bowl to make a colorful ring.

Variation

In step 3, replace the tomato mixture with 2 green onions, sliced; 2 stalks celery, thinly sliced; 1/4 cup (60 mL) black olives; 1 tbsp (15 mL) chopped parsley; 1 tbsp (15 mL) olive oil; and 2 tsp (10 mL) red wine vinegar. Combine in a small bowl, sprinkle over the lentil mixture and serve.

Greek Bean Salad

This salad can be whipped up in no time if you don't mind using canned beans. It tastes even better the next day!

2 cups	cooked white kidney beans	500 mL
1	onion, thinly slivered	1
1	tomato, cut into $1/2$-inch (1 cm) cubes	1
$1/4$ cup	extra virgin olive oil	60 mL
1 tbsp	red wine vinegar	15 mL
	Salt and freshly ground black pepper	
2	hard-cooked eggs, thinly sliced	2
2 cups	thinly sliced cucumber	500 mL
1 cup	drained pickled green peppers (pepperoncini)	250 mL
$1/4$ cup	kalamata olives (about 8)	60 mL
	A few sprigs fresh parsley, chopped	

1. Place beans in a bowl. Add slivered onion and cubed tomato. Fold gently into beans.

2. Whisk together oil and vinegar until emulsified. Add dressing to bean mixture; fold in gently but thoroughly. Season to taste with salt and pepper.

3. On a serving plate, spread out dressed beans, mounding them slightly. Decorate the borders with alternating rounds of egg and cucumber slices. Place the pickled green peppers inside this border to ring the beans. Dot the surface with the olives and garnish with chopped parsley.

4. Serve immediately or cover and let stand at room temperature for up to 1 hour before serving.

Nutrients per serving

Calories	221
Fat	13 g
Saturated Fat	2 g
Cholesterol	62 mg
Sodium	239 mg
Carbohydrate	20 g
Fiber	6 g
Sugars	4 g
Protein	8 g
Calcium	42 mg
Iron	2 mg

"Roasted" Garlic, Hemp and Parsley Dressing

Makes about 1 cup (250 mL)

Garlic is a rich source of inulin and a great antibacterial agent.

Tip

To store hemp seeds, place them in an airtight container and refrigerate. This will prevent the fats from turning rancid. Hemp seeds can also be frozen for up to 6 months. They are extremely high in protein, containing up to 5 grams per tablespoon (15 mL).

- Electric food dehydrator
- Blender

15 to 20	cloves garlic, peeled	15 to 20
3 tbsp	cold-pressed extra virgin olive oil	45 mL
2 cups	chopped fresh flat-leaf (Italian) parsley	500 mL
1/2 cup	cold-pressed hemp oil	125 mL
1/4 cup	freshly squeezed lemon juice	60 mL
1/4 cup	raw shelled hemp seeds	60 mL
1/2 tsp	fine sea salt	2 mL
1/4 tsp	sweet paprika	1 mL
1/4 cup	filtered water (approx.)	60 mL

1. In a shallow dish, combine garlic and olive oil. Toss well. Place in dehydrator, and spread evenly. Dehydrate at 105°F (41°C) for 10 to 12 hours or until brown (it should resemble traditional roasted garlic).

2. In blender, combine "roasted" garlic, parsley, hemp oil, lemon juice, hemp seeds, salt and paprika. Blend at high speed until smooth.

3. Scrape down the sides of the blender jar. With the motor running, slowly add enough water through the opening in the lid to create a creamy dressing. Serve immediately or cover and refrigerate for up to 5 days.

Variations

Substitute 1/4 cup (60 mL) freshly squeezed lime juice, 1 tbsp (15 mL) chopped gingerroot and 1 tsp (5 mL) ground coriander for the parsley and lemon juice.

Substitute an equal quantity of sesame seeds, soaked in 1/2 cup (125 mL) water for 20 minutes, for the hemp seeds. Drain and discard the soaking water and rinse under cold running water.

Nutrients per 1 tbsp (15 mL)	
Calories	102
Fat	10 g
Saturated Fat	1 g
Cholesterol	0 mg
Sodium	87 mg
Carbohydrate	2 g
Fiber	0 g
Sugars	0 g
Protein	1 g
Calcium	17 mg
Iron	1 mg

Tomato Basil Dressing

Makes about 1½ cups (375 mL)

Few things say "summer" more than tomatoes and basil.

Nutrients per 1 tbsp (15 mL)	
Calories	41
Fat	4 g
Saturated Fat	1 g
Cholesterol	0 mg
Sodium	121 mg
Carbohydrate	0 g
Fiber	0 g
Sugars	0 g
Protein	0 g
Calcium	2 mg
Iron	0 mg

• Blender

1 cup	chopped tomatoes	250 mL
½ cup	cold-pressed extra virgin olive oil	125 mL
¼ cup	filtered water	60 mL
3 tbsp	tamari	45 mL
2	cloves garlic	2
2	bunches fresh basil, roughly chopped	2

1. In blender, combine tomatoes, olive oil, water, tamari, garlic and basil. Blend at high speed until smooth. Serve immediately or cover and refrigerate for up to 4 days.

Creamy Miso Dressing

Makes about 1¾ cups (425 mL)

Nutrients per 1 tbsp (15 mL)	
Calories	44
Fat	4 g
Saturated Fat	1 g
Cholesterol	0 mg
Sodium	128 mg
Carbohydrate	2 g
Fiber	0 g
Sugars	1 g
Protein	0 g
Calcium	2 mg
Iron	0 mg

• Blender

1 cup	filtered water	250 mL
½ cup	cold-pressed extra virgin olive oil	125 mL
¼ cup	unpasteurized brown rice miso	60 mL
2 tbsp	raw agave nectar	30 mL
1 tbsp	tamari	15 mL
2	cloves garlic, peeled	2

1. In blender, combine water, olive oil, miso, agave nectar, tamari and garlic. Blend at high speed until smooth. Serve immediately or cover and refrigerate for up to 5 days.

Variation

For a healthy boost of omega-3 fatty acids, replace ¼ cup (60 mL) of the olive oil with ¼ cup (60 mL) cold-pressed flaxseed oil.

Pasta and Grains

Tomato Sauce. 246

Spaghetti and Soyballs 247

Smoked Gouda Mac and Cheese. 248

Green Macaroni and Cheese 249

Penne with Mushrooms, Sun-Dried Tomatoes
     and Artichokes. 250

Grilled Vegetable Lasagna 252

Fusilli with Leeks 254

Vegetarian Pad Thai 255

"Barbecue" Pulled Burdock Sandwich 256

Couscous Bake 258

Couscous with Cilantro, Tomatoes and Peas. 259

Polenta with Fried Tomato. 260

Cheesy Grits 262

Vegetable Fried Rice 263

Eggplant Pilaf 264

Tomato and Onion Rice Pilau. 266

Baked Springtime Risotto. 267

Squash-Laced Wild Rice and Barley Casserole. 268

Tomato Sauce

**Makes about
4 cups (1 L)**

*This tomato-basil-garlic
sauce works with any
recipe that calls for a
tomato enhancement. It
freezes well and is easy to
make in large batches.*

Tip

Canned whole plum
tomatoes can replace
fresh. Use 2 cans (each
28 oz/796 mL), reserving
2 cups (500 mL) of the
juice for use if the sauce
needs thinning.

3 lbs	ripe tomatoes	1.5 kg
1/3 cup	olive oil	75 mL
Pinch	salt	Pinch
8	cloves garlic, roughly chopped	8
1/2 tsp	hot pepper flakes	2 mL
1 1/2 tbsp	dried basil (or 1/4 to 1/2 cup/60 to 125 mL packed chopped fresh basil)	22 mL
1 tbsp	balsamic vinegar	15 mL
6	sun-dried tomatoes, finely chopped	6

1. Blanch tomatoes in boiling water for 30 seconds. Over a bowl, peel, core and deseed them. Chop tomatoes roughly and set aside. Strain any accumulated tomato juices from bowl; add half of the juices to the chopped tomatoes. Save or freeze the other half for recipes that call for tomato juice.

2. In a large, deep frying pan or pot, heat oil over high heat for 30 seconds. Add salt and stir. Add chopped garlic and stir-fry for 30 seconds. Add hot pepper flakes and stir-fry for 30 seconds.

3. Add chopped tomatoes and juices. Stir-cook until boiling. Add basil (if using dried), the vinegar and sun-dried tomatoes. Mix well, and reduce heat to medium-low. Cook for 20 to 25 minutes, maintaining a steady bubbling, stirring occasionally.

4. If using fresh basil, add it now to taste (no amount is too much). Stir in, and continue cooking for 5 minutes. Remove from heat and cover. Let rest for 5 to 10 minutes to develop flavor. Stir to redistribute the oil that has risen to the top, and serve immediately.

Nutrients per 1/2 cup
(125 mL)

Calories	122
Fat	9 g
Saturated Fat	1 g
Cholesterol	0 mg
Sodium	41 mg
Carbohydrate	9 g
Fiber	2 g
Sugars	5 g
Protein	2 g
Calcium	34 mg
Iron	1 mg

Spaghetti and Soyballs

*Here's an old standard
with a contemporary
vegan twist. You get the
health benefits of soy, the
great taste of tomato sauce
and the satisfaction of
comfort food.*

Tip

You can substitute 14 oz
(420 g) soy ground meat
alternative for the meatless
meatballs. Pinch off small
pieces and roll into balls
approximately 1 inch
(2.5 cm) in diameter. Soy
meat alternatives come in
a variety of textures. Those
found in the refrigerated
section of your supermarket
tend to be moister than
those found in the frozen
section. The moist versions
are easiest to work with
when forming soyballs.

Nutrients per serving (1 of 6)	
Calories	503
Fat	26 g
Saturated Fat	4 g
Cholesterol	0 mg
Sodium	431 mg
Carbohydrate	48 g
Fiber	8 g
Sugars	9 g
Protein	22 g
Calcium	80 mg
Iron	4 mg

8 oz	spaghetti	250 g
¼ cup	dry bread crumbs	60 mL
2 tbsp	coarsely chopped fresh oregano leaves (or 2 tsp/10 mL dried)	30 mL
1 tbsp	coarsely chopped fresh parsley (or 1 tsp/5 mL dried)	15 mL
1 tbsp	whole wheat or unbleached all-purpose flour	15 mL
1	package (14 oz/420 g) meatless meatballs	1
4 cups	tomato sauce (store-bought or see recipe, page 246)	1 L
3 tbsp	olive oil	45 mL
	Grated vegan Parmesan cheese alternative (optional)	

1. In a pot of boiling salted water, cook spaghetti for 8 minutes or until tender to the bite. Drain.

2. Meanwhile, in a bowl, combine bread crumbs, oregano, parsley and flour. Add meatballs and toss until evenly coated. Transfer to a plate, shaking off excess crumb mixture. Set aside.

3. In a pot, heat tomato sauce over low heat until heated through.

4. Meanwhile, in a large nonstick skillet, heat oil over medium-high heat for 30 seconds. Add meatballs and cook, turning, until lightly browned and crispy. Using a slotted spoon, transfer to tomato sauce. Simmer, uncovered, for 5 minutes or until heated through.

5. Divide hot spaghetti among plates. Spoon soyballs and sauce over top.

Smoked Gouda Mac and Cheese

You'll love this twist on an all-American classic: mac and cheese made with smoked Gouda. It's great as a side dish with barbecued meats.

Tip

Freshly grated or shaved Parmesan cheese is always best right off the wedge, but prepackaged containers can be found in the refrigerated specialty cheese section of your local supermarket.

- Preheat oven to 350°F (180°C)
- 8-cup (2 L) casserole dish, greased

2 cups	elbow macaroni	500 mL
1 tbsp	butter	15 mL
2	cloves garlic, minced	2
1/4 cup	thinly sliced green onions	60 mL
2 tbsp	all-purpose flour	30 mL
2 cups	milk	500 mL
1/2 tsp	salt	2 mL
1/4 tsp	freshly ground black pepper	1 mL
1/2 cup	shredded smoked Gouda cheese	125 mL
6 tbsp	freshly grated Parmesan cheese	90 mL
1/2 cup	dry bread crumbs	125 mL

1. In a large pot of boiling water, cook macaroni according to package directions. Drain and set aside.

2. Meanwhile, in a large saucepan, melt butter over medium heat. Sauté garlic and green onions for about 2 minutes or until tender. Whisk in flour and sauté for 1 minute.

3. Gradually whisk in milk, salt and pepper; reduce heat and simmer, whisking constantly, for 3 to 5 minutes or until thickened. Remove from heat and stir in Gouda and Parmesan until melted. Stir in macaroni. Spoon into prepared casserole dish and sprinkle with bread crumbs.

4. Bake in preheated oven for 20 minutes or until bubbling.

Nutrients per serving	
Calories	438
Fat	15 g
Saturated Fat	9 g
Cholesterol	53 mg
Sodium	725 mg
Carbohydrate	53 g
Fiber	2 g
Sugars	9 g
Protein	22 g
Calcium	472 mg
Iron	2 mg

Green Macaroni and Cheese

Makes 5 servings

Pasta made from 100% whole wheat flour maintains the three essential parts of the whole grain kernel: the bran, the germ and the endosperm.

- Food processor

1	bag (10 oz/300 g) baby spinach	1
2 tbsp	freshly squeezed lemon juice	30 mL
1 tbsp	extra virgin olive oil	15 mL
12 oz	whole wheat macaroni	375 g
1 cup	shredded white Cheddar cheese	250 mL
1/2 cup	slivered almonds, toasted	125 mL
	Freshly ground black pepper	

1. In food processor, pulse spinach, lemon juice and olive oil for 15 seconds, until roughly puréed (don't overdo it).

2. Cook macaroni according to package directions until al dente (tender to the bite). Drain and return to the pot. Add spinach mixture, tossing to coat evenly. Stir in cheese and almonds. Season to taste with pepper.

This recipe courtesy of Jody MacLean.

Nutrients per serving	
Calories	428
Fat	17 g
Saturated Fat	6 g
Cholesterol	24 mg
Sodium	191 mg
Carbohydrate	56 g
Fiber	8 g
Sugars	1 g
Protein	20 g
Calcium	275 mg
Iron	5 mg

Penne with Mushrooms, Sun-Dried Tomatoes and Artichokes

A little of this richly flavored sauce goes a long way.

Tips

If you don't have homemade portobello mushrooms or roasted red peppers, look for marinated portobello mushrooms and roasted red peppers in jars or in the deli section of major supermarkets. Both work fine for this recipe.

If you want a more liquidy sauce, add ¼ cup (60 mL) tomato juice before adding the soy creamer.

3 tbsp	olive oil	45 mL
1	large sweet onion (such as Vidalia), thinly sliced	1
2	cloves garlic, minced	2
3	Baked Portobello Mushrooms (see recipe, opposite), thinly sliced	3
2	roasted red bell peppers (see box, page 225), thinly sliced	2
¾ cup	drained canned artichoke hearts, quartered	175 mL
¼ cup	coarsely chopped drained oil-packed sun-dried tomatoes	60 mL
8 oz	penne	250 g
½ cup	soy creamer	125 mL
1 tbsp	finely chopped fresh oregano leaves (or 1 tsp/5 mL dried)	15 mL
	Salt and freshly ground black pepper	

1. In a large nonstick skillet, heat oil over medium-low heat for 30 seconds. Add onion and cook for 12 minutes or until very soft and lightly browned.

2. Add garlic and cook, stirring, for 1 minute. Add portobello mushrooms, roasted peppers, artichoke hearts and sun-dried tomatoes and cook, stirring, for 5 to 7 minutes or until vegetables are tender.

3. Meanwhile, in a large pot of boiling salted water, cook penne for 8 minutes or according to package instructions, until tender to the bite.

4. Add soy creamer and oregano to vegetable mixture and stir well. Cook for 5 minutes longer to blend flavors. Divide hot penne among serving bowls and spoon vegetable mixture over top. Season to taste with salt and pepper.

Nutrients per serving	
Calories	457
Fat	19 g
Saturated Fat	3 g
Cholesterol	0 mg
Sodium	135 mg
Carbohydrate	58 g
Fiber	4 g
Sugars	8 g
Protein	11 g
Calcium	32 mg
Iron	2 mg

Baked Portobello Mushrooms

Makes 4 servings

Baked portobello mushrooms have many uses. They can be sliced and added to salads and sauces or served whole on a bun for a satisfying sandwich.

Tip

When removing the mushroom stem, carefully cut it out with a paring knife to leave the mushroom cap intact.

- 13- by 9-inch (33 by 23 cm) glass baking dish, greased

¼ cup	olive oil	60 mL
2 tbsp	balsamic vinegar	30 mL
	Salt and freshly ground black pepper	
4	portobello mushrooms, stems removed (see tip, at left)	4

1. In a small bowl, whisk together olive oil, balsamic vinegar, and salt and pepper to taste.

2. Place mushrooms in prepared baking dish, gill side up, and pour marinade over top, making sure each mushroom cap is completely covered. Cover dish and refrigerate for 1 to 2 hours to allow mushrooms to absorb some of the marinade.

3. Preheat oven to 350°F (180°C).

4. Drain off excess marinade. Bake mushrooms for 35 minutes or until soft.

Variations

Portobello Mushroom Burgers: Serve whole baked mushrooms on a bun or soft roll.

Portobello Mushroom Burgers with Caramelized Onions: For a nice change, top burgers with caramelized onions. To caramelize onions, melt 2 tbsp (30 mL) soy margarine in a skillet over medium heat. Add 1 large onion, thinly sliced. Sprinkle with 1 tsp (5 mL) natural cane sugar and cook, stirring often, for 20 minutes or until onion is soft and lightly browned.

Nutrients per serving	
Calories	153
Fat	14 g
Saturated Fat	2 g
Cholesterol	0 mg
Sodium	8 mg
Carbohydrate	6 g
Fiber	1 g
Sugars	3 g
Protein	2 g
Calcium	9 mg
Iron	1 mg

Grilled Vegetable Lasagna

Makes 8 servings

Two simple changes give this lasagna a delicious new flavor — the vegetables are grilled first, and tofu is used as a layer with the cheese, making it rich in calcium.

- Preheat oven to 350°F (180°C)
- 13- by 9-inch (33 by 23 cm) baking pan, sprayed with nonstick cooking spray

1	small onion, chopped	1
1 tbsp	vegetable oil	15 mL
3	cloves garlic, chopped	3
1	carrot, diced	1
1	stalk celery, diced	1
2 cups	sliced mushrooms	500 mL
1	can (19 oz/540 mL) tomatoes	1
1	can (7½ oz/213 mL) tomato sauce	1
1 tsp	crushed dried basil	5 mL
1 tsp	crushed dried oregano	5 mL
½ tsp	salt	2 mL
¼ tsp	freshly ground black pepper	1 mL
1½ lbs	herb-flavored or plain tofu	750 g
2	zucchini, sliced lengthwise and grilled	2
½	eggplant, sliced and grilled	½
1	red bell pepper, quartered, grilled and peeled	1
1 cup	lower-fat cottage cheese	250 mL
3 cups	shredded part-skim mozzarella cheese	750 mL
⅓ cup	freshly grated Parmesan cheese	75 mL

1. In a Dutch oven, sauté onion in oil until tender. Stir in garlic, carrot, celery and mushrooms; sauté for 5 minutes. Add tomatoes, breaking up with fork; add tomato sauce, basil and oregano. Simmer, uncovered, for 15 to 20 minutes or until thickened and reduced to about 2½ cups (625 mL). Season with salt and pepper.

Nutrients per serving

Calories	328
Fat	17 g
Saturated Fat	6 g
Cholesterol	27 mg
Sodium	873 mg
Carbohydrate	17 g
Fiber	5 g
Sugars	7 g
Protein	33 g
Calcium	1282 mg
Iron	4 mg

Tips

Instead of using traditional noodles as a base, this lasagna uses tofu. For best results, use firm or extra-firm tofu.

To grill peppers, heat barbecue or broiler; place peppers on grill or broiling pan and cook until skins turn black. Keep turning peppers until skins are blistered and black. Place roasted peppers in large pot with lid. The steam will make them sweat and skin will be easier to peel off. Let peppers cool. Remove stems, seeds and skin.

2. Cut half of the tofu into $\frac{1}{4}$-inch (0.5 cm) thick slices. Line bottom of prepared pan with slices. Spread with half of the sauce. Cut zucchini, eggplant and red pepper into bite-size pieces; sprinkle half over sauce. Sprinkle with half each of the cottage and mozzarella cheeses.

3. Slice the remaining tofu and arrange in layer over cheese. Top with the remaining sauce, vegetables and cottage cheese. Blend the remaining mozzarella with Parmesan; sprinkle over top. Cover tightly with foil.

4. Bake in preheated oven for 15 minutes. Uncover and bake until hot and golden, 15 to 20 minutes. Let stand for 5 minutes before serving.

This recipe is courtesy of chef Bernard Casavant and dietitian Jane Thornthwaite.

Fusilli with Leeks

Take colorful ridged fusilli and a smooth pink sauce studded with green-and-white leeks. What have you got? A surefire crowd-pleaser — irresistible, even for the most fickle of appetites.

Tips

Be sure to wash leeks thoroughly, splitting down the middle and paying special care to the grit that hides where the green and white parts meet.

Double-strength stock or broth: For the enhanced flavor requirements of sauces (as opposed to soups), prepare a concentrated version of stock or broth by boiling it down to reduce its volume by half.

Nutrients per serving (1 of 4)	
Calories	388
Fat	14 g
Saturated Fat	3 g
Cholesterol	10 mg
Sodium	181 mg
Carbohydrate	57 g
Fiber	4 g
Sugars	6 g
Protein	10 g
Calcium	53 mg
Iron	3 mg

2	tomatoes	2
3 cups	three-color fusilli	750 mL
3 tbsp	olive oil, divided	45 mL
1/4 tsp	salt	1 mL
1/4 tsp	freshly ground black pepper	1 mL
2 cups	finely chopped leeks (white and light green parts only)	500 mL
Pinch	dried oregano	Pinch
1 tsp	chopped fresh sage (or a pinch dried)	5 mL
1/2 cup	double-strength Vegetable Stock (page 212) or ready-to-use vegetable broth (see tip, at left)	125 mL
2 tbsp	heavy or whipping (35%) cream	30 mL
	Grated Romano cheese	

1. Blanch tomatoes in boiling water for 30 seconds. Over a bowl, peel, core and deseed them. Chop tomatoes roughly and set aside. Strain any accumulated tomato juices from bowl; add to the chopped tomatoes.

2. In a large pot of boiling salted water, cook pasta according to package directions until tender but firm. Rinse pasta and drain. Add 1 tbsp (15 mL) olive oil and toss; cover and set aside.

3. Meanwhile, in a large frying pan, heat 2 tbsp (30 mL) oil over high heat for 30 seconds. Add salt and pepper and stir. Add chopped leeks and stir-fry until softened, about 2 to 3 minutes. Add oregano and sage and stir-fry for 30 seconds.

4. Stir in tomatoes and juice, mashing down the tomato. Add stock and bring to a boil, continuing to mash tomatoes and stirring for 2 to 3 minutes. Reduce heat to minimum; add cream, stirring to mix evenly, and cook for 2 to 3 minutes. Toss pasta with sauce; transfer to serving bowls. Top with grated cheese and serve immediately.

Vegetarian Pad Thai

Here's a vegetarian version of the popular noodle dish, with tofu replacing the chicken and shrimp. Omit the eggs, if desired.

Tip

You can add extra vegetables, such as thinly sliced asparagus, beans or shredded cabbage.

8 oz	dried medium or wide rice noodles	250 g
1/4 cup	soy sauce	60 mL
1/4 cup	ketchup	60 mL
2 tbsp	freshly squeezed lime juice	30 mL
1 tbsp	palm sugar or packed brown sugar	15 mL
1/4 cup	vegetable oil, divided	60 mL
8 oz	firm tofu, cut into 1/4-inch (0.5 cm) cubes	250 g
1/2	red bell pepper, thinly sliced	1/2
2	large eggs, beaten	2
3	cloves garlic, chopped	3
2 cups	bean sprouts, divided	500 mL
3	green onions, chopped	3
1 tsp	thinly sliced fresh red chile peppers	5 mL
1/4 cup	chopped peanuts	60 mL
2 tbsp	chopped fresh cilantro leaves	30 mL
1	lime, cut into wedges	1

1. Place noodles in a large bowl. Cover with very hot water and let stand for 10 to 12 minutes or until softened but firm. Rinse well with cold water and drain.

2. In a small bowl or measuring cup, combine soy sauce, ketchup, lime juice and sugar.

3. Heat a wok or large skillet over medium-high heat and add 2 tbsp (30 mL) oil. Add tofu and red pepper and stir-fry for 3 minutes. Remove and reserve.

4. Add the remaining oil to wok and heat. Add eggs and garlic and stir-fry to scramble eggs.

5. Add soy sauce mixture and noodles and toss to combine for 2 minutes or until noodles are softened but not mushy (if mixture becomes dry add a few spoonfuls of water or broth to prevent scorching).

6. Add tofu, red pepper and 1¾ cups (425 mL) bean sprouts and toss for 1 minute or until hot.

7. Transfer to a serving platter and top with the remaining bean sprouts, green onions, chiles, peanuts and cilantro. Garnish with lime wedges.

Nutrients per serving	
Calories	394
Fat	19 g
Saturated Fat	2 g
Cholesterol	62 mg
Sodium	820 mg
Carbohydrate	46 g
Fiber	3 g
Sugars	6 g
Protein	14 g
Calcium	312 mg
Iron	3 mg

"Barbecue" Pulled Burdock Sandwich

Burdock has a somewhat woody flavor that combines well with barbecue sauce. Be sure to start this recipe 2 to 3 days before you want to serve it, because the burdock needs time to pickle.

Tips

Burdock is fibrous in texture. You need to shred or slice it thinly in order to allow the marinade to penetrate.

Burdock will begin to oxidize (turn brown) as soon as it is cut. If you prefer it to remain light-colored, prepare your pickling solution before shredding. Transfer the burdock to the liquid immediately after it has been shredded.

You can use a box grater to shred the burdock, but it will be more difficult than using a food processor fitted with the shredding blade.

1 cup	filtered water	250 mL
1/4 cup	apple cider vinegar	60 mL
3 tbsp	raw agave nectar	45 mL
1 tsp	fine sea salt	5 mL
2 cups	shredded peeled burdock root (about 2 medium)	500 mL
1 1/2 cups	Sun-Dried Tomato Barbecue Sauce (see recipe, opposite)	375 mL
4	slices Buckwheat Toast (page 156)	

1. In a deep, non-reactive container, combine water, vinegar, agave nectar and salt. Add burdock and toss well. Cover and set aside for 2 to 3 days, until burdock has become soft enough to chew easily.

2. Transfer to a colander and drain. Rinse well under cold running water and transfer to a bowl.

3. Toss pickled burdock with Sun-Dried Tomato Barbecue Sauce. Place Buckwheat Toast on a serving plate and spoon burdock overtop. Serve immediately as an open-face sandwich.

Variation

Instead of the Buckwheat Toast, use 8 romaine lettuce leaves to make sandwiches.

Nutrients per serving	
Calories	290
Fat	8 g
Saturated Fat	1 g
Cholesterol	0 mg
Sodium	1243 mg
Carbohydrate	54 g
Fiber	5 g
Sugars	28 g
Protein	5 g
Calcium	58 mg
Iron	2 mg

Sun-Dried Tomato Barbecue Sauce

**Makes 2¹/₂ cups
(625 mL)**

*This tangy sauce makes
a delectable replacement
for traditional sugar-laden
barbecue sauces. It pairs
well with raw food recipes
where barbecuing would
be the traditional method
of preparation, such as
mock burgers or meat.*

Tips

To soak the sun-dried
tomatoes for this recipe,
place in a bowl and
add 2 cups (500 mL)
water. Cover and set
aside for 30 minutes.
Drain, discarding any
remaining water.

If you have a high-powered
blender, use it to make
this sauce. With a regular
blender, the texture is never
as creamy and smooth.

- Blender

1 cup	dry-packed sun-dried tomatoes, soaked (see tip, at left)	250 mL
1 cup	filtered water	250 mL
¹/₄ cup	apple cider vinegar	60 mL
¹/₄ cup	raw agave nectar	60 mL
3 tbsp	chopped green onion (green and white parts)	45 mL
3 tbsp	cold-pressed extra virgin olive oil	45 mL
2 tbsp	freshly squeezed lemon juice	30 mL
1 tbsp	tamari	15 mL
¹/₂ tsp	fine sea salt	2 mL
¹/₂ tsp	smoked sweet paprika (optional)	2 mL
Pinch	cayenne pepper	Pinch

1. In blender, combine soaked sun-dried tomatoes, water,
   vinegar, agave nectar, green onion, olive oil, lemon
   juice, tamari, salt, paprika (if using) and cayenne.
   Blend at high speed until smooth. Transfer to an
   airtight container or glass jar and refrigerate for up to
   4 days.

Nutrients per 1 tbsp (15 mL)	
Calories	18
Fat	1 g
Saturated Fat	0 g
Cholesterol	0 mg
Sodium	85 mg
Carbohydrate	2 g
Fiber	0 g
Sugars	2 g
Protein	0 g
Calcium	2 mg
Iron	0 mg

Couscous Bake

Makes 8 servings

This casserole is great hot, cold or at room temperature, served alone or in a lettuce wrap.

Tip

If you have homemade Vegetable Stock (page 212) on hand, use it in this recipe in place of store-bought broth.

- Preheat oven to 375°F (190°C)
- 10-cup (2.5 L) casserole dish

1½ cups	ready-to-use vegetable broth	375 mL
1 cup	couscous	250 mL
½ tsp	salt	2 mL
¼ cup	olive oil	60 mL
3	cloves garlic, minced	3
1	large onion, finely chopped	1
1	can (28 oz/796 mL) diced tomatoes, drained and ⅓ cup (75 mL) juice reserved	1
2 cups	loosely packed fresh spinach leaves, sliced	500 mL
⅓ cup	pine nuts	75 mL
1 tsp	dried basil	5 mL
½ tsp	freshly ground black pepper	2 mL
1 cup	shredded Muenster cheese	250 mL

1. In a medium saucepan, bring broth to a boil over high heat. Add couscous and salt; cover, remove from heat and let stand for 5 minutes or until liquid is absorbed. Fluff with a fork.

2. In a large skillet, heat oil over medium-high heat. Sauté garlic and onion for 5 to 7 minutes or until tender. Add tomatoes and cook, stirring often, for 10 minutes. Stir in couscous, reserved tomato juice, spinach, pine nuts, basil and pepper.

3. Spread half the couscous mixture in casserole dish. Sprinkle with cheese. Spread the remaining couscous over cheese.

4. Cover and bake in preheated oven for 25 to 30 minutes or until bubbling.

Nutrients per serving	
Calories	269
Fat	15 g
Saturated Fat	4 g
Cholesterol	14 mg
Sodium	649 mg
Carbohydrate	26 g
Fiber	4 g
Sugars	4 g
Protein	8 g
Calcium	157 mg
Iron	1 mg

Couscous with Cilantro, Tomatoes and Peas

Makes 4 servings

A tiny form of pasta with roots in North Africa, couscous cooks quickly and makes a satisfying companion to stir-fried dishes. In its quick-cooking form, couscous can be on your table in about 5 minutes' time.

Tip

To prepare the tomatoes, cut off stem end, quarter tomatoes lengthwise and chop crosswise into small chunks, discarding any seeds and liquid left after chopping.

2¾ cups	water	675 mL
1¾ cups	quick-cooking couscous	425 mL
1 cup	frozen tiny peas	250 mL
1 tsp	salt (or to taste)	5 mL
2 tbsp	vegetable oil	30 mL
¾ cup	chopped onion	175 mL
1 tbsp	chopped garlic	15 mL
¾ cup	coarsely chopped plum (Roma) tomatoes (see tip, at left)	175 mL
¼ cup	chopped fresh cilantro	60 mL

1. In a saucepan over high heat, bring water to a rolling boil. Stir in couscous, peas and salt. Cover pan and remove from heat. Set aside for 5 minutes.

2. Meanwhile, heat oil in a skillet over medium-high heat. Add onion and garlic, and cook, stirring once, until garlic is fragrant and onions are softened, about 1 minute. Add tomatoes, stirring well, and cook for 1 minute. Remove from heat.

3. Uncover couscous and, using a wooden spoon or a fork, stir gently and fluff into a soft, grainy mixture. Add tomato mixture and stir well. Add cilantro, stirring well. Serve hot or warm.

Nutrients per serving	
Calories	402
Fat	8 g
Saturated Fat	1 g
Cholesterol	0 mg
Sodium	635 mg
Carbohydrate	68 g
Fiber	6 g
Sugars	4 g
Protein	12 g
Calcium	41 mg
Iron	1 mg

Polenta with Fried Tomato

Polenta, a popular Italian dish, is made by boiling cornmeal into a thick, solidified porridge.

2½ cups	water	625 mL
½ tsp	salt	2 mL
1 cup	yellow cornmeal	250 mL
¼ cup	olive oil	60 mL
2 tbsp	butter	30 mL
¼ tsp	salt	1 mL
¼ tsp	freshly ground black pepper	1 mL
½ cup	sliced red onion	125 mL
½	green bell pepper, cut into strips	½
2	ripe tomatoes, cut into eighths	2
3	cloves garlic, thinly sliced	3
1 tsp	dried basil	5 mL
4 oz	soft goat cheese, crumbled	125 g
	A few sprigs fresh basil and/or parsley, chopped	
4	black olives, pitted and chopped	4

1. In a large saucepan, bring water to a rolling boil over high heat. Add salt. Add cornmeal in a thin but steady stream, stirring constantly (preferably with a wooden spoon). Reduce heat to medium-low, and continue stirring for 2 to 3 minutes, until the mixture is smooth and has thickened to the consistency of mashed potatoes.

2. Transfer the polenta to a medium bowl and cover with an inverted plate. Let set for about 5 minutes.

3. Holding the bowl and plate together, turn the polenta onto the plate. (A small tap on the bottom of the bowl will help to dislodge it from the bowl.) It will be soft but dense, holding the shape of a small cake. Quarter the cake, and cut each quarter into 3 slices.

Nutrients per serving

Calories	279
Fat	18 g
Saturated Fat	7 g
Cholesterol	19 mg
Sodium	385 mg
Carbohydrate	25 g
Fiber	2 g
Sugars	2 g
Protein	6 g
Calcium	47 mg
Iron	2 mg

To remove the skin from a clove of garlic, use the butt end of a chef's knife to press firmly but gently on the clove to loosen the skin. Using your index finger and thumb, carefully ease off the skin.

4. In a large frying pan, heat oil and butter over medium-high heat for 1 minute. Stir in salt and pepper. Add red onion and green pepper to pan in a single layer. Make another layer with polenta wedges and cook for 4 minutes, until starting to scorch. Flip the polenta over (the onion and pepper will turn over, too). Reduce heat to medium and fry this side for 4 minutes.

5. Flip polenta again and fry the first side for another 2 minutes, until all the ingredients are slightly browned. Push polenta and vegetables to the sides of the pan. Increase heat to medium-high and add the tomato wedges to the vacated center of the pan; fry for 2 to 3 minutes until tomatoes begin to soften. Sprinkle garlic and basil over everything and then gently fold the tomatoes and polenta together for 2 to 3 minutes until saucy, a little messy and luscious.

6. Sprinkle goat cheese crumbles evenly over the mixture, and fold into the polenta once or twice. Remove from heat when the cheese starts to melt, usually within 1 minute. Serve garnished with chopped herb(s) and bits of chopped olives.

Cheesy Grits

Feel great about eating your cheesy grits, knowing that the prebiotic-rich onions and garlic are keeping your gut happy.

Tips

If you have homemade Vegetable Stock (page 212) on hand, use it in this recipe in place of store-bought broth.

Choose a reduced-sodium broth to lower the amount of sodium to 319 mg per serving.

- 4-cup (1 L) baking dish, lightly greased
- Large (about 5-quart) oval slow cooker

1 tbsp	olive oil	15 mL
1	onion, finely chopped	1
4	cloves garlic, minced	4
1/2 tsp	cracked black peppercorns	2 mL
2 cups	ready-to-use chicken or vegetable broth	500 mL
1/2 cup	stone-ground grits	125 mL
1 1/2 cups	shredded old Cheddar cheese, divided	375 mL

1. In a large skillet, heat oil over medium heat. Add onion and cook, stirring, until softened, about 3 minutes. Add garlic and peppercorns and cook, stirring, for 1 minute. Add broth and bring to a boil. Gradually add grits, stirring constantly, until smooth and blended. Continue cooking and stirring until grits are slightly thickened, about 4 minutes. Stir in 1 cup (250 mL) cheese. Transfer to prepared baking dish. Cover tightly with foil and secure with a string.

2. Place in slow cooker stoneware and pour in enough boiling water to come 1 inch (2.5 cm) up the sides of the dish. Cover and cook on Low for 8 hours or on High for 4 hours. Stir well and let stand uncovered for 2 to 3 minutes to absorb any liquid.

3. Meanwhile, preheat broiler. Sprinkle the remaining cheese over top of grits and place under broiler until melted and lightly browned.

Variation

Chile-Spiked Cheesy Grits: If you like a little heat, finely mince 1 chipotle chile in adobo sauce. Stir in along with the peppercorns.

Nutrients per serving	
Calories	303
Fat	18 g
Saturated Fat	10 g
Cholesterol	42 mg
Sodium	1042 mg
Carbohydrate	22 g
Fiber	2 g
Sugars	2 g
Protein	12 g
Calcium	314 mg
Iron	1 mg

Vegetable Fried Rice

Fried rice originated in China but has become a worldwide favorite. Be generous with your garlic and onions, for additional prebiotics.

Tip

Many cooks prefer to use cold rice when making fried rice. Plan ahead and cook rice the day before or even several hours ahead of time. After fluffing cooked rice gently with a fork, turn out onto a baking sheet or shallow dish. Let cool and refrigerate without covering until very cold, then cover. Before cooking, break up large clumps before adding it to the pan.

2 tbsp	vegetable oil	30 mL
4	cloves garlic, chopped	4
1	onion, chopped	1
1 cup	sliced fresh mushrooms	250 mL
1 cup	chopped napa or savoy cabbage	250 mL
1/2 cup	chopped carrots	125 mL
1/2 cup	thinly sliced green beans	125 mL
1/2 cup	corn kernels	125 mL
1/4 cup	green peas	60 mL
2	large eggs, beaten (optional)	2
3 cups	cooked rice	750 mL
2 tbsp	soy sauce	30 mL
1	tomato, cut into wedges	1
12	English cucumber slices	12

1. Heat a wok or large skillet over medium-high heat and add oil. Add garlic and onion and stir-fry for 1 minute.

2. Add mushrooms, cabbage, carrots, beans, corn and peas. Stir-fry for 3 to 4 minutes or until just tender.

3. Add eggs (if using) and cook, stirring, for 2 minutes or until set. Stir in rice and toss to combine rice with all ingredients for 3 minutes or until heated through.

4. Add soy sauce and toss to combine for 2 minutes or until hot.

5. Serve garnished with tomato wedges and cucumber slices.

Nutrients per serving	
Calories	308
Fat	8 g
Saturated Fat	1 g
Cholesterol	0 mg
Sodium	523 mg
Carbohydrate	53 g
Fiber	3 g
Sugars	5 g
Protein	7 g
Calcium	40 mg
Iron	3 mg

Eggplant Pilaf

This enhanced rice dish will complement any number of vegetable side dishes. It can even make a nice lunch on its own, with cucumber raita.

Tip

This is a high-sodium recipe. Use half or even a quarter of the salt to reduce the sodium content.

4 cups	diced eggplant (unpeeled) (about 1 medium)	1 L
1 tbsp	salt	15 mL
2 tbsp	olive oil	30 mL
1 tsp	salt	5 mL
1/2 tsp	freshly ground black pepper	2 mL
1/2 tsp	ground turmeric	2 mL
2	whole cloves	2
Pinch	ground cumin	Pinch
1	onion, minced	1
1 cup	finely chopped leek (white and light green parts only)	250 mL
4	cloves garlic, minced	4
2 cups	rice (preferably basmati)	500 mL
3 cups	boiling water	750 mL
1/4 cup	olive oil	60 mL
	Cucumber raita (optional)	

1. Place the cubed eggplant and salt in bowl; add cold water to cover. Mix well and set aside.

2. In a heavy-bottomed pot with a tight-fitting lid, heat 2 tbsp (30 mL) oil over high heat for 30 seconds. Add salt, pepper, turmeric, cloves and cumin; stir for 30 seconds. Add onion and stir-fry for 1 minute. Add chopped leek and continue stir-frying for 1 minute. Add garlic and stir-fry for 30 seconds.

3. Add rice and stir-fry until grains are shiny, about 1 to 2 minutes. (Don't worry if the spices start to scorch on the bottom of the pan; the next addition will cure that.)

Nutrients per serving	
Calories	274
Fat	10 g
Saturated Fat	1 g
Cholesterol	0 mg
Sodium	1170 mg
Carbohydrate	42 g
Fiber	3 g
Sugars	2 g
Protein	4 g
Calcium	41 mg
Iron	1 mg

Be sure to wash leeks
thoroughly, splitting down
the middle and paying
special care to the grit that
hides where the green and
white parts meet.

4. Add boiling water, and pull pot off heat as it sizzles
and splutters for 30 seconds. Reduce heat to low;
return pot to heat, cover tightly and let it simmer
for 20 minutes. Then remove from heat but do not
uncover. Let rice mixture rest for 10 minutes to temper.

5. Meanwhile, in a large frying pan, heat $\frac{1}{4}$ cup (60 mL)
oil over high heat for 1 minute. Drain eggplant cubes
and add to oil (carefully: there will be spluttering). Fry
for 6 to 7 minutes, stirring and tossing actively, until
all the cubes have softened and have started to brown.
Remove from heat and set aside.

6. Fluff rice and add fried eggplant, folding from the
bottom up to distribute the eggplant, as well as the
onions and leeks that will have risen to the top of
the rice. Transfer to a presentation dish and serve
immediately with a side bowl of cucumber raita as
an accompaniment, if desired.

Tomato and Onion Rice Pilau

Rice is a chameleon, taking on the hues and taste nuances of whatever it is cooked in. In this recipe, it is tomato-tart and onion-sweet and spice-rich, and altogether a welcome addition to any curry meal.

Tip

Soaking the rice helps prevent it from breaking up and becoming mushy when you're making a pilau. It is an extra step, but well worth it.

1 cup	basmati rice	250 mL
	Cold water	
2 tbsp	vegetable oil	30 mL
2	bay leaves	2
1/2 tsp	cumin seeds	2 mL
1	small red onion, finely chopped	1
2	cloves garlic, minced	2
3/4 tsp	salt	3 mL
1 1/4 cups	water	300 mL
1 cup	canned diced tomatoes, with juice	250 mL

1. In a sieve, rinse rice under cool running water until water runs fairly clear. Transfer rice to a bowl and cover with cold water. Let soak for 20 minutes. Drain well.

2. In a saucepan, heat oil over medium heat until hot but not smoking. Add bay leaves and cumin seeds; cook, stirring, until seeds start to pop, about 1 minute. Add onion and cook, stirring, until very soft and starting to brown, about 5 minutes. Add garlic and salt; cook, stirring, for 1 minute.

3. Stir in rice until well coated with spices. Stir in water and tomatoes; bring to a boil. Reduce heat to low, cover and simmer until rice is tender and liquid is absorbed, about 15 minutes. Remove from heat and let stand, covered, for 5 minutes. Fluff with a fork. Discard bay leaves.

Nutrients per serving	
Calories	247
Fat	7 g
Saturated Fat	1 g
Cholesterol	0 mg
Sodium	580 mg
Carbohydrate	41 g
Fiber	2 g
Sugars	2 g
Protein	4 g
Calcium	53 mg
Iron	1 mg

Baked Springtime Risotto

Here's another great oven-baked rice dish that cooks unsupervised while you spend time with your family preparing the rest of the meal.

Tip

Using reduced-sodium broth will lower the sodium content of each serving to 213 mg.

- Preheat oven to 350°F (180°C)
- 12-cup (3 L) casserole dish with cover
- Baking sheet

1 tbsp	olive oil	15 mL
1	small onion, diced	1
1	clove garlic, minced	1
1 cup	Arborio rice	250 mL
3 cups	hot ready-to-use chicken broth, divided	750 mL
1/2 tsp	salt (or to taste)	2 mL
10	thin spears asparagus, cut into short pieces	10
1	red bell pepper, cut into thin strips	1
1/4 cup	freshly grated Parmesan cheese	60 mL
1/4 cup	minced fresh parsley	60 mL
	Freshly ground black pepper	

1. In a medium saucepan, heat oil over medium heat. Sauté onion and garlic for 5 minutes or until softened. Add rice and cook, stirring, for about 1 minute or until evenly coated. Add 2 cups (500 mL) broth and salt; bring to a simmer. Transfer to casserole dish, cover and place on baking sheet.

2. Bake in preheated oven for 15 minutes. Remove from oven and stir in the remaining broth, asparagus and red pepper. Cover and bake for 15 minutes or until rice is al dente (tender to the bite) and most of the liquid is absorbed.

3. Ladle into serving bowls and sprinkle each serving with cheese, parsley and pepper to taste.

This recipe courtesy of dietitian Andrea Holmes.

Variations

The first time you add broth, replace 1/2 cup (125 mL) of the broth with an equal amount of dry white wine.

This dish works well with other vegetable combinations. Try portobello mushrooms or butternut squash in the fall.

Nutrients per serving	
Calories	135
Fat	3 g
Saturated Fat	1 g
Cholesterol	6 mg
Sodium	764 mg
Carbohydrate	22 g
Fiber	2 g
Sugars	2 g
Protein	4 g
Calcium	40 mg
Iron	1 mg

Squash-Laced Wild Rice and Barley Casserole

Makes 6 servings

This hearty casserole is great winter fare. It's simple and very tasty. A tossed green salad is all you need to add.

Tips

To clean leeks, fill sink full of lukewarm water. Split leeks in half lengthwise and submerge in water, swishing them around to remove all traces of dirt. Transfer to a colander and rinse under cold water.

Use pearled, pot or whole barley in this recipe — whichever you prefer. Whole (also known as hulled) barley is the most nutritious form of the grain.

To make ahead, complete step 1. Cover and refrigerate for up to 2 days. When you're ready to cook, complete the recipe.

Nutrients per serving	
Calories	235
Fat	5 g
Saturated Fat	1 g
Cholesterol	0 mg
Sodium	439 mg
Carbohydrate	46 g
Fiber	8 g
Sugars	7 g
Protein	6 g
Calcium	115 mg
Iron	3 mg

- **Medium to large (3½- to 5-quart) slow cooker**

1 tbsp	vegetable oil	15 mL
2	leeks (white and light green parts only), thinly sliced (see tip, at left)	2
2	carrots, peeled and diced	2
2	stalks celery, diced	2
4	cloves garlic, minced	4
1 tsp	salt	5 mL
1 tsp	cracked black peppercorns	5 mL
½ tsp	dried thyme (or 2 sprigs fresh)	2 mL
1	bay leaf	1
½ cup	barley, rinsed (see tip, at left)	125 mL
½ cup	wild rice, rinsed	125 mL
4 cups	Vegetable Stock (page 212) or ready-to-use vegetable broth, divided	1 L
4 cups	diced butternut squash (½-inch/1 cm dice)	1 L

1. In a skillet, heat oil over medium heat. Add leeks, carrots and celery and cook, stirring, until softened, about 7 minutes. Add garlic, salt, peppercorns, thyme and bay leaf and cook, stirring, for 1 minute. Add barley and wild rice and toss until well coated. Add 2 cups (500 mL) stock, stir well and bring to a boil. Boil for 2 minutes. Transfer to slow cooker stoneware.

2. Stir in squash and the remaining stock. Cover and cook on Low for 8 hours or on High for 4 hours, until barley is tender. Discard bay leaf.

Legumes, Tofu and Tempeh

Lentils Bolognese 270

Black Lentil Sloppy Joes 271

Lentil Tagine 272

Tasty Chickpea Cakes 273

Easy Black Beans 274

Barbecue Baked Beans 275

Cilantro Black Bean Burgers 276

Baked Orzo and Beans 277

Jamaican Peas and Cauliflower "Rice" 278

Barbecue Barley and Sweet Potato Chili 279

Baked Plantain and Peanut Stew 280

Spicy Tofu with Vegetables 281

Baked Curried Tofu with Tomato Masala 282

Teriyaki Tempeh Satay with Peanut Sauce 284

Lentils Bolognese

This great recipe is easy to make and is a great vegetarian take on a traditional Italian dish. Serve on top of whole wheat spaghetti and sprinkle with freshly grated Parmesan cheese.

1 cup	dried brown or red lentils, picked through and rinsed	250 mL
2 cups	water	500 mL
1	bay leaf	1
2 tbsp	olive oil	30 mL
2	cloves garlic, crushed	2
1	onion, minced	1
1 cup	sliced mushrooms	250 mL
1 cup	chopped canned tomatoes	250 mL
1	can (5½ oz/156 mL) tomato paste	1
1	apple, diced	1
½ cup	cider vinegar	125 mL
1 tsp	dried oregano	5 mL
	Juice of 1 lemon	

1. In a medium saucepan, bring lentils, water and bay leaf to a boil over high heat. Reduce heat to medium and cook for about 20 minutes or until lentils are soft. Drain and rinse and discard bay leaf. Set aside.

2. In a large saucepan, heat oil over medium heat. Sauté garlic, onion and mushrooms until softened, about 5 minutes. Add cooked lentils, tomatoes, tomato paste, apple, vinegar, oregano and lemon juice; bring to a boil. Reduce heat, cover and simmer for 45 minutes.

This recipe courtesy of Elaine Bass.

Nutrients per serving	
Calories	316
Fat	8 g
Saturated Fat	1 g
Cholesterol	0 mg
Sodium	190 mg
Carbohydrate	48 g
Fiber	10 g
Sugars	12 g
Protein	15 g
Calcium	74 mg
Iron	5 mg

Black Lentil Sloppy Joes

Makes 4 to 5 servings

This recipe is the perfect potluck dish.

Tips

To soak the lentils, place in a bowl and add 2 cups (500 mL) water. Cover and set aside for 10 to 12 hours, changing the water every 3 to 4 hours (or place in the refrigerator for 18 hours, changing the water once). Drain and rinse under cold running water until the water runs clear.

To soak the walnuts, place in a bowl and add 4 cups (1 L) water. Cover and set aside for 30 minutes. Drain, discarding liquid.

To soak the sun-dried tomatoes, combine with 1 cup (250 mL) warm water. Set aside for 30 minutes. Drain, discarding liquid.

- Food processor

¹/₂ cup	dried black lentils, soaked (see tip, at left)	125 mL
2 cups	walnut pieces, soaked (see tip, at left)	500 mL
¹/₄ cup	dry-packed sun-dried tomatoes, soaked (see tip, at left)	60 mL
1 cup	chopped tomatoes	250 mL
¹/₂ cup	chopped red bell pepper	125 mL
¹/₄ cup	chopped green bell pepper	60 mL
3 tbsp	nutritional yeast	45 mL
4	cloves garlic	4
2 tbsp	freshly squeezed lemon juice	30 mL
1 tbsp	chopped fresh rosemary	15 mL
1 tbsp	ground cumin	15 mL
1 tsp	chili powder	5 mL
1 tsp	fine sea salt	5 mL
Pinch	cayenne pepper	Pinch

1. In food processor, process soaked sun-dried tomatoes, chopped tomatoes, red and green pepper, nutritional yeast, garlic, lemon juice, rosemary, cumin, chili powder, salt and cayenne until smooth, stopping the motor and scraping down the sides of the work bowl as necessary.

2. Add soaked walnuts and lentils and process until combined and no large pieces remain. Serve immediately or cover and refrigerate for up to 4 days.

Nutrients per serving (1 of 5)	
Calories	366
Fat	27 g
Saturated Fat	3 g
Cholesterol	0 mg
Sodium	633 mg
Carbohydrate	24 g
Fiber	7 g
Sugars	4 g
Protein	13 g
Calcium	75 mg
Iron	4 mg

Lentil Tagine

Lentils, prebiotic-rich whole-food legumes, provide over 13 grams of prebiotics in a 100-gram serving.

Tips

If using a tagine, be sure that the base is flameproof so it can sit directly on an electric or gas stovetop. If the tagine is clay and not flameproof, use a Dutch oven or enamel pan with a lid; or use a saucepan for steps 1 and 2 and transfer to the tagine to bake.

For this recipe, try Lundberg short-grain brown rice, which is soft and chewy when cooked. Long-grain brown rice, red rice or a blend of your favorites will also work.

- Preheat oven to 375°F (190°C)
- Flameproof tagine or Dutch oven

1 cup	dried red lentils	250 mL
1 tbsp	olive oil	15 mL
1	onion, chopped	1
1	carrot, finely chopped	1
2	cloves garlic, minced	2
1	1-inch (2.5 cm) slice or cube candied ginger, finely chopped	1
1 tbsp	garam masala	15 mL
1 tsp	curry powder	5 mL
½ cup	brown rice (see tip, at left)	125 mL
1	can (19 oz/540 mL) sliced peaches, with juice	1
3 cups	ready-to-use mushroom broth, vegetable broth or water	750 mL
¼ cup	red or white wine (optional)	60 mL
	Sea salt and freshly ground black pepper	

1. In a strainer, pick over and remove any small stones or grit from lentils. Rinse under cool water. Drain and set aside.

2. In base of tagine, heat oil over medium heat. Add onion and carrot. Cook, stirring frequently, for 5 minutes or until slightly softened. Add garlic and cook, stirring frequently, for 2 minutes or until onion and garlic are soft. Stir in ginger, garam masala and curry. Cook, stirring constantly, for 30 seconds.

3. Add lentils, rice, peaches, broth and red wine (if using). Bring to a boil. Cover and bake in preheated oven for 1 hour, stirring once halfway through cooking, until lentils and rice are soft. Season to taste with salt and pepper.

Nutrients per serving	
Calories	369
Fat	5 g
Saturated Fat	1 g
Cholesterol	0 mg
Sodium	127 mg
Carbohydrate	68 g
Fiber	9 g
Sugars	17 g
Protein	15 g
Calcium	62 mg
Iron	5 mg

Tasty Chickpea Cakes

Makes 5 servings

The combination of seasoning and oatmeal, which can't be detected in the final result, makes these cakes — a version of the Middle Eastern specialty falafel — a satisfying main dish.

Tips

In some locations, chickpeas are known as garbanzo beans.

If you prefer, you can use 2 tbsp (30 mL) chopped fresh mint leaves in place of the dried.

- Food processor

$\frac{1}{2}$ cup	rolled oats (quick-cooking or old-fashioned)	125 mL
1 tbsp	freshly squeezed lemon juice	15 mL
1	can (14 to 19 oz/398 to 540 mL) chickpeas, drained and rinsed	1
2 tbsp	coarsely chopped fresh flat-leaf (Italian) parsley	30 mL
1	small onion, coarsely chopped	1
3	cloves garlic, minced	3
2 tsp	cumin seeds	10 mL
2 tsp	dried mint (see tip, at left)	10 mL
1 tsp	chili powder	5 mL
$\frac{1}{2}$ tsp	salt	2 mL
$\frac{1}{4}$ tsp	freshly ground black pepper	1 mL
$\frac{1}{4}$ cup	olive or vegetable oil	60 mL
3 tbsp	cornmeal or bread crumbs	45 mL

1. In food processor, combine oats with lemon juice and pulse three or four times or until blended. Add chickpeas and parsley and pulse 10 times or until chickpeas are ground and mixture is blended but not puréed.

2. Add onion, garlic, cumin seeds, mint, chili powder, salt and pepper. Pulse 5 times or until mixed. (The large pieces of onion and the chickpeas should be broken down, but the mixture should have a coarse texture.)

3. With moistened hands, shape mixture into five cakes, each about $2\frac{1}{2}$ inches (6 cm) in diameter and $\frac{3}{4}$ inch (2 cm) thick. Sprinkle cornmeal on both sides.

4. In a large skillet, heat oil over high heat until hot but not smoking. Add cakes and fry for 1 minute. Reduce heat to medium and fry for 1 to 2 minutes longer or until browned. Flip cakes and fry for 2 to 3 minutes longer or until browned on both sides and hot in the center. Serve immediately.

Variations

Substitute sesame seeds for the cumin seeds.

Add a splash of sesame oil to the vegetable oil when frying the cakes.

Nutrients per serving	
Calories	260
Fat	13 g
Saturated Fat	2 g
Cholesterol	0 mg
Sodium	483 mg
Carbohydrate	31 g
Fiber	5 g
Sugars	1 g
Protein	6 g
Calcium	54 mg
Iron	3 mg

Easy Black Beans

This spicy recipe is great for those rushed days when you're not very organized and are wondering what to make for supper as you drive home.

Tip

If your family doesn't like heat, leave out the chipotle pepper.

1 tsp	vegetable oil	5 mL
1	small onion, chopped	1
1	can (19 oz/540 mL) black beans, drained and rinsed (about 2 cups/500 mL)	1
1½ cups	water	375 mL
½ cup	tomato paste	125 mL
1	chipotle pepper in adobo sauce	1
1	bay leaf	1
1 tsp	ground cumin	5 mL
2 tbsp	chopped fresh cilantro (optional)	30 mL

1. In a large skillet, heat oil over medium heat. Sauté onion until softened, about 5 minutes. Stir in beans, water, tomato paste, chipotle pepper, bay leaf and cumin; bring to a boil. Reduce heat and simmer for 15 minutes or until slightly thickened. Discard the chipotle and bay leaf. (If you leave the chipotle in, the dish will be too spicy!)

2. Ladle into bowls and garnish with cilantro, if desired.

This recipe courtesy of dietitian Chantal Saad Haddad.

Nutrients per serving	
Calories	302
Fat	4 g
Saturated Fat	0 g
Cholesterol	0 mg
Sodium	877 mg
Carbohydrate	52 g
Fiber	14 g
Sugars	11 g
Protein	16 g
Calcium	129 mg
Iron	6 mg

Barbecue Baked Beans

This dish is evidence that vegetarians can also enjoy the robust pleasures of down-home baked beans. The addition of dried mushrooms, miso and smoked paprika provides the rich flavors associated with Southern barbecue.

Tips

For this quantity of beans, use 2 cans (14 to 19 oz/398 to 540 mL) drained and rinsed, or cook 2 cups (500 mL) dried beans.

To make ahead, complete steps 1 and 2. Cover and refrigerate for up to 2 days. When you're ready to cook, complete the recipe.

* Medium (about 4-quart) slow cooker

1	package (¹/₂ oz/14 g) dried porcini mushrooms	1
1 cup	hot water	250 mL
1 tbsp	vegetable oil	15 mL
2	onions, finely chopped	2
4	stalks celery, diced	4
2	carrots, peeled and diced	2
2	cloves garlic, minced	2
1 tsp	minced gingerroot	5 mL
1 tsp	salt	5 mL
1 tsp	cracked black peppercorns	5 mL
1	bay leaf	1
1	2-inch (5 cm) cinnamon stick	1
1	can (14 oz/398 mL) crushed tomatoes	1
4 cups	drained cooked white beans (such as navy)	1 L
¹/₄ cup	pure maple syrup	60 mL
1 tbsp	dark miso	15 mL
1 to 2 tsp	smoked paprika	5 to 10 mL

1. In a bowl, combine dried mushrooms and hot water. Stir well and let stand for 30 minutes. Strain through a fine sieve, reserving mushrooms and liquid separately. Chop mushrooms finely. Set aside.

2. In a skillet, heat oil over medium heat. Add onions, celery and carrots and cook, stirring, until softened, about 7 minutes. Add garlic, ginger, salt, peppercorns, bay leaf, cinnamon stick and reserved mushrooms and cook, stirring, for 1 minute. Stir in crushed tomatoes and reserved mushroom soaking liquid. Transfer to slow cooker stoneware.

3. Add beans and stir well. Cover and cook on Low for 6 hours or on High for 3 hours, until beans are tender. Discard bay leaf and cinnamon.

4. In a small bowl, combine maple syrup, miso and paprika. Add to stoneware and stir well. Cover and cook on High for 20 minutes to meld flavors. Serve hot.

Nutrients per serving	
Calories	287
Fat	4 g
Saturated Fat	0 g
Cholesterol	0 mg
Sodium	623 mg
Carbohydrate	53 g
Fiber	16 g
Sugars	11 g
Protein	13 g
Calcium	155 mg
Iron	5 mg

Cilantro Black Bean Burgers

Just the thing when summer heats up and evening al fresco dining is tops on the schedule.

• Food processor

1/3 cup	rolled spelt flakes	75 mL
1 tsp	ground cumin	5 mL
1 tsp	dried oregano	5 mL
1 tsp	salt	5 mL
1 tsp	freshly ground black pepper	5 mL
1/2 tsp	chipotle pepper powder	2 mL
1/2 tsp	garlic powder	2 mL
2 cups	cooked black beans	500 mL
2 tbsp	grated onion	30 mL
2 tbsp	finely chopped fresh cilantro	30 mL
1/4 cup	cooked short-grain brown rice	60 mL
2 to 4 tbsp	olive oil	30 to 60 mL
1	large tomato, cut into 6 slices	1
1	avocado, sliced	1
1	small red onion, thinly sliced	1
6 to 12	romaine lettuce leaves	6 to 12
1/2 cup	vegan mayonnaise alternative	125 mL
6	burger buns, split and warmed	6

1. In food processor, combine spelt, cumin, oregano, salt, pepper, chipotle powder and garlic powder and pulse to combine, 3 or 4 times. Add beans, onion and cilantro and process until mixture is blended but still chunky, 10 to 20 seconds.

2. Transfer mixture to a bowl and, using your hands, mix in rice. Using clean wet hands, form mixture into 6 patties, about 1 inch (2.5 cm) thick. Place on a plate and let stand for 5 minutes.

3. Place a large, heavy-bottomed skillet over medium heat and let pan get hot. Add 2 tsp (10 mL) oil and tip pan to coat. Using a spatula, carefully place patties into hot oil, in batches as necessary, and cook until bottoms are well browned and slightly crisp, 3 to 4 minutes. Carefully flip burgers and cook until bottoms are browned and burgers are heated through, 2 to 3 minutes. Transfer cooked burgers to plate. Repeat with the remaining patties, adding oil and adjusting heat between batches, as necessary.

4. Place tomato, avocado, red onion and lettuce leaves on a large platter. Scoop chipotle mayonnaise into a small bowl. Serve burgers along with warm buns and pass condiments and spread.

Nutrients per burger	
Calories	376
Fat	16 g
Saturated Fat	3 g
Cholesterol	0 mg
Sodium	709 mg
Carbohydrate	49 g
Fiber	10 g
Sugars	6 g
Protein	11 g
Calcium	96 mg
Iron	3 mg

Baked Orzo and Beans

Makes 4 to 6 servings

Orzo — a jumbo rice lookalike — may be the most versatile of all pastas.

- Preheat oven to 350°F (180°C)
- 10-cup (2.5 L) casserole dish with lid

2½ cups	orzo	625 mL
1 tbsp	olive oil	15 mL
½ cup	sliced red onion	125 mL
2	tomatoes, roughly chopped	2
2 cups	Tomato Sauce (page 246)	500 mL
2 cups	cooked red kidney beans	500 mL
1 cup	tomato juice	250 mL
1 cup	shaved Parmesan cheese	250 mL
1 tbsp	extra virgin olive oil	15 mL
	A few sprigs fresh parsley, chopped	
	Grated Romano cheese (optional)	

1. In a large pot of boiling salted water, cook orzo until al dente, about 10 minutes.

2. Meanwhile, in a skillet, heat oil over high heat for 30 seconds; add onion and cook, stirring, for 1 or 2 minutes, until slightly charred. Remove from heat and set aside.

3. When orzo is cooked, drain well and transfer to casserole. Add sautéed onions to orzo and stir to combine. Add tomatoes and tomato sauce; mix thoroughly. Add cooked beans; fold until evenly distributed.

4. Cover orzo mixture and bake in preheated oven, covered, for 30 minutes. Remove from oven and mix in tomato juice. Top with Parmesan shavings and return to the oven, uncovered, for another 10 to 12 minutes, until the cheese is melted. Serve on pasta plates, making sure each portion is topped with some of the melted cheese. Drizzle a few drops of extra virgin olive oil on each portion and garnish with chopped parsley. Serve immediately, with Romano (if using) as an accompaniment.

Nutrients per serving (1 of 6)	
Calories	402
Fat	15 g
Saturated Fat	4 g
Cholesterol	12 mg
Sodium	350 mg
Carbohydrate	51 g
Fiber	8 g
Sugars	8 g
Protein	17 g
Calcium	207 mg
Iron	4 mg

Jamaican Peas and Cauliflower "Rice"

Makes 4 servings

Coconut oil, allspice and thyme, together with cauliflower "rice" and dark red kidney beans, give this oh-so-easy side dish its down-island flavor.

Tip

Instead of using a food processor, grate the cauliflower florets using the large holes of a cheese grater.

- Food processor

1	small to medium head cauliflower, ends trimmed	1
3 tbsp	virgin coconut oil	45 mL
2	cloves garlic, minced	2
1/2 tsp	ground allspice	2 mL
1 tsp	dried thyme	5 mL
1/2 tsp	fine sea salt	2 mL
1/2 tsp	hot pepper sauce	2 mL
1	can (14 to 19 oz/398 to 540 mL) dark red kidney beans, drained and rinsed	1
1/2 cup	chopped green onions	125 mL

1. Cut or break cauliflower into large florets. Place half the florets in food processor and process until the size and texture of rice. Transfer to a large bowl and repeat with the remaining cauliflower.

2. In a large skillet, melt coconut oil over low heat. Add garlic and allspice; cook, stirring, for 1 minute or until fragrant. Add cauliflower, thyme, salt and hot pepper sauce. Increase heat to medium-high and cook, stirring, for 3 to 4 minutes or until cauliflower is softened.

3. Stir in beans and green onions; cook, stirring, for 2 to 3 minutes or until beans are warmed through.

Nutrients per serving	
Calories	216
Fat	11 g
Saturated Fat	9 g
Cholesterol	0 mg
Sodium	668 mg
Carbohydrate	24 g
Fiber	9 g
Sugars	5 g
Protein	8 g
Calcium	75 mg
Iron	2 mg

Barbecue Barley and Sweet Potato Chili

Makes 6 servings

This unusual chili has great flavor. Serve with a simple green salad topped with sliced avocado.

Tips

Use the type of barley you prefer — pearled, pot or whole. Whole (also known as hulled) barley is the most nutritious form of the grain.

Use your favorite chili powder blend in this recipe or, if you prefer, ground ancho, New Mexico or guajillo peppers.

To make ahead, complete step 1. Cover and refrigerate for up to 2 days. When you're ready to cook, complete the recipe. Because the barley soaks up liquid on sitting, add an extra 1/2 cup (125 mL) stock or water before cooking.

Nutrients per serving	
Calories	257
Fat	4 g
Saturated Fat	0 g
Cholesterol	0 mg
Sodium	653 mg
Carbohydrate	49 g
Fiber	12 g
Sugars	4 g
Protein	10 g
Calcium	110 mg
Iron	5 mg

• Medium to large (3½- to 5-quart) slow cooker

1 tbsp	vegetable oil	15 mL
2	onions, finely chopped	2
2	cloves garlic, minced	2
1 tbsp	ground cumin (see tip, page 303)	15 mL
1 tsp	dried oregano, crumbled	5 mL
1 tsp	salt	5 mL
1/2 tsp	cracked black peppercorns	2 mL
1/2 cup	barley (see tip, at left)	125 mL
1	can (28 oz/796 mL) tomatoes, with juice, coarsely crushed	1
1 cup	Vegetable Stock (page 212) or ready-to-use vegetable broth	250 mL
2	sweet potatoes, peeled and cut into 1-inch (2.5 cm) cubes	2
2 cups	cooked red kidney or black beans	500 mL
1 tbsp	chili powder, dissolved in 2 tbsp (30 mL) freshly squeezed lime juice	15 mL
1	jalapeño pepper, minced (or 1/2 to 1 canned chipotle pepper in adobo sauce, minced)	1
1	green bell pepper, finely chopped (optional)	1
	Sliced roasted bell peppers (optional)	
	Finely chopped fresh cilantro	

1. In a large skillet, heat oil over medium heat. Add onions and cook, stirring, until softened, about 3 minutes. Add garlic, cumin, oregano, salt and peppercorns and cook, stirring, for 1 minute. Add barley and toss to coat. Add tomatoes and bring to a boil. Transfer to slow cooker stoneware.

2. Add stock, sweet potatoes and beans. Cover and cook on Low for 6 to 8 hours or on High for 3 to 4 hours, until barley and sweet potatoes are tender. Stir in chili powder solution, jalapeño pepper and green pepper (if using). Cover and cook on High for 20 to 30 minutes, until flavors have melded and green pepper is tender. To serve, ladle into soup plates and garnish with roasted peppers (if using) and cilantro.

Baked Plantain and Peanut Stew

Makes 6 servings

Here is another great stuffing for wraps and vegetables. Once baked and cooked in the stew, the plantains or bananas lose their characteristic banana taste. They are an excellent stew ingredient because they thicken the mixture.

Tips

Plantains usually arrive at supermarkets green and hard. Store in a paper bag for 1 or 2 days to ripen quickly. Plantains turn yellow with solid black splotches when ripe.

For this recipe, try Lundberg short-grain brown rice, which is soft and chewy when cooked. Long-grain brown rice, red rice or a blend of your favorites will also work.

- Preheat oven to 375°F (190°C)
- Baking sheet

2	large ripe plantains (or 3 large ripe bananas)	2
2 tbsp	olive oil	30 mL
1	onion, chopped	1
2	cloves garlic, minced	2
1	jalapeño pepper, finely chopped	1
1/2 cup	brown rice (see tip, at left)	125 mL
1 tbsp	grated gingerroot	15 mL
1 tsp	ground cumin	5 mL
1 to 2 tsp	garam masala	5 to 10 mL
1 tsp	sea salt	5 mL
1/4 tsp	ground nutmeg	1 mL
2 cups	ready-to-use mushroom broth, vegetable broth or water	500 mL
1	can (28 oz/796 mL) stewed or crushed tomatoes, with juice	1
1/2 cup	chunky peanut butter	125 mL
1/2 cup	coarsely chopped peanuts	125 mL

1. Trim tops off plantains and place on baking sheet. Bake in preheated oven for 15 minutes or until peel is charred and puffy. Let cool. Slice in half lengthwise and peel off skin. Coarsely chop flesh and set aside.

2. In a saucepan, heat oil over medium heat. Add onion and cook, stirring occasionally, for 5 minutes or until slightly softened. Add garlic and jalapeño and cook, stirring frequently, for 3 minutes or until vegetables are tender. Add rice, ginger, cumin, garam masala to taste, salt and nutmeg and cook, stirring constantly, for 1 minute.

3. Stir in broth and tomatoes and bring to a boil. Add baked plantains and peanut butter and stir well. Cover, reduce heat to low and simmer for 45 minutes or until rice is tender. Ladle into bowls and garnish with peanuts.

Nutrients per serving	
Calories	416
Fat	22 g
Saturated Fat	3 g
Cholesterol	0 mg
Sodium	830 mg
Carbohydrate	49 g
Fiber	7 g
Sugars	17 g
Protein	12 g
Calcium	85 mg
Iron	4 mg

Spicy Tofu with Vegetables

Vegetarian festivals are celebrated in Thailand, with a large one held in Phuket around October. Spicy tofu is often one of the specialties on offer.

3 tbsp	vegetable oil, divided	45 mL
12 oz	firm tofu, patted dry, cut into 1/2-inch (1 cm) cubes	375 g
3	shallots, thinly sliced	3
2	cloves garlic, thinly sliced	2
1	carrot, cut into matchstick pieces	1
1/2	red bell pepper, cut into thin strips	1/2
1 cup	sliced asparagus or green beans, cut into 1-inch (2.5 cm) pieces	250 mL
2 tbsp	soy sauce	30 mL
2 tbsp	freshly squeezed lime juice	30 mL
2 1/2 tsp	chopped fresh red chile pepper	12 mL
2 tsp	granulated sugar	10 mL
1/2 tsp	freshly ground black pepper	2 mL

1. Heat a wok or large skillet over medium-high heat and add 2 tbsp (30 mL) oil. Add tofu and stir-fry for 4 minutes, turning carefully, until golden brown. Remove with a slotted spoon and reserve.

2. Add the remaining oil to wok. Add shallots and garlic and stir-fry for 1 minute.

3. Add carrot, red pepper and asparagus and stir-fry for 2 minutes.

4. Add soy sauce, lime juice, chile, sugar and pepper and cook, stirring, for 1 minute.

5. Return tofu to wok and cook for 1 minute or until combined and heated through.

Nutrients per serving	
Calories	250
Fat	18 g
Saturated Fat	2 g
Cholesterol	0 mg
Sodium	527 mg
Carbohydrate	11 g
Fiber	3 g
Sugars	4 g
Protein	15 g
Calcium	598 mg
Iron	3 mg

Baked Curried Tofu with Tomato Masala

Two stages of cooking infuse the tofu with deep flavor and a jammy-textured curry coating. They also make it look very appetizing, elevating humble tofu into a dish fit for company.

• Baking sheet, lined with parchment paper

12 oz	firm or extra-firm tofu, drained	375 g
1 tbsp	vegetable oil	15 mL
1 or 2	hot green chile peppers, minced	1 or 2
10	curry leaves	10
½ tsp	garam masala	2 mL
1 cup	Basic Gravy (page 153)	250 mL
1 cup	canned crushed (ground) tomatoes	250 mL
½ cup	water	125 mL
1 tbsp	soy sauce	15 mL
	Chopped fresh cilantro	
	Plain yogurt (optional)	

1. On a cutting board, stand block of tofu on one long, narrow side. Cut lengthwise into 3 slices. Cut each slice in half to make 2 squares and cut each square diagonally to make triangles. Set aside.

2. In a large nonstick skillet, heat oil over medium heat until hot but not smoking. Add chiles, curry leaves and garam masala; cook, stirring, until fragrant, about 1 minute. Add gravy and cook, stirring, for 1 minute. Add tomatoes, water and soy sauce; bring to a boil, stirring.

3. Add tofu and turn to coat in sauce. Reduce heat and simmer, turning tofu once, until sauce is very thick, about 15 minutes. Discard curry leaves, if desired.

4. Meanwhile, preheat oven to 400°F (200°C).

Nutrients per serving	
Calories	212
Fat	13 g
Saturated Fat	2 g
Cholesterol	0 mg
Sodium	613 mg
Carbohydrate	14 g
Fiber	4 g
Sugars	2 g
Protein	16 g
Calcium	636 mg
Iron	4 mg

5. Using a slotted spatula, transfer tofu pieces, with sauce clinging to them, to prepared baking sheet, placing them at least 1 inch (2.5 cm) apart. Set any remaining sauce aside.

6. Bake until tofu is glazed and sauce is lightly browned, about 15 minutes. Serve sprinkled with cilantro and reserved sauce and topped with yogurt (if using).

Variations

Add shredded mozzarella cheese on top of tofu for the last 5 minutes of baking in step 6.

To grill tofu instead of baking, preheat grill to medium. Place tofu and sauce on a large piece of greased foil on grill. Cover and grill until sauce is lightly browned, about 10 minutes.

Teriyaki Tempeh Satay with Peanut Sauce

Makes 4 to 6 servings

Crispy teriyaki tempeh provides just the right crunch drizzled with a smooth and spicy peanut sauce. Super easy and very festive, this dish is perfect piled high on rice and served with bright sautéed pea greens and garlic.

Tip

Peanut sauce can be made ahead and refrigerated in an airtight container for up to 1 week. Bring to room temperature before using.

- Blender

Peanut Sauce

1 cup	unsweetened natural peanut butter	250 mL
2 tbsp	coconut milk	30 mL
2 tbsp	tamari	30 mL
2 tbsp	agave nectar	30 mL
1 tbsp	freshly squeezed lime juice	15 mL
1 tsp	garlic chile sauce	5 mL
1/4 to 1/2 cup	hot water	60 to 125 mL

Teriyaki Tempeh Satay

2 cups	peanut oil	500 mL
2	packages (each 8 oz/250 g) teriyaki tempeh, cut lengthwise into 1/2-inch (1 cm) strips	2

1. *Peanut Sauce:* In blender, combine peanut butter, coconut milk, tamari, agave, lime juice and garlic chile sauce and purée until smooth, drizzling in hot water as needed to thin sauce. Set aside.

2. *Satay:* In a large, heavy-bottomed saucepan, heat oil over high heat. When a small crumb of tempeh dropped into oil immediately sizzles, oil is ready. Working in batches, carefully place tempeh in hot oil and fry until light brown and crispy, 3 to 4 minutes. Using a slotted spoon, remove from oil and transfer to a plate lined with paper towels. Serve hot with peanut sauce for dipping.

Nutrients per serving (1 of 6)

Calories	513
Fat	35 g
Saturated Fat	6 g
Cholesterol	0 mg
Sodium	388 mg
Carbohydrate	34 g
Fiber	9 g
Sugars	8 g
Protein	22 g
Calcium	127 mg
Iron	2 mg

Vegetables

Jerusalem Artichoke Stew 286

Yummy Asparagus 287

Garlic-Spiked Bok Choy 287

Spicy Kimchi 288

Eggplant with Green Chiles 289

Curried Green Beans Masala 290

Cheesy Shoestring Jicama Fries 291

Leek and Tomato Cobbler 292

Stir-Fried Shiitakes with Garlic 293

Mushroom, Tomato and Asparagus Toss 294

Green Pea and Asparagus Curry 295

Sugar Snap Peas with Cherry Tomatoes 296

Creamed Garlic Spinach 297

Calabrese Swiss Chard. 298

Stuffed Zucchini 299

Stir-Fried Mixed Vegetables 300

Veggie Kabobs 301

Curried Root Vegetables Masala 302

Squash with Quinoa and Apricots 303

Green Thai Curry with Spinach and Sweet Potatoes 304

Curried Spinach and Potatoes with Yogurt. 305

Garlic Mashed Potatoes. 306

Layered Artichokes and Potatoes 307

Crispy Coconut French Fries. 308

Jerusalem Artichoke Stew

Makes 4 to 6 servings

While most stews are robust and full of texture and flavor, this one is delicate, with a subtle yet no less complex taste. It takes advantage of the autumn harvest of Jerusalem artichokes, native to eastern North America. These root vegetables are also known as sunchokes, earth apples or Canadian potatoes.

Tips

If you have homemade Vegetable Stock (page 212) on hand, use it in this recipe in place of store-bought broth.

Using reduced-sodium broth will lower the sodium content of each serving to 313 mg.

You can use 2 cups (500 mL) cooked white beans, drained and rinsed, instead of canned.

Nutrients per serving (1 of 6)	
Calories	146
Fat	3 g
Saturated Fat	0 g
Cholesterol	0 mg
Sodium	846 mg
Carbohydrate	25 g
Fiber	5 g
Sugars	9 g
Protein	5 g
Calcium	51 mg
Iron	3 mg

1 tbsp	olive oil	15 mL
1	onion, chopped	1
2	stalks celery, chopped	2
2	cloves garlic, finely chopped	2
4 cups	ready-to-use vegetable broth or water	1 L
2 cups	diced Jerusalem artichokes or potatoes	500 mL
1	carrot, diced	1
1/2 cup	shredded rutabaga or green cabbage	125 mL
1/4 cup	dry white wine	60 mL
1	can (14 to 19 oz/398 to 540 mL) cannellini beans or flageolets, drained and rinsed	1
3 tbsp	chopped fresh parsley	45 mL
2 tbsp	freshly squeezed lemon juice	30 mL
	Sea salt and freshly ground black pepper	

1. In a large saucepan, heat oil over medium heat. Add onion and celery and cook, stirring occasionally, for 6 to 8 minutes or until soft. Add garlic and cook, stirring frequently, for 2 minutes. Add broth. Increase heat to high and bring to a boil. Add Jerusalem artichokes, carrot, rutabaga and white wine. Cover, reduce heat to medium-low and simmer, stirring once or twice, for 15 minutes or until vegetables are tender when pierced with the tip of a knife.

2. Add beans, parsley and lemon juice and heat through. Season to taste with salt and pepper. Using a potato masher, mash some of the vegetables to thicken the stew.

Yummy Asparagus

1 tbsp	butter	15 mL
1	bunch asparagus, ends trimmed	1
1	clove garlic, minced	1
1 tbsp	freshly grated Parmesan cheese	15 mL

Makes 2 to 4 servings

1. In a medium saucepan, melt butter over medium heat. Sauté asparagus and garlic, shaking pan constantly, until just tender, about 5 minutes. Sprinkle with cheese and allow it to melt before serving.

This recipe courtesy of dietitian Roberta Lowcay.

Nutrients per serving (1 of 4)

Calories	47
Fat	3 g
Saturated Fat	2 g
Cholesterol	9 mg
Sodium	21 mg
Carbohydrate	3 g
Fiber	2 g
Sugars	1 g
Protein	2 g
Calcium	34 mg
Iron	2 mg

Garlic-Spiked Bok Choy

Makes 4 servings

This simple, traditional stir-fry might inspire you to include bok choy on your weekly grocery list.

1	head bok choy (about 1¼ lbs/625 g)	1
2 tbsp	vegetable oil	30 mL
1 tbsp	chopped garlic	15 mL
1 tsp	salt (or to taste)	5 mL
2 tbsp	water	30 mL

1. Trim 2 to 3 inches (5 to 7.5 cm) from the base of bok choy (discard any wilted outer leaves). Halve bok choy lengthwise and place each half cut side down on a cutting board. Cut it crosswise into 2-inch (5 cm) pieces. Transfer to a large bowl and toss with your hands to separate into individual pieces. (You will need about 6 cups/1.5 L.)

2. Heat a wok or a large, deep skillet over medium-high heat. Add oil and swirl to coat pan. Add garlic and salt and toss well, until garlic is fragrant, about 30 seconds. Add bok choy and cook, undisturbed, about 1 minute. Toss well.

3. Add water and continue cooking, tossing occasionally, until bok choy is tender-crisp, 1 to 2 minutes more. Transfer to a serving plate. Serve hot, warm or at room temperature.

Nutrients per serving

Calories	92
Fat	8 g
Saturated Fat	1 g
Cholesterol	0 mg
Sodium	674 mg
Carbohydrate	4 g
Fiber	1 g
Sugars	2 g
Protein	2 g
Calcium	149 mg
Iron	1 mg

Spicy Kimchi

Makes 6 to 8 servings

This fermented Korean side dish lends a spicy crunch to any meal. The healthy bacteria created in this process make it great for the digestion. Indulge your health and eat it daily. It's great with salads, rice, beans, mashed potatoes and eggs.

Tips

You want to make sure that you don't have large chunks of salt remaining after rinsing. Gently grinding the salt in a mortar, or with a rolling pin on a cutting board, will achieve this result.

Look for Korean chili powder in well-stocked Asian markets. If you can't find it, substitute 2 tsp (10 mL) paprika and 1 tsp (5 mL) hot pepper flakes.

- Sealable glass container (about 16 cups/4 L)

8 cups	packed chopped napa cabbage (2-inch/2.5 cm squares)	2 L
1 cup	coarse sea salt, gently ground (see tip, at left)	250 mL
¼ cup	chopped green onions (white and green parts)	60 mL
3 tbsp	Korean chili powder (see tip, at left)	45 mL
2 tbsp	tamari	30 mL
2 tbsp	raw agave nectar	30 mL
2 tsp	chopped gingerroot	10 mL
2	cloves garlic, minced	2

1. In a bowl, combine cabbage and salt and toss until well combined. Cover and set aside at room temperature for 2 to 4 hours, until wilted. Transfer to a colander and rinse well under cold running water. Drain well and use your hands to squeeze out any excess liquid.

2. Transfer to a clean bowl and add green onions, chili powder, tamari, agave nectar, ginger and garlic. Toss until well combined.

3. Transfer to a sealable glass container and pack down tightly, using your hands or a wooden spoon to press out as much air as possible. Place plastic wrap directly on the surface of the kimchi to prevent contact with air and seal the lid tightly. Store in a cool, dry place for 4 to 5 days or until the mixture begins to take on a slightly sour taste. Transfer to the refrigerator and store for up to a month.

Nutrients per serving (1 of 8)	
Calories	39
Fat	1 g
Saturated Fat	0 g
Cholesterol	0 mg
Sodium	309 mg
Carbohydrate	8 g
Fiber	2 g
Sugars	4 g
Protein	2 g
Calcium	38 mg
Iron	1 mg

Eggplant with Green Chiles

Coddled in a fiery sauce, this eggplant turns out tender and flavorful.

Tip

The long, tender Asian-style eggplant works best for this recipe. Cut crosswise into thin slices of even thickness for even cooking.

3 tbsp	vegetable oil	45 mL
1	onion, diced	1
½ tsp	salt	2 mL
½ tsp	hot pepper flakes	2 mL
½ tsp	freshly ground black pepper	2 mL
½ tsp	ground cumin	2 mL
2	hot green chile peppers, thickly sliced	2
1 tsp	ground turmeric	5 mL
½ cup	water	125 mL
2 cups	thinly sliced eggplant	500 mL
8	curry leaves	8
	Chopped fresh cilantro	

1. In a large skillet, heat oil over medium heat. Add onion, salt, hot pepper flakes, black pepper and cumin; cook, stirring, until onion starts to soften, about 2 minutes. Add chiles and turmeric; cook, stirring, for 30 seconds.

2. Stir in water and bring to a simmer. Gently fold in eggplant and curry leaves until coated in sauce. Cover, reduce heat to medium-low and simmer, without stirring, until eggplant is tender, about 6 minutes. Season to taste with salt. Serve sprinkled with cilantro.

Nutrients per serving	
Calories	124
Fat	11 g
Saturated Fat	1 g
Cholesterol	0 mg
Sodium	296 mg
Carbohydrate	7 g
Fiber	2 g
Sugars	3 g
Protein	1 g
Calcium	26 mg
Iron	1 mg

Curried Green Beans Masala

Makes 4 to 6 servings

Cooked through but still textured green beans in a fragrant sauce make for an easy side course to more substantial curries. The beans will get softer the longer they wait in their sauce, so they should be served as soon as they are ready.

Tips

Blanching the beans before adding them to the sauce ensures that they will have a nice, tender-crisp texture. The acid in the tomato can prevent the beans from softening.

If you want to blanch the beans ahead of time, rinse immediately in cold water until chilled after step 1. Drain, cover and refrigerate for up to 1 day.

8 oz	green beans, trimmed	250 g
1 tbsp	vegetable oil	15 mL
1 tsp	mustard seeds	5 mL
1/2 tsp	cumin seeds	2 mL
1	large tomato, diced	1
10	fresh curry leaves	10
1/2 cup	Basic Gravy (page 153)	125 mL
1/4 cup	water	60 mL
	Salt	

1. In a saucepan of boiling salted water, cook green beans just until bright green and slightly tender, about 3 minutes. Drain and set aside.

2. In a large skillet, heat oil over medium heat until hot but not smoking. Add mustard seeds and cumin seeds; cook, stirring, until toasted and fragrant but not yet popping, about 30 seconds. Add tomato and curry leaves; cook, stirring, until tomato is softened, about 2 minutes.

3. Add gravy and cook, stirring, for 1 minute. Add water and bring to a boil, stirring. Reduce heat and boil gently for 3 minutes. Add green beans and cook, stirring often, just until tender-crisp, about 3 minutes. Season to taste with salt.

Nutrients per serving (1 of 6)	
Calories	51
Fat	3 g
Saturated Fat	0 g
Cholesterol	0 mg
Sodium	91 mg
Carbohydrate	5 g
Fiber	2 g
Sugars	3 g
Protein	1 g
Calcium	34 mg
Iron	1 mg

Cheesy Shoestring Jicama Fries

Makes 4 to 6 servings

The marinade for this recipe not only helps break down the texture of the jicama but also provides a rich, cheesy flavor.

Tips

Jicama tastes like a blend of apple, potato and celery. It is mildly sweet and has a high water content.

To trim the jicama, use a chef's knife to remove a small slice from all four sides to square it off before peeling.

If you prefer fatter fries, after cutting the jicama into slices, cut it into strips approximately 1 inch (2.5 cm) wide.

- Mandoline
- Blender

1	large jicama, peeled (see tips, at left)	1
1/2 cup	whole raw cashews	125 mL
1/2 cup	nutritional yeast	125 mL
1/4 cup	filtered water	60 mL
1/4 cup	cold-pressed extra virgin olive oil	60 mL
3 tbsp	freshly squeezed lemon juice	45 mL
1/2 tsp	fine sea salt	2 mL

1. Using mandoline, slice jicama lengthwise into pieces approximately 1/4 inch (0.5 cm) thick. Stack the slices on top of each other and, using a sharp chef's knife, cut lengthwise into strips approximately 1/4 inch (0.5 cm) wide. Cover and set aside.

2. In blender, combine cashews, nutritional yeast, water, olive oil, lemon juice and salt. Blend at high speed until smooth.

3. In a bowl, toss jicama strips with sauce until well coated. Serve immediately or cover and refrigerate for up to 2 days.

Nutrients per serving (1 of 6)	
Calories	238
Fat	15 g
Saturated Fat	2 g
Cholesterol	0 mg
Sodium	244 mg
Carbohydrate	24 g
Fiber	11 g
Sugars	4 g
Protein	5 g
Calcium	30 mg
Iron	2 mg

Leek and Tomato Cobbler

If you like tomatoes, you'll enjoy this cobbler. The addition of sun-dried tomatoes intensifies the tomato flavor. Combined with sweet, mild leeks and a hint of Italian seasoning, this makes a very tasty main course.

Tips

Use no-salt-added canned tomatoes to reduce the sodium content of this recipe.

Sun-dried tomatoes packed in olive oil are already reconstituted. If you are using the packaged dry variety, reconstitute them according to the package directions — they usually need to be blanched for about 5 minutes in boiling water.

To make ahead, complete step 1. Cover and refrigerate for up to 2 days. When you're ready to cook, complete the recipe.

Nutrients per serving	
Calories	150
Fat	6 g
Saturated Fat	1 g
Cholesterol	1 mg
Sodium	784 mg
Carbohydrate	22 g
Fiber	3 g
Sugars	5 g
Protein	3 g
Calcium	106 mg
Iron	1 mg

• Small to medium (2- to 4-quart) slow cooker

2 tbsp	olive oil	30 mL
3	leeks (white and light green parts only), cleaned (see tip, page 268) and sliced	3
4	cloves garlic, minced	4
1 tsp	salt	5 mL
1 tsp	dried Italian seasoning	5 mL
1/2 tsp	cracked black peppercorns	2 mL
2 tbsp	all-purpose flour	30 mL
1	can (28 oz/796 mL) diced tomatoes, with juice	1
2 tbsp	finely chopped reconstituted sun-dried tomatoes (see tip, at left)	30 mL
1 cup	shredded Swiss cheese (optional)	250 mL

Topping

3/4 cup	all-purpose flour	175 mL
1/4 tsp	salt	1 mL
1 tsp	baking soda	5 mL
1/3 cup	buttermilk	75 mL
1 tbsp	olive oil	15 mL

1. In a skillet, heat oil over medium heat. Add leeks and cook, stirring, until softened, about 5 minutes. Add garlic, salt, Italian seasoning and peppercorns and cook, stirring, for 1 minute. Add flour and cook, stirring, for 1 minute. Add diced tomatoes and sun-dried tomatoes and cook, stirring, until mixture comes to a boil and thickens, about 5 minutes. Transfer to slow cooker stoneware.

2. Cover and cook on Low for 4 hours or on High for 1 1/2 hours. Stir in cheese (if using) and turn heat to High, if necessary.

3. *Topping:* In a bowl, combine flour and salt. Make a well in the middle. In a cup or bowl with a pouring spout, combine baking soda, buttermilk and olive oil. Pour into well and mix until blended. Drop batter by spoonfuls over hot vegetable mixture. Cover and cook on High for 45 minutes, until a tester inserted in the center comes out clean.

Stir-Fried Shiitakes with Garlic

Mushrooms develop deep flavor and a pleasing texture when stir-fried. This dish goes especially well with a main course of grilled salmon or steak and a salad tossed with a bright and tangy dressing.

Tip

If you have homemade Vegetable Stock (page 212) on hand, use it in this recipe in place of store-bought broth.

¼ cup	ready-to-use vegetable broth or water	60 mL
1 tsp	granulated sugar	5 mL
1 tsp	salt (or to taste)	5 mL
8 oz	shiitake mushrooms	250 g
8 oz	button mushrooms	250 g
3	green onions	3
2 tbsp	vegetable oil	30 mL
2 tbsp	coarsely chopped garlic	30 mL
2 tbsp	thinly sliced shallots or finely chopped onion	30 mL
½ tsp	freshly ground black pepper	2 mL

1. In a small bowl, combine broth, sugar and salt and stir well. Set aside.

2. Prepare shiitakes by removing and discarding stems. Slice caps crosswise into ½-inch (1 cm) strips. Slice button mushrooms, including stems, crosswise into thin slices. Trim green onions and chop white parts coarsely. Chop green tops into 1-inch (2.5 cm) lengths. Set green onions aside separately from mushrooms.

3. Heat a wok or a large, deep skillet over high heat. Add oil and swirl to coat pan. Add garlic and shallots and toss well, until garlic is fragrant, about 15 seconds.

4. Add shiitake and button mushrooms and spread into a single layer. Cook, undisturbed, for 1 minute. Toss well. Cook, tossing once or twice, until mushrooms start to release their liquid and soften, 1 minute more.

5. Add broth mixture and toss well. Cook, tossing once, until mushrooms are tender, 1 to 2 minutes more.

6. Add pepper and green onions and cook for 1 minute more. Toss once. Transfer to a serving plate. Serve hot or warm.

Nutrients per serving	
Calories	126
Fat	8 g
Saturated Fat	1 g
Cholesterol	0 mg
Sodium	649 mg
Carbohydrate	10 g
Fiber	2 g
Sugars	4 g
Protein	3 g
Calcium	9 mg
Iron	1 mg

Mushroom, Tomato and Asparagus Toss

Colorful and delicious, this dish is especially fine served over grilled or fried polenta, buttered grits or a rice pilaf.

Tips

If you have homemade Vegetable Stock (page 212) on hand, use it in this recipe in place of store-bought broth.

Before slicing portobello mushroom caps for this recipe, scrape out the dark gills lining the cap. Use a spoon to scoop them out, starting at the stem area and pulling outward to the edge of the cap.

3 tbsp	dry sherry or Shaoxing rice wine	45 mL
2 tbsp	soy sauce	30 mL
1 tbsp	ready-to-use vegetable broth or water	15 mL
1/2 tsp	granulated sugar	2 mL
1/2 tsp	salt (or to taste)	2 mL
1 lb	fresh asparagus	500 g
8 oz	portobello mushroom caps (see tip, at left)	250 g
2 tbsp	vegetable oil	30 mL
1 tbsp	chopped onion	15 mL
1 tbsp	chopped gingerroot	15 mL
2 tsp	chopped garlic	10 mL
3/4 cup	halved cherry tomatoes	175 mL
3 tbsp	chopped fresh cilantro	45 mL
2 tsp	Asian sesame oil	10 mL

1. In a small bowl, combine sherry, soy sauce, broth, sugar and salt and stir well. Set aside.

2. Trim asparagus by snapping off ends. Cut each asparagus spear on the diagonal into 1/4-inch (0.5 cm) pieces, leaving the tips whole. You should have about 3 cups (750 mL) chopped asparagus. Set aside.

3. Quarter mushrooms and then thinly slice each section into 1/4-inch (0.5 cm) thick pieces. Set aside.

4. Heat a wok or a large deep skillet over high heat. Add vegetable oil and swirl to coat pan. Add onion, ginger and garlic and toss well, until fragrant, about 15 seconds.

5. Add mushrooms and toss well. Spread into a single layer and cook, undisturbed, for 30 seconds. Add asparagus and toss well. Cook, tossing often, until both vegetables have begun to wilt, 1 minute.

6. Add sherry mixture, pouring in around sides of pan. Toss well. Cook, tossing occasionally, until asparagus is tender-crisp, 1 to 2 minutes more.

7. Add cherry tomatoes, cilantro and sesame oil and toss well. Transfer to a serving plate. Serve hot or warm.

Nutrients per serving (1 of 6)	
Calories	104
Fat	7 g
Saturated Fat	1 g
Cholesterol	0 mg
Sodium	584 mg
Carbohydrate	7 g
Fiber	2 g
Sugars	4 g
Protein	3 g
Calcium	23 mg
Iron	2 mg

Green Pea and Asparagus Curry

Makes 4 to 6 servings

The onions melt into a sweet, spicy sauce for the fresh peas and asparagus.

Tip

To chop the onions for this sauce, use a food processor, not a blender, which will liquefy them. The onions should be chopped into a fine mash but not liquefied, because the water will separate out at that point. Yellow cooking onions are best for this purpose (sweet varieties have a higher water content).

• Food processor

4	onions, cut in half, divided	4
2 tbsp	vegetable oil	30 mL
1 to 2 tbsp	curry powder	15 to 30 mL
2 tsp	natural cane sugar (optional)	10 mL
2	tomatoes, chopped	2
2 cups	fresh or frozen green peas	500 mL
2 cups	fresh or frozen asparagus pieces	500 mL
1 tbsp	freshly squeezed lemon juice	15 mL
¼ cup	chopped fresh cilantro or flat-leaf (Italian) parsley	60 mL

1. Thinly slice $1\frac{1}{2}$ onions and set aside. Using food processor, chop the remaining onions into a coarse pulp (see tip, at left).

2. In a saucepan or skillet, heat oil over medium-high heat. Add sliced onions. Cover, reduce heat to low and sweat onions for 8 to 10 minutes or until very soft. Add onion pulp and curry powder. Cook over medium-high heat, stirring frequently, for 5 minutes or until any liquid has disappeared. Add sugar (if using) and stir until dissolved. Add tomatoes, green peas, asparagus and lemon juice. Reduce heat and simmer, stirring once or twice, for 8 to 10 minutes or until vegetables are tender when pierced with the tip of a knife. Garnish with cilantro.

Variation

Substitute shelled fresh or frozen edamame (green soybeans) for the peas.

Nutrients per serving (1 of 6)	
Calories	119
Fat	5 g
Saturated Fat	0 g
Cholesterol	0 mg
Sodium	8 mg
Carbohydrate	15 g
Fiber	5 g
Sugars	7 g
Protein	5 g
Calcium	43 mg
Iron	2 mg

Sugar Snap Peas with Cherry Tomatoes

Makes 4 servings

Sugar snap peas burst with sweet, juicy flavor. Here they're cooked quickly with ginger and garlic. Cherry tomatoes tossed in at the end of cooking need only a quick turn in the hot pan to complete this pleasing dish.

8 oz	sugar snap peas (about 3 cups/750 mL)	250 g
¼ cup	water	60 mL
2 tsp	soy sauce	10 mL
1 tsp	granulated sugar	5 mL
½ tsp	salt (or to taste)	2 mL
2 tbsp	vegetable oil	30 mL
2 tsp	finely chopped gingerroot	10 mL
1 tsp	coarsely chopped garlic	5 mL
1 cup	halved cherry tomatoes	250 mL
1 tsp	Asian sesame oil	5 mL

1. Trim sugar snap peas, cutting off stem end and pulling it along straight edge to remove any strings.

2. In a small bowl, combine water, soy sauce, sugar and salt and stir well. Set aside.

3. Heat a wok or a large, deep skillet over high heat. Add vegetable oil and swirl to coat pan. Add ginger and garlic and toss well Add sugar snap peas and cook, undisturbed, for 1 minute.

4. Add soy sauce mixture to pan and toss once. Reduce heat to medium. Continue cooking, tossing occasionally, until peas are vivid green and tender-crisp, about 2 minutes more.

5. Add cherry tomatoes and sesame oil and toss once. Transfer to a serving plate. Serve hot or warm.

Nutrients per serving	
Calories	126
Fat	8 g
Saturated Fat	1 g
Cholesterol	0 mg
Sodium	461 mg
Carbohydrate	12 g
Fiber	3 g
Sugars	5 g
Protein	3 g
Calcium	46 mg
Iron	1 mg

Creamed Garlic Spinach

Creamy, garlicky spinach is a classic flavor combination. This healthier raw version retains all the nutritional content of the baby spinach and garlic while sacrificing none of the original dish's taste.

Tips

You may substitute 2 bunches roughly chopped field or bunched spinach for the baby spinach.

Garlic cloves come in all sizes. If the cloves you are using are large, reduce the amount called for in this recipe to 2 cloves. If they are small, increase to 8 cloves. Remember, you can always add more but you can't take away, so be careful not to overdo it.

To reduce the sodium content of this recipe, use less salt.

- Blender

4 cups	packed baby spinach	1 L
2 tbsp	cold-pressed extra virgin olive oil	30 mL
3 tbsp	freshly squeezed lemon juice, divided	45 mL
1 tsp	fine sea salt, divided	5 mL
1 cup	whole raw cashews	250 mL
¾ cup	filtered water	175 mL
6	cloves garlic (see tip, at left)	6

1. In a bowl, combine spinach, olive oil, 1 tbsp (15 mL) lemon juice and ½ tsp (2 mL) salt. Toss until well combined. Cover and set aside for 10 minutes, until softened.

2. In blender, combine cashews, water, garlic and the remaining lemon juice and salt. Blend at high speed until smooth. Transfer 1 cup (250 mL) marinated spinach to blender. Blend at high speed until smooth.

3. Pour spinach-cashew purée over the remaining marinated spinach and mix well. Serve immediately or cover and refrigerate for up to 2 days.

Nutrients per serving	
Calories	275
Fat	23 g
Saturated Fat	4 g
Cholesterol	0 mg
Sodium	747 mg
Carbohydrate	16 g
Fiber	2 g
Sugars	2 g
Protein	6 g
Calcium	43 mg
Iron	3 mg

Calabrese Swiss Chard

Makes 4 servings

Earthy, grassy Swiss chard makes a gorgeous, incredibly tasty side dish.

Tip

An equal amount of kale or mustard greens can be used in place of the Swiss chard.

1½ lbs	Swiss chard (about 1 large bunch)	750 g
1½ tbsp	virgin coconut oil	22 mL
3	cloves garlic, minced	3
3 tbsp	dried currants or coarsely chopped raisins	45 mL
¼ tsp	fine sea salt	1 mL
¼ tsp	hot pepper flakes	1 mL
1 tbsp	red wine vinegar	15 mL

1. Trim stems and center ribs from Swiss chard, then cut stems and ribs crosswise into 1-inch (2.5 cm) pieces. Stack chard leaves, roll them up crosswise into a tight cylinder and cut the cylinder crosswise into 1-inch (2.5 cm) thick slices.

2. In a large, heavy pot, melt coconut oil over low heat. Add garlic and cook, stirring, for 1 to 2 minutes or until golden. Stir in chard stems and ribs; increase heat to medium, cover and cook, stirring occasionally, for 8 to 10 minutes or until stems are tender.

3. Add half the chard leaves and cook, stirring, for 1 minute or until slightly wilted. Add the remaining chard leaves, currants, salt and hot pepper flakes; cover and cook, stirring occasionally, for 4 to 6 minutes or until leaves are tender. Stir in vinegar.

4. Using a slotted spoon, transfer Swiss chard mixture to plates or a serving bowl.

Nutrients per serving	
Calories	100
Fat	5 g
Saturated Fat	4 g
Cholesterol	0 mg
Sodium	539 mg
Carbohydrate	12 g
Fiber	3 g
Sugars	6 g
Protein	4 g
Calcium	97 mg
Iron	3 mg

Stuffed Zucchini

Makes 4 servings

Here's a unique presentation for a versatile vegetable.

Tip

If you have homemade Vegetable Stock (page 212) on hand, use it in this recipe in place of store-bought broth.

- Preheat oven to 350°F (180°C)
- Baking sheet

³⁄₄ cup	ready-to-use vegetable broth	175 mL
2	small zucchini, halved lengthwise	2
2	green onions, chopped	2
2	cloves garlic, minced	2
1	tomato, diced	1
¹⁄₂ tsp	dried basil	2 mL
¹⁄₂ tsp	dried thyme	2 mL
¹⁄₄ tsp	hot pepper sauce	1 mL
³⁄₄ cup	shredded Cheddar cheese	175 mL

1. In a large skillet, over medium-high heat, bring broth to a boil. Reduce heat to medium and add zucchini halves, skin side up. Cook for 2 to 3 minutes or until tender. Remove zucchini and let cool. Discard excess liquid.

2. Using a spoon, scoop out zucchini flesh, leaving a shell. Chop zucchini flesh. In a large bowl, combine zucchini flesh, green onions, garlic, tomato, basil, thyme and hot pepper sauce. Fill zucchini shells with mixture and top with cheese. Place filled shells on baking sheet.

3. Bake in preheated oven for 10 minutes or until heated through and cheese is melted.

This recipe courtesy of dietitian Laurie Evans.

Nutrients per serving	
Calories	107
Fat	7 g
Saturated Fat	5 g
Cholesterol	22 mg
Sodium	323 mg
Carbohydrate	5 g
Fiber	1 g
Sugars	3 g
Protein	6 g
Calcium	174 mg
Iron	1 mg

Stir-Fried Mixed Vegetables

Makes 6 servings

Practically any combination of vegetables can be stir-fried. The longer a vegetable takes to cook, the smaller the pieces should be (e.g., carrots should be cut into matchsticks or very thinly sliced). Try not to overload the wok, otherwise cooking will be slowed and some vegetables will overcook.

Tips

If you have homemade Vegetable Stock (page 212) on hand, use it in this recipe in place of store-bought broth.

To toast sesame seeds, place seeds in a dry skillet. Place over medium heat and cook for 2 to 3 minutes, stirring occasionally, until golden brown. Tip onto a plate and cool completely. Store toasted sesame seeds in a small container and freeze for up to 4 weeks.

Nutrients per serving	
Calories	106
Fat	7 g
Saturated Fat	1 g
Cholesterol	0 mg
Sodium	483 mg
Carbohydrate	10 g
Fiber	3 g
Sugars	4 g
Protein	4 g
Calcium	64 mg
Iron	2 mg

2 tbsp	vegetable oil	30 mL
3	cloves garlic, chopped	3
1 tbsp	chopped gingerroot	15 mL
1/2	bunch broccoli (about 8 oz/250 g), cut into small florets	1/2
1	carrot, cut into matchstick pieces	1
1/2	red bell pepper, cut into bite-size pieces	1/2
1 cup	sliced green beans	250 mL
1 cup	sliced asparagus	250 mL
1 cup	snow peas, trimmed	250 mL
1 cup	quartered mushrooms	250 mL
1/4 cup	ready-to-use vegetable broth or water	60 mL
2 tbsp	soy sauce	30 mL
1 tbsp	oyster sauce	15 mL
1 tsp	sesame oil	5 mL
1 tbsp	sesame seeds, toasted (see tip, at left)	15 mL
	Fresh cilantro leaves	

1. Heat a large wok or skillet over medium-high heat and add oil. Add garlic and ginger and stir-fry for 30 seconds.

2. Add broccoli, carrot, red pepper, beans, asparagus, snow peas and mushrooms and toss to combine.

3. Add broth and bring to a boil. Cover and cook for 2 minutes or until vegetables are just tender.

4. Add soy sauce, oyster sauce and sesame oil and cook, stirring, for 30 seconds.

5. Garnish with sesame seeds and cilantro.

Veggie Kabobs

In summer and early fall, when fresh vegetables are in season, this dish is a standby. The kabobs are equally delicious served hot or at room temperature.

Tips

The longer the marinating time, the deeper the flavors.

Any leftover veggies from these kabobs make a perfect beginning for tasty pasta dishes or salads.

For convenience, cook the vegetables in a nonstick grill basket, being aware that some may cook more quickly than others.

Nutrients per serving (1 of 8)	
Calories	99
Fat	7 g
Saturated Fat	1 g
Cholesterol	0 mg
Sodium	8 mg
Carbohydrate	8 g
Fiber	2 g
Sugars	5 g
Protein	2 g
Calcium	24 mg
Iron	1 mg

- Preheat grill or broiler
- 16 bamboo or metal skewers

1/3 cup	freshly squeezed lemon juice	75 mL
1/4 cup	olive oil	60 mL
1	clove garlic, minced	1
2 tsp	dried oregano (or 2 tbsp/30 mL finely chopped fresh)	10 mL
	Salt and freshly ground black pepper	
2	bell peppers (any color), cut into 1-inch (2.5 cm) strips	2
2	small zucchini, cut into 1-inch (2.5 cm) thick slices	2
2 cups	grape or cherry tomatoes (about 16)	500 mL
2 cups	whole button mushrooms (about 16)	500 mL
1	large onion, cut into 8 wedges and halved crosswise, separated into single layers	1
1	yellow summer squash (such as golden zucchini) cut into 1-inch (2.5 cm) cubes	1

1. In a large bowl or resealable plastic bag, combine lemon juice, olive oil, garlic, oregano, and salt and pepper to taste. Add bell peppers, zucchini, tomatoes, mushrooms, onion and squash and stir to evenly coat. Marinate at room temperature for 15 to 20 minutes or in the refrigerator for up to 12 hours.

2. Thread vegetables onto skewers, alternating to form an attractive pattern and leaving a bit of space between the pieces to allow air to circulate.

3. Grill or broil, turning and basting often with the remaining marinade, for 8 to 10 minutes or until vegetables are browned on all sides and tender. While cooking, rotate location of the skewers on the grill or broiler to ensure even cooking.

Variation

The vegetables (unskewered) can also be spread in a single layer on two greased rimmed baking sheets and baked in a preheated 400°F (200°C) oven for 30 to 35 minutes. Turn the vegetables and rotate the pans after 20 minutes.

Curried Root Vegetables Masala

Makes 4 to 6 servings

Earthy and substantial, this curry relies on root vegetables for those late-autumn and winter days when more fragile vegetables are at a premium.

Tip

Traditionally, whole spices are left in curries when serving, but they aren't meant to be eaten. Be sure to let your guests know not to eat the whole cloves in this dish.

1/4 cup	vegetable oil, divided	60 mL
1	small sweet potato, cut into 1/2-inch (1 cm) cubes	1
1	boiling or all-purpose potato, cut into 1/2-inch (1 cm) cubes	1
1	large carrot, cut into 1/2-inch (1 cm) thick slices	1
1	beet, cut into 1/2-inch (1 cm) cubes	1
1	small onion, thinly sliced	1
1/4 cup	minced garlic (about 8 cloves)	60 mL
1 tsp	ground cumin	5 mL
1 tsp	hot pepper flakes	5 mL
1/2 tsp	whole cloves	2 mL
2 tbsp	raisins	30 mL
2 cups	canned or fresh diced tomatoes, with juice	500 mL
1/2 cup	water	125 mL
2 tbsp	freshly squeezed lemon juice	30 mL
	Salt	

1. In a large skillet, heat half the oil over high heat. Add sweet potato, potato, carrot and beet, in batches as necessary; cook, stirring, until vegetables start to brown and soften, about 5 minutes. Using a slotted spoon, transfer to a bowl, leaving as much oil in the pan as possible and adding more oil between batches as necessary. Set vegetables aside.

2. Return pan to medium-high heat. Add onion and cook, stirring, until starting to brown, about 2 minutes. Add garlic, cumin, hot pepper flakes and cloves; cook, stirring, for 1 minute.

3. Stir in raisins, tomatoes, water and lemon juice; bring to a simmer. Simmer, stirring often, until tomatoes are softened, about 2 minutes.

4. Stir in reserved vegetables and cook, stirring occasionally, until vegetables are tender and sauce is slightly thickened, about 20 minutes. Season to taste with salt.

Nutrients per serving (1 of 6)	
Calories	173
Fat	10 g
Saturated Fat	1 g
Cholesterol	0 mg
Sodium	221 mg
Carbohydrate	20 g
Fiber	3 g
Sugars	8 g
Protein	3 g
Calcium	43 mg
Iron	1 mg

Squash with Quinoa and Apricots

Banish the blahs with this robust combination of fruits, vegetables and a nutritious whole grain seasoned with ginger, orange and a hint of cinnamon.

Tips

If you prefer, use frozen chopped butternut squash in this recipe. Reduce the quantity to 2 cups (500 mL).

For best results, toast and grind the cumin yourself. Place seeds in a dry skillet and cook, stirring, until fragrant, about 3 minutes. Immediately transfer to a mortar or a spice grinder and grind.

To make ahead, complete step 1. Cover and refrigerate overnight or for up to 2 days. When you're ready to cook, continue with steps 2 and 3.

Nutrients per serving

Calories	226
Fat	4 g
Saturated Fat	1 g
Cholesterol	0 mg
Sodium	316 mg
Carbohydrate	44 g
Fiber	6 g
Sugars	11 g
Protein	6 g
Calcium	68 mg
Iron	3 mg

- Medium to large (3½- to 5-quart) slow cooker

1 tbsp	vegetable oil	15 mL
2	onions, finely chopped	2
2	cloves garlic, minced	2
1 tbsp	minced gingerroot	15 mL
1 tbsp	ground cumin (see tip, at left)	15 mL
2 tsp	finely grated orange zest	10 mL
1	2-inch (5 cm) cinnamon stick	1
1 tsp	ground turmeric	5 mL
1 tsp	salt	5 mL
½ tsp	cracked black peppercorns	2 mL
1 cup	Vegetable Stock (page 212) or ready-to-use vegetable broth	250 mL
½ cup	freshly squeezed orange juice	125 mL
4 cups	cubed peeled winter squash (1-inch/2.5 cm cubes)	1 L
2	apples, peeled, cored and sliced	2
½ cup	chopped dried apricots	125 mL
1½ cups	quinoa, rinsed	375 mL

1. In a skillet, heat oil over medium heat. Add onions and cook, stirring, until softened, about 3 minutes. Add garlic, ginger, cumin, orange zest, cinnamon stick, turmeric, salt and peppercorns and cook, stirring, for 1 minute. Add stock and orange juice and bring to a boil. Transfer to slow cooker stoneware.

2. Add squash, apples and apricots to stoneware and stir well. Cover and cook on Low for 6 hours or on High for 3 hours, until vegetables are tender. Discard cinnamon stick.

3. In a pot, bring 3 cups (750 mL) of water to a boil. Add quinoa in a steady stream, stirring to prevent lumps, and return to a boil. Cover, reduce heat to low and simmer for 15 minutes, until tender and liquid is absorbed. Add to slow cooker and stir well. Serve immediately.

Green Thai Curry with Spinach and Sweet Potatoes

Makes 8 servings

This vegetarian take on Thai green curry tickles your taste buds with flavors from Southeast Asia.

Tip

If you can only find a 19-oz (540 mL) can of chickpeas, use about three-quarters of the can (about $1\frac{1}{2}$ cups/375 mL drained).

1 tbsp	virgin coconut oil	15 mL
1	large onion, thinly sliced	1
2 tbsp	Thai green curry paste	30 mL
2 lbs	sweet potatoes, peeled and cut into 1-inch (2.5 cm) chunks	1 kg
$1\frac{1}{2}$ cups	coconut water or water	375 mL
	Fine sea salt	
1	can (14 to 15 oz/398 to 425 mL) chickpeas, drained and rinsed	1
1	can (14 oz/398 mL) coconut milk (full-fat), well-stirred	1
8 cups	packed baby spinach (about 6 oz/175 g)	2 L
2 tbsp	freshly squeezed lime juice	30 mL
	Cayenne pepper	

1. In a large saucepan, melt coconut oil over low heat. Add onion, increase heat to medium-high and cook, stirring, for 6 to 8 minutes or until softened. Add curry paste and cook, stirring, for 30 seconds.

2. Stir in sweet potatoes, coconut water and 1 tsp (5 mL) salt; bring to a boil. Reduce heat and simmer, stirring occasionally, for 12 minutes.

3. Stir in chickpeas and coconut milk; reduce heat and simmer, stirring occasionally, for 3 to 7 minutes or until sweet potatoes are tender.

4. Stir in spinach and lime juice; simmer for 1 to 2 minutes or until spinach is wilted. Season to taste with salt and cayenne.

Nutrients per serving	
Calories	296
Fat	13 g
Saturated Fat	11 g
Cholesterol	0 mg
Sodium	304 mg
Carbohydrate	42 g
Fiber	8 g
Sugars	7 g
Protein	6 g
Calcium	92 mg
Iron	4 mg

Curried Spinach and Potatoes with Yogurt

Makes 4 to 6 servings

This healthy, delicious curry is a balanced meal all on its own.

Tip

Full-fat yogurt provides the best texture in this recipe. A lower-fat yogurt will work, but avoid fat-free yogurt and any with added gelatin. When cooked, gelatin in yogurt can cause the yogurt to split and create a curdled texture.

1 tbsp	cornstarch	15 mL
1 cup	plain yogurt (preferably full-fat)	250 mL
2 tbsp	vegetable oil	30 mL
1 tbsp	mustard seeds	15 mL
1 tsp	cumin seeds	5 mL
1/2 cup	chopped red onion	125 mL
2	cloves garlic, minced	2
1/2 tsp	salt	2 mL
1 tbsp	Indian yellow curry paste or masala blend	15 mL
2	boiling or all-purpose potatoes, cut into 1/2-inch (1 cm) cubes	2
1/2 cup	water	125 mL
6 cups	fresh spinach, trimmed (about 6 oz/175 g)	1.5 L

1. In a bowl, stir cornstarch and yogurt until blended and smooth. Set aside at room temperature.

2. In a large skillet, heat oil over medium heat until hot but not smoking. Add mustard seeds and cumin seeds; cook, stirring, until toasted and fragrant but not yet popping, about 30 seconds. Add red onion and cook, stirring, until softened and starting to brown, about 5 minutes. Add garlic, salt and curry paste; cook, stirring, until blended and fragrant, about 1 minute.

3. Stir in potatoes until coated with spices. Pour in water and cover pan quickly. Reduce heat to medium-low and boil gently, stirring occasionally, until potatoes are tender and most of the liquid is absorbed, about 20 minutes.

4. Stir in yogurt mixture. Gradually add spinach to skillet, one handful at a time, stirring just until wilted. Season to taste with salt.

Nutrients per serving (1 of 6)	
Calories	144
Fat	6 g
Saturated Fat	1 g
Cholesterol	3 mg
Sodium	65 mg
Carbohydrate	18 g
Fiber	3 g
Sugars	4 g
Protein	5 g
Calcium	121 mg
Iron	2 mg

Garlic Mashed Potatoes

Makes 6 servings

Eight cloves of garlic may seem overpowering, but when roasted, garlic assumes a mellow and gentle flavor, which complements the subtle taste of the potatoes. The herbs add additional flavor to this tasty mixture.

Tips

If desired, use 1 tsp (5 mL) fresh tarragon instead of the dried.

When mashing potatoes, be sure to use a potato masher or a ricer, not a food processor. A food processor quickly overprocesses the potatoes, breaking down their starch content and producing an unappetizing, gluey result.

- Preheat oven to 350°F (180°C)
- Small ovenproof dish

8	cloves garlic	8
1/2 tsp	olive oil	2 mL
4	potatoes (russet or Yukon Gold)	4
1/2 cup	2% evaporated milk	125 mL
2 tsp	chopped fresh parsley	10 mL
1 tsp	chopped fresh chives or green onions	5 mL
1/4 tsp	crumbled dried tarragon	1 mL
1/2 tsp	salt	2 mL
1/4 tsp	freshly ground white pepper	1 mL

1. In ovenproof dish, toss garlic with olive oil; roast in preheated oven for 20 to 25 minutes or until lightly browned.

2. Peel potatoes; boil or microwave until tender. Mash potatoes with garlic. Add milk, parsley, chives, tarragon, salt and pepper; mash until soft and creamy. (Add more milk if necessary for desired consistency.)

This recipe courtesy of chef Larry DeVries and dietitians Jackie Kopilas, Rachel Barkley and Heather Duncan.

Nutrients per serving	
Calories	105
Fat	1 g
Saturated Fat	0 g
Cholesterol	3 mg
Sodium	236 mg
Carbohydrate	21 g
Fiber	3 g
Sugars	3 g
Protein	4 g
Calcium	72 mg
Iron	1 mg

Layered Artichokes and Potatoes

Fresh artichokes and potatoes combine with Parmesan cheese in this tasty casserole.

Tips

If you have homemade Vegetable Stock (page 212) on hand, use it in this recipe in place of store-bought broth.

Never throw away stale bread; instead, make fresh bread crumbs! Trim off the crusts, then tear bread into pieces. Process in a food processor to coarse crumbs. One slice of bread makes about $\frac{1}{3}$ cup (75 mL) crumbs.

- Preheat oven to 375°F (190°C)
- 11- by 7-inch (28 by 18 cm) glass baking dish, greased

2	cloves garlic, chopped	2
$\frac{2}{3}$ cup	freshly grated Parmesan cheese	150 mL
6 tbsp	freshly squeezed lemon juice, divided	90 mL
4	artichokes (each about 12 oz/375 g)	4
$1\frac{1}{2}$ lbs	potatoes, peeled and cut into $\frac{1}{4}$-inch (0.5 cm) thick slices	750 g
$\frac{1}{2}$ tsp	salt	2 mL
$\frac{1}{4}$ tsp	freshly ground black pepper	1 mL
$\frac{1}{2}$ cup	ready-to-use vegetable broth	125 mL
$\frac{1}{3}$ cup	fresh bread crumbs	75 mL

1. In a small bowl, combine garlic and Parmesan. Set aside.

2. Fill a large bowl with water and add $\frac{1}{4}$ cup (60 mL) lemon juice. For each artichoke, peel away all outer leaves. Remove leaves at the base until the fuzzy choke is visible. Trim the leaves with a paring knife, removing any fibrous green portions. Trim the bottom $\frac{1}{4}$ inch (0.5 cm) from the stem and pare away the tough outer skin. Remove the choke. Cut the stem and heart into thin slices and place in lemon water while you continue preparing the remaining artichokes.

3. Arrange half the potatoes in prepared baking dish. Drain artichokes and layer on top of potatoes. Sprinkle with the remaining lemon juice, salt, pepper and half the garlic mixture. Arrange the remaining potatoes on top. Pour broth over potatoes.

4. Cover and bake in preheated oven for 1 to $1\frac{1}{4}$ hours or until potatoes are tender.

5. In a bowl, combine bread crumbs and the remaining garlic mixture. Sprinkle over potatoes. Bake, uncovered, for 10 to 15 minutes or until topping is golden.

Nutrients per serving (1 of 8)	
Calories	149
Fat	2 g
Saturated Fat	1 g
Cholesterol	6 mg
Sodium	396 mg
Carbohydrate	28 g
Fiber	6 g
Sugars	2 g
Protein	7 g
Calcium	122 mg
Iron	1 mg

Crispy Coconut French Fries

Makes 6 servings

Giving the vitamin C–packed potato wedges a bath in hot water removes some of their starch, allowing them to become brown and crispy like oil-cooked fries.

Tip

Coconut oil can be stored at room temperature, and it has the longest shelf life of any plant oil. The oil will fluctuate from liquid to solid; this is completely normal and does not affect the oil's quality.

- Preheat oven to 475°F (240°C)
- Large rimmed baking sheet, lined with parchment paper

1½ lbs	russet potatoes, peeled and cut lengthwise into 3-inch (7.5 cm) long by ¼-inch (0.5 cm) thick sticks	750 g
	Hot water	
2 tbsp	virgin coconut oil	30 mL
¾ tsp	fine sea salt	3 mL
½ tsp	cracked black peppercorns	2 mL

1. Place potatoes in a large bowl and add enough hot (not boiling) water to cover. Let stand for 10 minutes. Drain, pat dry and return to dry bowl.

2. Meanwhile, in a small skillet, melt coconut oil over low heat.

3. Pour oil over potatoes, tossing to coat. Add salt and peppercorns, tossing to coat. Spread in a single layer on prepared baking sheet.

4. Bake in preheated oven for 18 to 20 minutes or until golden on the bottom. Turn potatoes over and bake for 10 minutes or until golden and crisp. Serve immediately.

Variations

Garlicky French Fries: In step 2, add 4 cloves coarsely chopped garlic to melted oil. Cook, stirring, for 2 to 3 minutes or until garlic is golden. Using a slotted spoon, transfer garlic to a small bowl and set aside. Prepare fries as directed; sprinkle reserved garlic over finished fries.

Sweet Potato Fries: Preheat oven to 425°F (225°C). Use sweet potatoes instead of russet potatoes and skip step 1. Bake for 20 minutes. Gently turn sweet potatoes over and bake for 12 to 17 minutes or until crisp.

Parsnip Fries: Preheat oven to 400°F (200°C). Use parsnips instead of russet potatoes and skip step 1. Bake for 15 minutes. Gently turn parsnips over and bake for 12 to 17 minutes or until crisp.

Nutrients per serving	
Calories	131
Fat	5 g
Saturated Fat	4 g
Cholesterol	0 mg
Sodium	355 mg
Carbohydrate	21 g
Fiber	2 g
Sugars	1 g
Protein	2 g
Calcium	10 mg
Iron	0 mg

Desserts

Caramel Lime Bananas 310

Strawberry Freeze 311

Spiced Banana Walnut Pudding 312

Apple Rice Pudding 313

Coconut Rice Pudding with Flambéed Bananas 314

Banana Orange Yogurt 315

Strawberry Yogurt Pie 316

Winter Fruit Crisp 317

Greek Honey Cake 318

Buttermilk Oat-Branana Cake 319

Coconut Black Bean Brownies 320

Layered Rocky Road Bars 321

Strawberry Sesame Banana Chews 322

Fruity Oatmeal Cookies 323

Caramel Lime Bananas

Makes 4 to 6 servings

This is a simple, quick dessert that can also be served as a snack.

Tips

Select bananas that are ripe but firm.

To toast coconut, place it on a baking sheet and bake in a preheated 300°F (150°C) oven for 8 to 10 minutes or until coconut is lightly colored. Stir once or twice to ensure even toasting. Let cool on pan. Coconut can be toasted, cooled, packaged in a freezer bag and frozen for up to 2 weeks.

- Preheat oven to 400°F (200°C)
- 8-inch (20 cm) square non-metallic baking dish (or another dish just big enough to hold bananas in a single layer)

¼ cup	butter, melted	60 mL
⅓ cup	freshly squeezed lime juice	75 mL
4	regular bananas, cut into 2-inch (5 cm) lengths (or 8 small sugar bananas)	4
⅓ cup	palm sugar or packed brown sugar	75 mL
2 tbsp	shredded coconut, toasted (see tip, at left)	30 mL

1. In a small bowl, combine butter and lime juice. Pour into baking dish.

2. Add bananas to baking dish and turn to coat all sides. Sprinkle sugar over bananas.

3. Bake in preheated oven for 15 to 17 minutes or until mixture starts to bubble and bananas are just tender. Sprinkle with coconut before serving.

Nutrients per serving (1 of 6)	
Calories	194
Fat	9 g
Saturated Fat	5 g
Cholesterol	20 mg
Sodium	6 mg
Carbohydrate	31 g
Fiber	2 g
Sugars	22 g
Protein	1 g
Calcium	19 mg
Iron	0 mg

Strawberry Freeze

**Makes 6 to
8 servings**

*Full-fat yogurt (at least
3.5%) is needed to ensure
the smooth, creamy
texture. You can make
other flavors with any
kind of frozen or fresh
fruit — just adjust the
sugar to taste.*

- Blender
- 9-inch (23 cm) square metal baking pan

2 cups	strawberries	500 mL
1/4 cup	liquid honey	60 mL
1 1/2 cups	vanilla-flavored yogurt	375 mL
1/3 cup	heavy or whipping (35%) cream	75 mL

1. In blender, on high speed, purée strawberries and honey. Blend in yogurt. Add cream and blend until well combined. Pour into baking pan, cover and freeze until almost solid, about 1 hour.

2. Break up frozen strawberry mixture. Scrape a few chunks at a time into clean blender and purée on high speed.

3. Scrape into an airtight container, cover and freeze for at least 4 hours, until firm, or for up to 3 days. Soften at room temperature for 15 minutes before serving.

Nutrients per serving (1 of 8)	
Calories	118
Fat	4 g
Saturated Fat	3 g
Cholesterol	16 mg
Sodium	35 mg
Carbohydrate	18 g
Fiber	1 g
Sugars	17 g
Protein	3 g
Calcium	92 mg
Iron	0 mg

Spiced Banana Walnut Pudding

**Makes 4 to
6 servings**

*The combination of
dates and bananas in this
recipe adds a toffee flavor
that is sure to satisfy any
sweet tooth.*

Tips

Coconut oil is solid at
room temperature but has
a melting point of 76°F
(24°C), so it is easy to
liquefy. To melt it, place in
a shallow glass bowl over a
pot of simmering water.

Get the freshest flavor by
grinding whole cinnamon
sticks in a spice grinder.

- **Food processor**

1½ cups	chopped banana	375 mL
½ cup	raw agave nectar	125 mL
½ cup	melted virgin coconut oil (see tip, at left)	125 mL
2 tsp	ground cinnamon	10 mL
½ cup	raw walnut pieces or halves	125 mL

1. In food processor, combine banana, agave nectar, coconut oil and cinnamon. Process until smooth. Add walnuts and pulse 8 to 10 times or until roughly chopped. Transfer to a bowl. Serve immediately or cover and refrigerate for up to 3 days.

Variations

Add a dash of vanilla extract.

Chocolate Banana Walnut Pudding: Substitute 2 tbsp (30 mL) raw cacao powder for the ground cinnamon.

Nutrients per serving (1 of 6)	
Calories	336
Fat	25 g
Saturated Fat	16 g
Cholesterol	0 mg
Sodium	1 mg
Carbohydrate	32 g
Fiber	2 g
Sugars	26 g
Protein	2 g
Calcium	20 mg
Iron	0 mg

Apple Rice Pudding

Yogurts with probiotics will list "live and active cultures" on the label. Enjoy not only the taste but the gut health benefits.

Tip

Strain the yogurt through a cheesecloth-lined sieve.

2 cups	soy milk	500 mL
³⁄₄ cup	short-grain white rice	175 mL
1 cup	apple pulp	250 mL
¹⁄₂ cup	apple juice	125 mL
3 tbsp	liquid honey	45 mL
¹⁄₂ cup	strained yogurt (see tip, at left)	125 mL
1 tbsp	finely chopped candied ginger	15 mL
¹⁄₂ tsp	ground cinnamon	2 mL
¹⁄₄ tsp	ground nutmeg	1 mL

1. In a saucepan, combine soy milk and rice. Bring to a light boil over medium-high heat. Cover, reduce heat and simmer gently for 20 minutes or until rice is cooked but still firm.

2. Increase heat slightly and stir in apple pulp, apple juice and honey. Simmer gently for 10 minutes or until liquid is slightly reduced, rice is tender and mixture is thick. Remove from heat and stir in yogurt, ginger, cinnamon and nutmeg.

Nutrients per serving	
Calories	296
Fat	3 g
Saturated Fat	1 g
Cholesterol	2 mg
Sodium	82 mg
Carbohydrate	62 g
Fiber	2 g
Sugars	28 g
Protein	7 g
Calcium	216 mg
Iron	2 mg

Coconut Rice Pudding with Flambéed Bananas

It is hard to believe that something this easy to make can taste so delicious.

Tip

To toast coconut, spread it on a baking sheet and place in a preheated 350°F (180°C) oven, stirring once or twice, for 7 to 8 minutes.

- Small to medium (2- to 3½-quart) slow cooker, stoneware lightly greased

³/₄ cup	short-grain brown rice	175 mL
1	can (14 oz/400 mL) coconut milk	1
1 cup	water	250 mL
½ cup	coconut sugar	125 mL
1 tsp	almond extract	5 mL
Pinch	sea salt	Pinch

Banana Topping

3 tbsp	butter or vegan butter substitute	45 mL
3 tbsp	coconut sugar	45 mL
4	bananas, sliced	4
¼ cup	amaretto liqueur	60 mL
¼ cup	toasted shredded unsweetened coconut (see tip, at left)	60 mL

1. In prepared slow cooker stoneware, combine rice, coconut milk, water, sugar, almond extract and salt. Cover and cook on High for 3 to 4 hours, until rice is tender. Uncover and stir well. Serve hot or transfer to a bowl, cover tightly and chill for up to 2 days.

2. *Topping:* In a skillet over medium heat, combine butter and sugar. Cook, stirring, until butter melts and mixture is smooth. Add bananas and cook, stirring, until tender, about 5 minutes. Sprinkle amaretto evenly over top and, standing well back, ignite. Allow liqueur to burn off. To serve, spoon pudding into bowls, top with bananas and garnish with toasted coconut.

Nutrients per serving	
Calories	367
Fat	17 g
Saturated Fat	14 g
Cholesterol	11 mg
Sodium	19 mg
Carbohydrate	52 g
Fiber	2 g
Sugars	31 g
Protein	3 g
Calcium	20 mg
Iron	3 mg

Banana Orange Yogurt

Makes 4 to 6 servings

This delicious yogurt packs a double whammy of pre- and probiotics.

Tip

When preparing the fruit for the C-Blend juice, remove the white pith and seeds from the citrus fruits before juicing.

- 9- by 5-inch (23 by 12.5 cm) metal loaf pan

2 cups	pulp from C-Blend juice (see recipe, page 169, and tip, at left)	500 mL
1 cup	plain yogurt	250 mL
1	ripe banana, mashed	1
2 tbsp	liquid honey	30 mL

1. In loaf pan combine pulp, yogurt, banana and honey. Freeze for 1 to 2 hours or until firm. If consistency is too hard, ripen in the refrigerator to soften.

Nutrients per serving
(1 of 6)

Calories	93
Fat	1 g
Saturated Fat	0 g
Cholesterol	2 mg
Sodium	30 mg
Carbohydrate	20 g
Fiber	2 g
Sugars	14 g
Protein	3 g
Calcium	95 mg
Iron	0 mg

Strawberry Yogurt Pie

Makes 8 servings

A fluffy filling with a crunchy crust makes this pie a light, refreshing ending to a special meal. This recipe is best when served the same day it is made.

Tip

This recipe can also be made with unsweetened raspberries, which would increase the fiber content to 4 g per serving. Substitute raspberry gelatin for the strawberry, for a change of taste.

• 9-inch (23 cm) pie plate, lightly greased

Crust

3 tbsp	butter or margarine	45 mL
3 tbsp	corn syrup	45 mL
3 tbsp	firmly packed brown sugar	45 mL
2½ cups	bran flakes cereal	625 mL

Filling

1	package (3 oz/85 g) strawberry gelatin	1
1 cup	boiling water	250 mL
1 cup	whole strawberries, slightly thawed if frozen	250 mL
1 cup	low-fat plain yogurt	250 mL

1. *Crust:* In a saucepan over medium-high heat, melt butter, corn syrup and brown sugar; bring mixture to a full boil, stirring constantly. Remove from heat; stir in cereal, mixing until cereal is completely coated. Press firmly around sides and bottom of prepared pie plate. Place in freezer while preparing filling.

2. *Filling:* Dissolve gelatin in boiling water. Cut strawberries into small pieces; stir into jelly mixture. Chill until mixture reaches the consistency of egg whites. Whisk in yogurt. Chill briefly until mixture is thick but not set. Pour into chilled pie crust. Refrigerate for about 2 hours before serving.

This recipe courtesy of Kellogg Canada Inc.

Nutrients per serving	
Calories	182
Fat	5 g
Saturated Fat	3 g
Cholesterol	13 mg
Sodium	172 mg
Carbohydrate	34 g
Fiber	2 g
Sugars	22 g
Protein	4 g
Calcium	72 mg
Iron	8 mg

Winter Fruit Crisp

Using several fruits instead of just one makes a crisp more colorful and adds flavor. Depending on the natural sweetness of each fruit, more or less sugar may be required. Large-flake rolled oats give this crisp a deliciously old-fashioned crunchy topping.

Tip

If desired, replace the cranberries in this recipe with 2 tbsp (30 mL) dried cranberries that have been soaked in 1 tbsp (15 mL) orange juice for 10 to 15 minutes.

- Preheat oven to 400°F (200°C)
- Shallow baking pan

3	large apples, peeled and sliced	3
2	large pears, peeled and sliced	2
1/2 cup	cranberries (fresh or frozen)	125 mL
2 tbsp	granulated sugar	30 mL
1 cup	large-flake (old-fashioned) rolled oats	250 mL
1/4 cup	packed brown sugar	60 mL
1/4 cup	natural wheat bran	60 mL
1/2 tsp	ground cinnamon	2 mL
1/3 cup	butter or margarine	75 mL

1. Place apples, pears and cranberries in baking pan. Sprinkle with granulated sugar.

2. In a medium bowl, combine oats, brown sugar, bran and cinnamon. Using a pastry blender or two knives, cut in butter until crumbly. Sprinkle over fruit mixture.

3. Bake in preheated oven for about 40 minutes or until mixture is bubbling and fruit is barely tender.

This recipe courtesy of dietitian Laurie A. Wadsworth.

Nutrients per serving	
Calories	307
Fat	11 g
Saturated Fat	7 g
Cholesterol	27 mg
Sodium	6 mg
Carbohydrate	52 g
Fiber	8 g
Sugars	33 g
Protein	3 g
Calcium	36 mg
Iron	1 mg

Greek Honey Cake

Makes 12 slices

Also known as revani, *this semolina-based cake is easy to concoct, and this version is light and lively. It works spectacularly with serious dairy accompaniments, such as whipped cream, clotted cream or ice cream.*

- Preheat oven to 350°F (180°C)
- Deep 12-inch (30 cm) round cake pan, lightly oiled and dusted with flour

8	large eggs, separated	8
½ cup	granulated sugar	125 mL
1 tbsp	finely chopped lemon zest	15 mL
1 cup	ground almonds	250 mL
½ cup	semolina	125 mL
1 tsp	baking powder	5 mL
3 tbsp	freshly squeezed lemon juice, divided	45 mL
1 cup	water	250 mL
1 cup	liquid honey	250 mL

1. In a large bowl, beat egg yolks, sugar and lemon zest until pale yellow and thickened. Add ground almonds and semolina; do not mix. Sprinkle baking powder on top of semolina; pour 1 tbsp (15 mL) lemon juice on top of the powder to make it froth. Mix together just until combined.

2. In another bowl, beat egg whites until stiff. Stir about one-quarter of the egg whites into the batter. Add the rest of the egg whites and fold into the batter with circular motions from the bottom up, until mixed thoroughly but not deflated (do not beat). Transfer to prepared cake pan.

3. Bake in preheated oven for 30 minutes or until browned, risen to twice its original height and a tester comes out clean. Remove from oven; cool completely on a wire rack.

4. In a small saucepan, bring 1 cup (250 mL) water to a boil. Stir in honey and the remaining lemon juice until dissolved. Return to a boil; reduce heat to medium and cook for 5 minutes, stirring occasionally. Pour hot syrup evenly over surface of cooled cake.

5. Let syrup absorb into the cake; cool once again. Do not unmold. Lift portions directly from the pan onto plates and serve either on its own or garnished with whipped cream or ice cream.

Nutrients per slice	
Calories	237
Fat	7 g
Saturated Fat	1 g
Cholesterol	124 mg
Sodium	50 mg
Carbohydrate	39 g
Fiber	1 g
Sugars	32 g
Protein	7 g
Calcium	62 mg
Iron	1 mg

Buttermilk Oat-Branana Cake

The glaze poured over this fabulous cake makes it extra moist and delicious.

Tips

This recipe is a great way to use overripe bananas. If you can't use bananas that are becoming ripe, pop them into a resealable plastic bag and freeze them. They will turn black, but once they are thawed and the skins are removed, they will be perfect for this recipe.

This recipe makes about 2 cups (500 mL) of glaze.

- Preheat oven to 350°F (180°C)
- 8-inch (20 cm) square metal baking pan, lightly greased and floured

1 cup	buttermilk	250 mL
2/3 cup	large-flake (old-fashioned) rolled oats	150 mL
1/3 cup	oat bran or wheat bran	75 mL
1/4 cup	butter or margarine	60 mL
1 cup	granulated sugar	250 mL
1	large egg	1
1 tsp	vanilla extract	5 mL
2	ripe bananas, mashed	2
1 1/2 cups	all-purpose flour	375 mL
1 tsp	baking soda	5 mL
1 tsp	baking powder	5 mL

Glaze

1/2 cup	granulated sugar	125 mL
1/2 cup	buttermilk	125 mL
1/4 cup	butter or margarine	60 mL
1/2 tsp	baking soda	2 mL

1. In a small bowl, pour buttermilk over rolled oats and oat bran. Let stand for 10 minutes.

2. In a medium bowl, cream butter and sugar. Beat in egg and vanilla. Combine bananas and buttermilk mixture with creamed ingredients. Sift together flour, baking soda and baking powder. Stir dry ingredients into banana mixture; blend well. Pour batter into prepared pan.

3. Bake in preheated oven for 45 minutes or until tester inserted in center comes out clean. Let stand for 5 minutes.

4. *Glaze:* In a small saucepan over medium heat, combine ingredients; bring just to a boil. (Watch closely; mixture will foam.)

5. Poke holes with a tester all over cake surface; pour glaze over cake while still warm. Let cake cool before cutting.

This recipe courtesy of Helen Sutton.

Nutrients per slice	
Calories	287
Fat	10 g
Saturated Fat	6 g
Cholesterol	39 mg
Sodium	192 mg
Carbohydrate	48 g
Fiber	2 g
Sugars	29 g
Protein	5 g
Calcium	111 mg
Iron	1 mg

Coconut Black Bean Brownies

Black beans add instant richness to brownies, but no one (especially children!) will ever guess they are there.

Tips

If you can only find a 19-oz (540 mL) can of beans, use about three-quarters of the can (about 1½ cups/375 mL drained).

Store the cooled brownies in an airtight container in the refrigerator for up to 5 days or in the freezer for up to 3 months.

Select natural cocoa powder rather than Dutch process. Natural cocoa powder has a deep, true chocolate flavor. The packaging should state whether it is Dutch process or not, but you can also tell by sight: if it is dark to almost black, it is Dutch process; natural cocoa powder is much lighter and is typically reddish brown in color.

Nutrients per brownie	
Calories	164
Fat	7 g
Saturated Fat	5 g
Cholesterol	0 mg
Sodium	180 mg
Carbohydrate	25 g
Fiber	4 g
Sugars	15 g
Protein	3 g
Calcium	57 mg
Iron	3 mg

- Preheat oven to 350°F (180°C)
- Food processor or high-speed blender
- 12-cup muffin pan, greased with virgin coconut oil

2 tbsp	psyllium husk	30 mL
⅔ cup	coconut water or water	150 mL
1	can (14 to 15 oz/398 to 425 mL) black beans, drained and rinsed	1
¾ cup	unsweetened natural cocoa powder (see tip, at left)	175 mL
⅔ cup	coconut sugar	150 mL
¼ tsp	fine sea salt	1 mL
¼ cup	melted virgin coconut oil	60 mL
1 tsp	vanilla extract	5 mL
1½ tsp	baking powder	7 mL
⅓ cup	miniature semisweet chocolate chips	75 mL

1. In a small cup or bowl, whisk together psyllium and coconut water. Let stand for 5 minutes to thicken.

2. In food processor, combine psyllium mixture, beans, cocoa powder, coconut sugar, salt, coconut oil and vanilla; process until completely smooth. Sprinkle with baking powder and process for 20 seconds or until combined.

3. Divide batter equally among prepared muffin cups. Sprinkle with chocolate chips.

4. Bake in preheated oven for 25 to 30 minutes or until tops are dry and edges start to pull away from the sides. Let cool completely in pan on a wire rack.

Layered Rocky Road Bars

Makes 25 bars

This recipe is so yummy-good, and individual bars are great reheated in the microwave.

- Preheat oven to 350°F (180°C)
- 8-inch (20 cm) square metal baking pan, greased and floured

1 cup	all-purpose flour	250 mL
3/4 cup	quick-cooking rolled oats	175 mL
1/2 cup	granulated sugar	125 mL
1/2 cup	butter, softened	125 mL
1/2 tsp	baking soda	2 mL
1/4 tsp	salt	1 mL
1/4 cup	salted peanuts, chopped	60 mL
1/2 cup	caramel ice cream topping	125 mL
1/2 cup	whole salted peanuts	125 mL
1 1/2 cups	mini marshmallows	375 mL
1/2 cup	semisweet chocolate chips	125 mL

1. In a medium bowl, using an electric mixer on low speed, beat flour, oats, sugar, butter, baking soda and salt for 1 to 2 minutes, stopping often to scrape down bowl, until mixture resembles coarse crumbs. Mix in chopped peanuts for 15 seconds. Reserve 3/4 cup (175 mL) of the oat mixture. Press the remaining oat mixture into bottom of prepared baking pan.

2. Bake in preheated oven for 12 to 15 minutes or until lightly browned. Remove from oven, leaving oven on.

3. Spread caramel topping evenly over hot crust. Sprinkle with whole peanuts, marshmallows and chocolate chips. Sprinkle the reserved oat mixture on top.

4. Bake for 20 to 25 minutes or until lightly browned. Let cool completely, then refrigerate for 2 hours or until firm. Cut into bars.

Variation

It is very hard to improve on this, but try pecans in place of the peanuts.

Nutrients per bar	
Calories	133
Fat	7 g
Saturated Fat	3 g
Cholesterol	11 mg
Sodium	68 mg
Carbohydrate	16 g
Fiber	1 g
Sugars	8 g
Protein	2 g
Calcium	22 mg
Iron	1 mg

Strawberry Sesame Banana Chews

Makes 16 to 20 cookies

These chewy treats are simple to prepare and taste quite heavenly.

Tip

Dehydrated foods will pick up moisture from the air unless they are stored in an airtight container away from sunlight. If the food was crispy when removed from the dehydrator but has become soft again, simply return it to the dehydrator until crisp.

- Food processor
- Electric food dehydrator

3 cups	chopped bananas	750 mL
2 cups	chopped hulled strawberries	500 mL
3 tbsp	raw agave nectar	45 mL
2 tbsp	sesame seeds	30 mL

1. In food processor, process bananas, strawberries and agave nectar until smooth (no visible pieces of fruit should remain). Transfer to a bowl and stir in sesame seeds.

2. Transfer mixture to a nonstick dehydrator sheet and, using your hands, spread evenly in a thin layer approximately ½ inch (1 cm) thick. Using a small knife, score into 16 to 20 equal portions. Dehydrate at 105°F (41°C) for 8 to 10 hours or until firm enough to handle. Serve immediately or allow to cool and transfer to an airtight container. Store, refrigerated, for up to 5 days.

Variation

Substitute 2 cups (500 mL) blueberries, 1 tsp (5 mL) ground cinnamon and a dash of vanilla extract for the strawberries.

Nutrients per cookie	
Calories	39
Fat	1 g
Saturated Fat	0 g
Cholesterol	0 mg
Sodium	0 mg
Carbohydrate	9 g
Fiber	1 g
Sugars	6 g
Protein	1 g
Calcium	13 mg
Iron	0 mg

Fruity Oatmeal Cookies

Makes 36 cookies

These make a tasty, healthy snack any time of the day.

Tips

When using margarine, choose a non-hydrogenated version to limit consumption of trans fats.

For the dried fruit, try raisins, chopped apricots and/or cranberries.

- Preheat oven to 350°F (180°C)
- Baking sheets, lightly greased or lined with parchment paper

2 cups	large-flake (old-fashioned) rolled oats	500 mL
1¼ cups	whole wheat flour	300 mL
1 cup	semisweet chocolate chips	250 mL
1 cup	dried fruit (see tip, at left)	250 mL
¾ cup	ground flax seeds (flaxseed meal)	175 mL
1 tsp	baking soda	5 mL
½ tsp	salt	2 mL
2	large bananas, mashed	2
¾ cup	liquid honey	175 mL
½ cup	margarine	125 mL

1. In a large bowl, combine oats, flour, chocolate chips, dried fruit, flax seeds, baking soda and salt.

2. In another large bowl, combine bananas, honey and margarine. Fold in oats mixture.

3. Drop dough by tablespoonfuls (15 mL), about 2 inches (5 cm) apart, onto prepared baking sheets. Flatten with a fork.

4. Bake in preheated oven for about 10 minutes or until lightly browned. Let cool on baking sheets on a wire rack for 5 minutes, then remove to rack to cool completely.

This recipe courtesy of Eileen Campbell.

Variations

Replace the semisweet chocolate chips with white chocolate or butterscotch chips, or leave them out entirely for a fruitier cookie.

Try rice syrup or light (fancy) molasses instead of honey.

Nutrients per cookie	
Calories	133
Fat	5 g
Saturated Fat	1 g
Cholesterol	0 mg
Sodium	95 mg
Carbohydrate	21 g
Fiber	2 g
Sugars	13 g
Protein	2 g
Calcium	16 mg
Iron	1 mg

References

Allen SJ, Martinez EG, Gregorio GV, Dans LF. Probiotics for treating acute infectious diarrhoea. *Cochrane Database Syst Rev*, 2010 Nov 10; 11: CD003048.

Barnard ND, Levin SM, Yokoyama Y. A systematic review and meta-analysis of changes in body weight in clinical trials of vegetarian diets. *J Acad Nutr Diet*, 2015 Jun; 115 (6): 954–69.

Beck L. Why you should add fermented foods — and their friendly bacteria — to your diet. *The Globe and Mail*, 2015 Aug 3. Available at: http://www.theglobeandmail.com/life/health-and-fitness/health/fermented-foods-that-are-full-of-friendly-bacteria/article25818633/.

Berg D, Clemente JC, Colombel JF. Can inflammatory bowel disease be permanently treated with short-term interventions on the microbiome? *Expert Rev Gastroenterol Hepatol*, 2015 Jun; 9 (6): 781–95.

Chisholm AH. Probiotics in preventing recurrent urinary tract infections in women: A literature review. *Urol Nurs*, 2015 Jan–Feb; 35 (1): 18–21.

Daniel H, Moghaddas Gholami A, Berry D, et al. High fat diet alters gut microbiota physiology in mice. *ISME J*, 2014 Feb; 8 (2): 295–308.

David LA, Maurice CF, Carmody RN, et al. Diet rapidly and reproducibly alters the human gut microbiome. *Nature*, 2014 Jan 23; 505 (7484): 559–63.

Devkota S, Wang Y, Musch MW, et al. Dietary-fat-induced taurocholic acid promotes pathobiont expansion and colitis in IL10-/- mice. *Nature*, 2012 Jul 5; 487 (7405):104–8.

Didari T, Mozaffari S, Nikfar S, Abdollahi M. Effectiveness of probiotics in irritable bowel syndrome: Updated systematic review with meta-analysis. *World J Gastroenterol*, 2015 Mar 14; 21 (10): 3072–84.

Estruch R, Ros E, Salas-Salvadó J, et al. Primary prevention of cardiovascular disease with a Mediterranean diet. *N Engl J Med*, 2013 Feb 25; 368: 1279–90.

Fava F, Gitau R, Griffin BA, et al. The type and quantity of dietary fat and carbohydrate alter faecal microbiome and short-chain fatty acid excretion in a metabolic syndrome "at risk" population. *Int J Obes* (Lond.), 2013 Feb; 37 (2): 216–23.

Forgie S, Zhanel G, Robinson J. Management of acute otitis media. *Paediatr Child Health*, 2009 Sep; 14 (7): 457–64.

Frolkis A, Dielman LA, Barkema HW, et al. Environment and the inflammatory bowel diseases. *Can J Gastroenterol*, 2013 Mar; 27 (3): e18–24.

Ginter E. Vegetarian diets, chronic diseases and longevity. *Bratisl Lek Listy*, 2008; 109 (10): 463–66.

Harvard Women's Health Watch. Becoming a vegetarian. Harvard Health Publications, Harvard Medical School, 2009 Oct 1. Available at: http://www.health.harvard.edu/staying-healthy/becoming-a-vegetarian.

Jandhyala SM, Talukdar R, Subramanyam C, et al. Role of the normal gut microbiota. *World J Gastroenterol*, 2015 Aug 7; 21 (29): 8787–803.

Jernberg C, Löfmark S, Edlund C, Jansson JK. Long-term impacts of antibiotic exposure on the human intestinal microbiota. *Microbiology*, 2010 Nov; 156 (Pt 11): 3216–23.

Lee D, Albenberg L, Compher C, et al. Diet in the pathogenesis and treatment of inflammatory bowel diseases. *Gastroenterology*, 2015 May; 148 (6): 1087–106.

Martínez I, Stegen JC, Maldonado-Gómez MX, et al. The gut microbiota of rural Papua New Guineans: Composition, diversity patterns, and ecological processes. *Cell Rep*, 2015 Apr 28; 11 (4): 527–38.

McFarland LV. Meta-analysis of probiotics for the prevention of antibiotic-associated diarrhea and the treatment of *Clostridium difficile* disease. *Am J Gastroenterol*, 2006 Apr; 101 (4): 812–22.

Orel R, Kamhi Trop T. Intestinal microbiota, probiotics and prebiotics in inflammatory bowel disease. *World J Gastroenterol*, 2014 Sep 7; 20 (33): 11505–24.

Orlich MJ, Singh PN, Sabaté J, et al. Vegetarian dietary patterns and the risk of colorectal cancers. *JAMA Intern Med*, 2015 May; 175 (5): 767–76.

Quigley EM. Gut bacteria in health and disease. *Gastroenterol Hepatol* (NY), 2013 Sep; 9 (9): 560–69.

Roberfroid M, Gibson GR, Hoyles L, et al. Prebiotic effects: Metabolic and health benefits. *Br J Nutr*, 2010 Aug; 104 Suppl 2: S1–63.

Smith MW. Probiotics and prebiotics: Ask the nutritionist. WebMD, 2012. Available at: http://www.webmd.com/vitamins-and-supplements/nutrition-vitamins-11/probiotics.

Surawicz CM, Brandt LJ, Binion DG, et al. Guidelines for diagnosis, treatment, and prevention of *Clostridium difficile* infections. *Am J Gastroenterol*, 2013 Apr; 108 (4): 478–98.

Szajewska H, Horvath A, Kołodziej M. Systematic review with meta-analysis: *Saccharomyces boulardii* supplementation and eradication of *Helicobacter pylori* infection. *Aliment Pharmacol Ther*, 2015 Jun; 41 (12): 1237–45.

Szajewska H, Kołodziej M. Systematic review with meta-analysis: *Saccharomyces boulardii* in the prevention of antibiotic-associated diarrhoea. *Aliment Pharmacol Ther*, 2015 Oct; 42 (7): 793–801.

Vegetarian Nutrition. What is a vegetarian diet? Available at: http://vegetariannutrition.net/vegetarian-diets/.

Vitetta L, Briskey D, Alford H, et al. Probiotics, prebiotics and the gastrointestinal tract in health and disease. *Inflammopharmacology*, 2014 Jun; 22 (3): 135–54.

Wright EK, Kamm MA, Teo SM, et al. Recent advances in characterizing the gastrointestinal microbiome in Crohn's disease: A systematic review. *Inflamm Bowel Dis*, 2015 Jun; 21 (6): 1219–28.

Wu GD, Chen J, Hoffmann C, et al. Linking long-term dietary patterns with gut microbial enterotypes. *Science*, 2011 Oct 7; 334 (6052): 105–8.

Yatsunenko T, Rey FE, Manary MJ, et al. Human gut microbiome viewed across age and geography. *Nature*, 2012 May 9; 486 (7402): 222–27.

Contributing Authors

Byron Ayanoglu with contributions from Algis Kemezys
125 Best Vegetarian Recipes
Recipes from this book are found on pages 222, 231, 234, 242, 246, 254, 260, 264, 277 and 318.

Byron Ayanoglu and Jennifer MacKenzie
Complete Curry Cookbook
Recipes from this book are found on pages 152–53, 207, 224, 266, 282, 289, 290, 302 and 305.

Andrew Chase and Nicole Young
The Blender Bible
Recipes from this book are found on pages 165, 193, 214–16, 240 and 311.

Tiffany Collins
300 Best Casserole Recipes
Recipes from this book are found on pages 151, 154, 184, 248, 258, 307 and 321.

Pat Crocker
The Juicing Bible
Recipes from this book are found on pages 169 (bottom), 170–72, 313 and 315.

Pat Crocker
The Smoothies Bible, Second Edition
Recipes from this book are found on pages 163 (top), 164 (bottom) and 165 (top).

Pat Crocker
The Vegan Cook's Bible
Recipes from this book are found on pages 185, 200, 230, 237, 238, 272, 280, 286 and 295.

Pat Crocker
The Vegetarian Cook's Bible
Recipes from this book are found on pages 168, 169 (top), 178, 195 (bottom), 212, 226 and 232.

Dietitians of Canada
Cook Great Food
Recipes from this book are found on pages 174, 176, 180, 233, 236, 252, 306, 316, 317 and 319.

Dietitians of Canada
Simply Great Food
Recipes from this book are found on pages 155, 181, 249, 267, 270, 274, 287 (top), 299 and 323.

Maxine Effenson-Chuck and Beth Gurney
125 Best Vegan Recipes
Recipes from this book are found on pages 196, 208, 241, 247, 250, 273 and 301.

Judith Finlayson
The Healthy Slow Cooker, Second Edition
Recipes from this book are found on pages 202, 209, 262 and 314.

Judith Finlayson
The Vegetarian Slow Cooker
Recipes from this book are found on pages 149, 175, 217, 220, 221, 268, 279, 292 and 303.

Judith Finlayson and Jordan Wagman
750 Best Appetizers
Recipes from this book are found on pages 190, 191, 198–99, 203, 204 and 206.

Nancie McDermott
300 Best Stir-Fry Recipes
Recipes from this book are found on pages 259, 287 (bottom), 293, 294 and 296.

Douglas McNish
Eat Raw, Eat Well
Recipes from this book are found on pages 148, 156, 160, 167, 243, 256–57, 271, 288 and 322.

Douglas McNish
Raw, Quick & Delicious!
Recipes from this book are found on pages 188, 189, 228, 244, 291, 297 and 312.

Lynn Roblin, Nutrition Editor
500 Best Healthy Recipes
A recipe from this book is found on page 197 (top).

Deb Roussou
350 Best Vegan Recipes
Recipes from this book are found on pages 147, 150, 158, 163, 166, 194–95 (top), 201, 276 and 284.

Camilla V. Saulsbury
500 Best Quinoa Recipes
Recipes from this book are found on pages 146, 182, 186 and 239.

Camilla V. Saulsbury
Complete Coconut Cookbook
Recipes from this book are found on pages 157, 162 (bottom), 177, 223, 229, 278, 298, 304, 308 and 320.

Andrew Schloss with Ken Bookman
2500 Recipes
Recipes from this book are found on pages 155, 159, 162, 179, 197 (bottom), 205 and 210.

Carla Snyder and Meredith Deeds
300 Sensational Soups
Recipes from this book are found on pages 218, 219 and 225.

Linda Stephen
Complete Book of Thai Cooking
Recipes from this book are found on pages 164 (top), 192, 255, 263, 281, 300 and 310.

Index

A

acacia gum, 67, 68
Align (*Bifidobacterium infantis*), 49
allergies, 20, 37
almond milk, 102
almonds, 98, 99. *See also* nut butters
  Asparagus Salsa, 206
  Bulgur Asparagus Salad, 237
  Coconut Quinoa Oat Granola, 146
  Greek Honey Cake, 318
  Green Macaroni and Cheese, 249
  Pantry Muesli, 147
amino acids, 95
aminoglycoside antibiotics, 47
ammonia, 26
amoxicillin, 47, 50
anemia, 91–92
antibiotics, 31–32
  for children, 30, 37–39
  diarrhea caused by, 36, 44–45, 47
  and microbiome, 10, 30–39
  and microbiota, 32–33, 34
  resistance to, 32, 33, 36
  use with probiotics, 50, 55
antioxidants, 80
apples and applesauce
  Apple Cranberry Bread, 175
  Apple Mint Smoothie, 163
  Apple Rice Pudding, 313
  Artichoke Eight, 170
  Banana Flapjacks (variation), 157
  Double Cheese, Apple and Maple Bagels, 155
  Lentils Bolognese, 270
  Mixed Fruit, Chia and Flaxseed Porridge, 148
  Squash with Quinoa and Apricots, 303
  Vegetable Stock, 212
  Winter Fruit Crisp, 317
apricots. *See also* fruit, dried
  Apricot Bran Bread, 176
  Orange Apricot Oatmeal Scones, 180
  Squash with Quinoa and Apricots, 303
arthritis, 89

artichokes. *See also* Jerusalem artichokes
  Artichoke and White Bean Spread, 209
  Artichoke Cheddar Squares, 184
  Artichoke Quiche, 154
  Artichoke Salsa, 205
  Layered Artichokes and Potatoes, 307
  Penne with Mushrooms, Sun-Dried Tomatoes and Artichokes, 250
  Spinach Artichoke Bread, 179
  Stuffed Mushroom Caps, 191
  Summer Artichoke Salad, 231
Arugula, Apricot and Crispy Chickpea Salad, 229
asparagus, 109
  Asparagus Mango Smoothie, 165
  Asparagus Salsa, 206
  Baked Springtime Risotto, 257
  Bulgur Asparagus Salad, 237
  Cream of Leek and Asparagus on Toast Points, 200
  Garden Vegetable Frittata, 151
  Green Pea and Asparagus Curry, 295
  Mushroom, Tomato and Asparagus Toss, 294
  Spicy Tofu with Vegetables, 281
  Stir-Fried Mixed Vegetables, 300
  Yummy Asparagus, 287
autism, 54
avocado
  Asparagus Mango Smoothie, 165
  Cheesy Avocado Dip, 204
  Cilantro Black Bean Burgers, 276
  Malibu Tofu Scramble, 149

B

bacteria. *See also* microbiome; probiotics; *specific species*
beneficial, 40–56
in colon, 15, 17
colonization by, 18–19, 22
diet and, 27–28
harmful, 35–36
hygiene practices and, 20, 37
types, 21–22
vs. viruses, 34

Bacteroides species, 27, 82, 83
  B. fragilis, 54
Bacteroidetes bacteria, 17, 18. *See also individual species*
bananas and plantains, 67, 113
  Baked Plantain and Peanut Stew, 280
  Banana Berry Kefir, 162
  Banana Bread, 177
  Banana Flapjacks, 157
  Banana Orange Yogurt, 315
  Buttermilk Oat-Branana Cake, 319
  Caramel Lime Bananas, 310
  Chilled Curried Banana Coconut Soup, 224
  Cocoa Banana Mini Muffins, 182
  Coconut Rice Pudding with Flambéed Bananas, 314
  Crunchy Chocolate Banana Pops, 189
  Fruity Oatmeal Cookies, 323
  Green Goddess, 164
  Mixed Fruit, Chia and Flaxseed Porridge, 148
  Peanut Butter and Banana Bread, 178
  Purple Power Shake, 162
  Spiced Banana Walnut Pudding, 312
  Strawberry Sesame Banana Chews, 322
  Sweet Tart Smoothie, 163
  Triple B Health Muffins, 181
Barbecue Baked Beans, 275
Barbecue Barley and Sweet Potato Chili, 279
"Barbecue" Pulled Burdock Sandwich, 256
Barbecued Tofu Nuggets, 196
barley
  Barbecue Barley and Sweet Potato Chili, 279
  Green Barley Water, 168
  Mushroom Barley Soup with Miso, 221
  Orange-Flavored Breakfast Barley with Cranberries and Pecans, 149
  Squash-Laced Wild Rice and Barley Casserole, 258
  Turkish-Style Barley Soup, 220
bars and squares, 185, 320–22

Basic Gravy, 153
   Baked Curried Tofu with
      Tomato Masala, 282
   Curried Green Beans Masala,
      290
   Spicy Tomato Curry with
      Poached Eggs, 152
basil. See also herbs
   Malibu Tofu Scramble, 149
   Pasta Salad with Yellow Tomato
      Sauce, 240
   Tomato Basil Dressing, 244
bean sprouts. See sprouts
beans, 71. See also beans, green;
      chickpeas
   Artichoke and White Bean
      Spread, 209
   Baked Orzo and Beans, 277
   Barbecue Baked Beans, 275
   Barbecue Barley and Sweet
      Potato Chili, 279
   Black Bean Coconut Soup, 223
   Cilantro Black Bean Burgers,
      276
   Coconut Black Bean Brownies,
      320
   Easy Black Beans, 274
   Greek Bean Salad, 242
   Jamaican Peas and Cauliflower
      "Rice," 278
   Jerusalem Artichoke Stew, 286
   Soy Milk, 166
beans, green
   Curried Green Beans Masala,
      290
   Spicy Tofu with Vegetables, 281
   Stir-Fried Mixed Vegetables,
      300
   Vegetable Fried Rice, 263
Benefibre, 61
berries. See also specific types of
      berries
   Mixed Fruit, Chia and Flaxseed
      Porridge, 148
   Purple Power Shake, 162
   Tropical Smoothie (variation),
      164
Bifidobacterium species, 25, 41, 65
   B. infantis (Align), 49
   prebiotics and, 68
Bilophilia wadsworthia, 24
bioavailability, 89
biotin, 16
bladder infections, 51–53
blood pressure, 63, 80, 101
blood sugar, 64, 71
blueberries. See also berries
   Strawberry Sesame Banana
      Chews (variation), 322
   Triple B Health Muffins, 181

Bok Choy, Garlic-Spiked, 287
bowel. See gastrointestinal tract
bowel movements, 63
brain–gut axis, 16
bran (oat or wheat), 113
   Apricot Bran Bread, 176
   Buttermilk Oat-Branana Cake,
      319
   Pantry Muesli, 147
   Super Health Bread, 174
   Triple B Health Muffins, 181
   Winter Fruit Crisp, 317
breads, 174–79
breads (as ingredient)
   Cheese Straws, 190
   Cream of Leek and Asparagus
      on Toast Points, 200
   Double Cheese, Apple and
      Maple Bagels, 155
   French Lentil Dip with Herbed
      Crostini, 201
   French Onion Soup, Classic,
      217
   Grilled Herb Crostini, 199
   Quick Zucchini and Jerusalem
      Artichoke on Grilled
      Crostini, 198
   Refried Pumpkin, 210
   Spinach Artichoke Bread, 179
   Whole Wheat Buttermilk
      French Toast, 155
breakfast and brunch dishes,
      145–60
broccoli, 99
   Brocco-Artichoke, 170
   Stir-Fried Mixed Vegetables,
      300
buckwheat and buckwheat flour
   Buckwheat Blinis, 193
   Buckwheat Toast, 156
   Crispy Buckwheat Tempehacon
      Waffles, 158
   Sweet Vanilla Buckwheat
      Almond Clusters, 188
bulgur
   Bulgur Asparagus Salad, 237
   Tabbouleh, 236
burdock root
   "Barbecue" Pulled Burdock
      Sandwich, 256
   Easy Root Coffee, 172
   Root Coffee Blend, 171
   Spring Tonic, 169
   Vegetable Stock, 212
buttermilk
   Buttermilk Oat-Branana Cake,
      319
   Orange Apricot Oatmeal
      Scones, 180
   Super Health Bread, 174

   Whole Wheat Buttermilk
      French Toast, 155
butyrate, 17, 24, 25, 68, 83

C

cabbage
   Artichoke Eight, 170
   Jerusalem Artichoke Stew, 286
   Spicy Kimchi, 288
   Vegetable Fried Rice, 263
   Vegetable Stock, 212
cacao. See chocolate
Calabrese Swiss Chard, 298
calcium, 102–4
cancer, 9, 81
   of colon, 57, 70
candida infections, 117
Caramel Lime Bananas, 310
carbohydrates, 11, 23, 24–25
cardiovascular disease, 9
   prebiotics and, 70–71
   vegetarian diet and, 80, 84
carnitine, 84
carrots. See also juices; vegetables
   Artichoke Eight, 170
   Barbecue Baked Beans, 275
   North African Carrot Quinoa
      Salad, 239
   Squash-Laced Wild Rice and
      Barley Casserole, 258
   Warm Pear and Snow Pea Salad
      with Miso Dressing, 230
cashews, 98, 99
   Cheesy Shoestring Jicama
      Fries, 291
   Creamed Garlic Spinach, 297
cauliflower
   Cauliflower and Cheese Soup,
      215
   Jamaican Peas and Cauliflower
      "Rice," 278
C-Blend, 169
celery. See also vegetables
   Artichoke Eight, 170
   Barbecue Baked Beans, 275
   Lentil Salad with Tomatoes and
      Tarragon (variation), 241
   Pasta Salad with Yellow Tomato
      Sauce, 240
   Squash-Laced Wild Rice and
      Barley Casserole, 258
cephalosporins, 47
cereals, 146–49
cereals (as ingredient)
   Apricot Bran Bread, 176
   Cilantro Black Bean Burgers, 276
   Pantry Muesli, 147
   Peanut Butter and Banana
      Bread, 178
   Strawberry Yogurt Pie, 316

Super Health Bread, 174
Whole-Grain Power Bars, 185
cheese. *See also specific types of cheese (below)*
  Caramelized Onion Dip, 202
  Cauliflower and Cheese Soup, 215
  Cheesy Avocado Dip, 204
  Couscous Bake, 258
  Double Cheese, Apple and Maple Bagels, 155
  French Onion Soup, Classic, 217
  Garlic Cheese, 197
  Grilled Vegetable Lasagna, 252
  Polenta with Fried Tomato, 260
  Smoked Gouda Mac and Cheese, 248
  Stuffed Mushroom Caps, 191
cheese, Cheddar
  Artichoke Cheddar Squares, 184
  Artichoke Quiche, 154
  Cheese Straws, 190
  Cheesy Grits, 262
  Green Macaroni and Cheese, 249
  Stuffed Zucchini, 299
cheese, mozzarella
  Baked Curried Tofu with Tomato Masala (variation), 282
  Pasta Salad with Yellow Tomato Sauce, 240
  Tomato Mozzarella Salad, 233
cheese, Parmesan
  Artichoke and White Bean Spread, 209
  Baked Orzo and Beans, 277
  Garden Vegetable Frittata, 151
  Layered Artichokes and Potatoes, 307
  Quick Zucchini and Jerusalem Artichoke on Grilled Crostini, 198
Cheesy Shoestring Jicama Fries, 291
chia seeds, 99
  Mixed Fruit, Chia and Flaxseed Porridge, 148
  Sweet Vanilla Buckwheat Almond Clusters, 188
  Whole-Grain Power Bars, 185
chickpea flour
  Banana Bread, 177
  Banana Flapjacks, 157
chickpeas. *See also* chickpea flour
  Arugula, Apricot and Crispy Chickpea Salad, 229
  Green Thai Curry with Spinach and Sweet Potatoes, 304

Hummus with Roasted Red Pepper, 208
Tasty Chickpea Cakes, 273
Tofu and Chickpea Garlic Dip, 197
chicory root, 110
  Easy Root Coffee, 172
  Root Coffee Blend, 171
children
  and antibiotic use, 30, 37–39
  diet effects on, 29
  fevers in, 30, 38–39
  microbiome of, 12, 54
Chilled Curried Banana Coconut Soup, 224
Chilled Fruited Gazpacho, 226
Chilled Yogurt Soup with Roasted Red Pepper and Pesto Swirls, 225
chocolate
  Cocoa Banana Mini Muffins, 182
  Coconut Black Bean Brownies, 320
  Coconut Milk (variation), 167
  Crunchy Chocolate Banana Pops, 189
  Fruity Oatmeal Cookies, 323
  Layered Rocky Road Bars, 321
  Spiced Banana Walnut Pudding (variation), 312
  Sweet Vanilla Buckwheat Almond Clusters (variation), 188
cholesterol, 63, 80
cilantro
  Cilantro Black Bean Burgers, 276
  Couscous with Cilantro, Tomatoes and Peas, 259
  Mushroom, Tomato and Asparagus Toss, 294
  North African Carrot Quinoa Salad, 239
ciprofloxacin, 34
Citrus Dressing, 232
clarithromycin, 47, 50
Classic French Onion Soup, 217
clindamycin, 34, 47
Clostridium species, 54
  C. difficile, 32, 35–36, 45–47
cocoa powder. *See* chocolate
coconut. *See also* coconut milk/water; coconut oil
  Arugula, Apricot and Crispy Chickpea Salad, 229
  Caramel Lime Bananas, 310
  Coconut Milk, 167
  Coconut Quinoa Oat Granola, 146

Pantry Muesli, 147
Sweet Vanilla Buckwheat Almond Clusters (variation), 188
coconut milk/water, 102
  Banana Bread, 177
  Banana Flapjacks, 157
  Black Bean Coconut Soup, 223
  Chilled Curried Banana Coconut Soup, 224
  Coconut Black Bean Brownies, 320
  Coconut Rice Pudding with Flambéed Bananas, 314
  Green Thai Curry with Spinach and Sweet Potatoes, 304
  Mixed Fruit, Chia and Flaxseed Porridge, 148
  Teriyaki Tempeh Satay with Peanut Sauce, 284
coconut oil
  Crispy Buckwheat Tempehacon Waffles, 158
  Crispy Coconut French Fries, 308
  Spiced Banana Walnut Pudding, 312
coffee substitutes, 171–72
colds, 38
colitis
  C. difficile, 32, 35–36, 45–47
  ulcerative, 21
colon, 15, 16, 67. *See also* gut
  bacteria in, 15, 17
  cancer of, 57, 70
commensal bacteria, 21–22
cookies, 186, 323
corn
  Asparagus Salsa, 206
  Roasted Summer Vegetable Soup, 219
  Vegetable Fried Rice, 263
cornmeal and grits
  Cheesy Grits, 262
  Polenta with Fried Tomato, 260
coughs, 38
couscous
  Couscous Bake, 258
  Couscous with Cilantro, Tomatoes and Peas, 259
  Roasted Red Peppers with Moroccan Couscous, 238
cranberries. *See also* fruit, dried
  Apple Cranberry Bread, 175
  Asparagus Salsa, 206
  C-Blend, 169
  Orange-Flavored Breakfast Barley with Cranberries and Pecans, 149
  Winter Fruit Crisp, 317

Cream of Leek and Asparagus on Toast Points, 200
Creamed Garlic Spinach, 297
Creamy Miso Dressing, 244
Crispy Buckwheat Tempehacon Waffles, 158
Crispy Coconut French Fries, 308
Crohn's disease, 18, 20, 21, 76. *See also* inflammatory bowel disease
Crunchy Chocolate Banana Pops, 189
Crunchy Tempehacon Bits, 159
cucumber
    Chilled Fruited Gazpacho, 226
    Gazpacho Salsa, 205
    Gazpacho Smoothie, 165
    Greek Bean Salad, 242
    Vegetable Fried Rice, 263
Curried Green Beans Masala, 290
Curried Root Vegetables Masala, 302
Curried Spinach and Potatoes with Yogurt, 305

D

dairy products, 90, 100–102, 105. *See also specific items*
dandelion greens, 110
    Dandelion Salad with Citrus Dressing, 232
    Spring Tonic, 169
dandelion root
    Easy Root Coffee, 172
    Root Coffee Blend, 171
    Spring Tonic, 169
    Vegetable Stock, 212
dehydrating, 154
depression, 29
desserts, 309–23
diabetes, 9, 56, 107
    diet and, 81, 101
diarrhea
    antibiotic-associated, 36, 44–45, 47
    infectious, 43, 69–70
    prebiotic treatment of, 69–70
    probiotic prevention of, 45
diet. *See also* 8-Step Biotic-Balanced Program; vegan diet; vegetarian diet
    ancient, 12
    Asian, 11–12
    bacterial response to, 27–28
    balanced, 81, 115
    and diabetes, 81, 101
    health effects, 29, 53
    high-fat, 27–28
    high-fiber, 63–64
    meat vs. plant, 24

Mediterranean, 11–12, 29, 78
    and microbiome, 11–12, 22–29
    modifying, 8
    North American, 11, 12, 77, 115
    plant-based foods in, 24, 126–27
    research on, 28–29, 80
    SMART goals for, 133–34
dips and spreads, 158, 197–210
disaccharides, 24–25
disease (chronic), 9, 18, 56. *See also specific conditions*
    prebiotics and, 69–72
    probiotics and, 40, 42
duodenum, 15
dysbiosis, 12

E

ear infections, 38
Easy Black Beans, 274
Easy Root Coffee, 172
eggplant
    Eggplant Pilaf, 264
    Eggplant with Green Chiles, 289
    Grilled Vegetable Lasagna, 252
    Roasted Summer Vegetable Soup, 219
    Sautéed Eggplant Salad, 234
    Smoky Eggplant Dip with Yogurt, 203
eggs, 99
    Artichoke Cheddar Squares, 184
    Artichoke Quiche, 154
    Garden Vegetable Frittata, 151
    Greek Bean Salad, 242
    Greek Honey Cake, 318
    Spicy Tomato Curry with Poached Eggs, 152
    Whole Wheat Buttermilk French Toast, 155
8-Step Biotic-Balanced Program, 124–32
    14-day meal plan, 135–39
    overview, 125
Enhanced Broth, 217
Escherichia coli (*E. coli*), 18, 48, 52

F

Faecalibacterium prausnitzii, 18, 83
fats (dietary), 11, 12, 23, 27–28. *See also* SCFAs
fatty liver disease, nonalcoholic (NAFLD), 71–72
fennel (bulb)
    Brocco-Artichoke, 170
    Lentil Soup Italian-Style, 222
fevers, 30, 38–39

fiber (dietary), 58–59. *See also* prebiotics
    benefits, 63–64
    food sources, 61
    forms, 60–63
    history, 108–9
    insoluble, 63
    and microbiota, 57–73
    recommended intake, 59–60, 113, 128–30
    soluble, 60–62
    supplements, 61–62, 130–31
fibromyalgia, 29
Firmicutes bacteria, 17, 18, 83
fish, 84
Flagyl (metronidazole), 36, 47, 50, 53
flax seeds
    Apple Cranberry Bread, 175
    Buckwheat Toast, 156
    Fruity Oatmeal Cookies, 323
    Mixed Fruit, Chia and Flaxseed Porridge, 148
    Pantry Muesli, 147
    Whole-Grain Power Bars, 185
fluoroquinolone antibiotics, 47
food diary, 126
food guides, 126–27
foods
    functional, 40–41
    iron sources, 131
    labels on, 114, 128–30, 132
    prebiotic sources, 108–9, 130
    probiotic sources, 101, 117–20, 127, 128
    quality of, 11
    quantity eaten, 127
French Lentil Dip with Herbed Crostini, 201
French Onion Soup, Classic, 217
fructo-oligosaccharides (FOS), 66, 108
fruit, 93, 105. *See also* berries; fruit, dried; juices; *specific fruits*
    C-Blend, 169
    Green Goddess, 164
    Lentil Tagine, 272
    Summer Artichoke Salad, 231
    Sweet Tart Smoothie, 163
    Tropical Smoothie, 164
fruit, dried. *See also specific fruits*
    Arugula, Apricot and Crispy Chickpea Salad, 229
    Calabrese Swiss Chard, 298
    Coconut Quinoa Oat Granola, 146
    Fruity Oatmeal Cookies, 323
    Orange Apricot Oatmeal Scones, 180

Pantry Muesli, 147
Superpower Breakfast Cookies, 186
Whole-Grain Power Bars, 185
Fusilli with Leeks, 254
Fusobacterium species, 67

G

galacto-oligosaccharides (GOS), 66, 67, 108
Garden Vegetable Frittata, 151
Gardnerella vaginalis, 53
garlic, 111–12. *See also* vegetables
   Caramelized Onion Dip, 202
   Cheesy Grits, 262
   Creamed Garlic Spinach, 297
   Creamy Miso Dressing, 244
   Crispy Coconut French Fries (variation), 308
   Garlic Cheese, 197
   Garlic Mashed Potatoes, 306
   Garlic Soup, 216
   Garlic-Spiked Bok Choy, 287
   "Roasted" Garlic, Hemp and Parsley Dressing, 243
   Roasted Garlic Sour Cream Dip, 199
   Roasted Summer Vegetable Soup, 219
   Stir-Fried Shiitakes with Garlic, 293
   Tomato Basil Dressing, 244
   Tomato Garlic Raita, 207
   Tomato Sauce, 246
gastrointestinal (GI) tract, 13–15, 17
   probiotic treatment for, 43–51
Gazpacho Salsa, 205
Gazpacho Smoothie, 165
ginger
   Apple Rice Pudding, 313
   Baked Plantain and Peanut Stew, 280
   Barbecue Baked Beans, 275
   Basic Gravy, 153
   Chilled Curried Banana Coconut Soup, 224
   Lentil Tagine, 272
   "Roasted" Garlic, Hemp and Parsley Dressing (variation), 243
   Squash with Quinoa and Apricots, 303
   Stir-Fried Mixed Vegetables, 300
   Sugar Snap Peas with Cherry Tomatoes, 296
   Vegetable Stock, 212

ginseng
   Easy Root Coffee, 172
   Root Coffee Blend, 171
   Spring Tonic, 169
grains (whole), 25. *See also specific grains*
   and microbiome, 59
   as nutrient source, 93, 97, 105
Greek Bean Salad, 242
Greek Honey Cake, 318
Green Barley Water, 168
Green Goddess, 164
Green Macaroni and Cheese, 249
Green Thai Curry with Spinach and Sweet Potatoes, 304
greens, 90. *See also* lettuce
   Arugula, Apricot and Crispy Chickpea Salad, 229
   Calabrese Swiss Chard, 298
   Dandelion Salad with Citrus Dressing, 232
   Spring Tonic, 169
Grits, Cheesy, 262
gut, 16, 25, 42. *See also* gastrointestinal tract; microbiome

H

Healthy Eating Index (HEI), 78
heart disease. *See* cardiovascular disease
Helicobacter pylori (*H. pylori*), 49–51
hemp seeds, 99
   "Roasted" Garlic, Hemp and Parsley Dressing, 243
   Sweet Vanilla Buckwheat Almond Clusters (variation), 188
herbs. *See also specific herbs*
   Cheesy Avocado Dip, 204
   Citrus Dressing, 232
   French Lentil Dip with Herbed Crostini, 201
   Green Barley Water, 168
   Quick Zucchini and Jerusalem Artichoke on Grilled Crostini, 198
   Spaghetti and Soyballs, 247
   Sunflower Seed Miso Butter (variation), 160
Homemade Yogurt, 159
honey
   Fruity Oatmeal Cookies, 323
   Greek Honey Cake, 318
Hummus with Roasted Red Pepper, 208
hydrogen sulfide, 26
hygiene practices, 20, 37

I

ileum, 15
immune system, 42, 68
inflammation, 83
inflammatory bowel disease (IBD), 48
   Crohn's disease, 18, 20, 21, 76
   ulcerative colitis, 21
insulin-like growth factor 1 (IGF-1), 81
intestines, 15. *See also* colon
inulin, 61, 66, 67, 108, 131
   for diarrhea, 69–70
iron (dietary), 89–94
   absorption of, 90–91, 92
   deficiency of, 91–92
   food sources, 93–94, 131
   supplements, 94
irritable bowel syndrome (IBS), 29, 48–49, 76
   managing, 116
   prebiotics and, 70

J

Jamaican Peas and Cauliflower "Rice," 278
jejunum, 15
Jerusalem artichokes (sunchokes), 110
   Artichoke Eight, 170
   Brocco-Artichoke, 170
   Jerusalem Artichoke Soup, 214
   Jerusalem Artichoke Stew, 286
   Quick Zucchini and Jerusalem Artichoke on Grilled Crostini, 198
jicama
   Cheesy Shoestring Jicama Fries, 291
   Mexican Jicama Slaw, 228
juices, 168–70
juices (as ingredient)
   Asparagus Mango Smoothie, 165
   Banana Berry Kefir, 162
   Chilled Fruited Gazpacho, 226
   Citrus Dressing, 232
   Green Goddess, 164
   Purple Power Shake, 162
   Tropical Smoothie, 164

K

kefir, 118
kidney infections, 51–53
kimchi, 120, 288
kiwifruit
   Apple Mint Smoothie, 163
   Green Goddess, 164
kombucha tea, 120

L

Lactobacillus species, 52, 53, 65
  L. acidophilus, 44
  L. casei, 44
  L. gasseri, 50
  L. plantarum (Tuzen), 44, 49
  L. reuteri, 55
  L. rhamnosus, 43, 44, 55
  prebiotics and, 68
lactose intolerance, 100
leeks, 112
  Artichoke Eight, 170
  Cream of Leek and Asparagus
    on Toast Points, 200
  Eggplant Pilaf, 264
  Fusilli with Leeks, 254
  Leek and Tomato Cobbler, 292
  Spinach Artichoke Bread, 179
  Squash-Laced Wild Rice and
    Barley Casserole, 258
  Turkish-Style Barley Soup, 220
  Vegetable Stock, 212
legumes, 90, 96. *See also* beans;
    chickpeas; lentils
lemon
  Arugula, Apricot and Crispy
    Chickpea Salad, 229
  Citrus Dressing, 232
  Greek Honey Cake, 318
  Hummus with Roasted Red
    Pepper (variation), 208
  "Roasted" Garlic, Hemp and
    Parsley Dressing, 243
lentils
  Black Lentil Sloppy Joes, 271
  French Lentil Dip with Herbed
    Crostini, 201
  Lentil Salad with Tomatoes and
    Tarragon, 241
  Lentils Bolognese, 270
  Lentil Soup Italian-Style, 222
  Lentil Tagine, 272
lettuce
  "Barbecue" Pulled Burdock
    Sandwich (variation), 256
  Cilantro Black Bean Burgers,
    276
  Tomato Mozzarella Salad, 233
lime
  Arugula, Apricot and Crispy
    Chickpea Salad (variation),
    229
  Black Bean Coconut Soup, 223
  Caramel Lime Bananas, 310
  C-Blend, 169
  Chilled Curried Banana
    Coconut Soup, 224
  Green Goddess, 164
  Mexican Jicama Slaw, 228

"Roasted" Garlic, Hemp and
    Parsley Dressing (variation),
    243
  Spicy Tofu with Vegetables,
    281
  Sweet Tart Smoothie, 163
  Tropical Smoothie, 164
liver disease, 71–72

M

macrolides antibiotics, 47
macronutrients, 22–28. *See also*
    carbohydrates; fats; protein
Malibu Tofu Scramble, 149
mango
  Asparagus Mango Smoothie,
    165
  Tropical Smoothie, 164
maple syrup/sap
  Barbecue Baked Beans, 275
  Double Cheese, Apple and
    Maple Bagels, 155
  Spring Tonic, 169
meat alternatives, 94, 98, 106.
    See also tempeh; tofu
  Spaghetti and Soyballs, 247
Metamucil, 61
metronidazole (Flagyl), 36, 47,
    50, 53
Mexican Jicama Slaw, 228
microbiome, 8. *See also* bacteria
  antibiotics and, 10, 30–39
  in children, 12, 54
  diet and, 11–12, 22–29, 81–84
  and disease, 18, 56
  functions, 16–17
  historical changes, 10, 20–21
  iron and, 90
  protein and, 95
microbiota, 13, 18–19. *See also*
    microbiome
  antibiotics and, 32–33, 34
  fiber and, 57–73
migraines, 29
milk and cream, 101–2. *See also*
    specific non-dairy milks
  Buckwheat Blinis, 193
  Cream of Leek and Asparagus
    on Toast Points, 200
  Homemade Yogurt, 159
  Jerusalem Artichoke Soup, 214
  Strawberry Freeze, 311
  Tropical Smoothie, 164
mint
  Apple Mint Smoothie, 163
  Green Goddess, 164
  Tabbouleh, 236
  Turkish-Style Barley Soup, 220
miso, 119, 128
  Barbecue Baked Beans, 275

Caramelized Onion Dip, 202
  Creamy Miso Dressing, 244
  Mushroom Barley Soup with
    Miso, 221
  Sunflower Seed Miso Butter,
    160
  Toasted Tofu with Onion Miso
    Jam, 194
  Warm Pear and Snow Pea Salad
    with Miso Dressing, 230
monosaccharides, 24–25
MRSA (methicillin-resistant
    Staphylococcus aureus), 32
muffins and scones, 180–83
mushrooms. *See also* vegetables
  Artichoke Quiche, 154
  Baked Portobello Mushrooms,
    251
  Baked Springtime Risotto
    (variation), 257
  Barbecue Baked Beans, 275
  Garden Vegetable Frittata, 151
  Grilled Vegetable Lasagna,
    252
  Lentils Bolognese, 270
  Malibu Tofu Scramble, 149
  Mushroom, Tomato and
    Asparagus Toss, 294
  Mushroom Barley Soup with
    Miso, 221
  Penne with Mushrooms,
    Sun-Dried Tomatoes and
    Artichokes, 250
  Stir-Fried Shiitakes with Garlic,
    293
  Stuffed Mushroom Caps, 191
Mycobacterium tuberculosis, 32

N

nitrosamines, 26
nonalcoholic fatty liver disease
    (NAFLD), 71–72
noodles. *See* pasta and noodles
North African Carrot Quinoa
    Salad, 239
nut butters, 99. *See also* tahini
  Baked Plantain and Peanut
    Stew, 280
  Peanut Butter and Banana
    Bread, 178
  Sweet Vanilla Buckwheat
    Almond Clusters, 188
  Teriyaki Tempeh Satay with
    Peanut Sauce, 284
nutritional yeast
  Black Lentil Sloppy Joes, 271
  Cheesy Shoestring Jicama
    Fries, 291
nuts, 98–99. *See also* nut butters;
    specific types of nuts

O

oats. *See also* bran
  Buttermilk Oat-Branana Cake, 319
  Chickpea Cakes, Tasty, 273
  Cocoa Banana Mini Muffins, 182
  Coconut Quinoa Oat Granola, 146
  Fruity Oatmeal Cookies, 323
  Layered Rocky Road Bars, 321
  Orange Apricot Oatmeal Scones, 180
  Pantry Muesli, 147
  Super Health Bread, 174
  Superpower Breakfast Cookies, 186
  Winter Fruit Crisp, 317
obesity, 9, 83, 107. *See also* weight loss
  prebiotics and, 65, 71
oligofructose, 68, 131
oligosaccharides, 24–25
olives
  Greek Bean Salad, 242
  Hummus with Roasted Red Pepper (variation), 208
  Lentil Salad with Tomatoes and Tarragon (variation), 241
  Polenta with Fried Tomato, 260
  Tofu and Chickpea Garlic Dip, 197
omega-3 fatty acids, 102
onions, 112. *See also* vegetables
  Baked Portobello Mushrooms (variation), 251
  Barbecue Baked Beans, 275
  Basic Gravy, 153
  Caramelized Onion Dip, 202
  French Onion Soup, Classic, 217
  Green Pea and Asparagus Curry, 295
  Toasted Tofu with Onion Miso Jam, 194
  Tomato and Onion Rice Pilau, 266
  Tomato Mozzarella Salad, 233
orange
  Apple Cranberry Bread, 175
  Apricot Bran Bread, 176
  Banana Orange Yogurt, 315
  C-Blend, 169
  Citrus Dressing, 232
  Mixed Fruit, Chia and Flaxseed Porridge, 148
  Orange Apricot Oatmeal Scones, 180

Orange-Flavored Breakfast Barley with Cranberries and Pecans, 149
Squash with Quinoa and Apricots, 303
osteoporosis, 70
otitis media (ear infection), 38

P

Pantry Muesli, 147
parsley. *See also* herbs
  Artichoke and White Bean Spread, 209
  Brocco-Artichoke, 170
  "Roasted" Garlic, Hemp and Parsley Dressing, 243
  Spring Tonic, 169
  Tabbouleh, 236
parsnips
  Artichoke Eight, 170
  Crispy Coconut French Fries (variation), 308
pasta and noodles
  Baked Orzo and Beans, 277
  Fusilli with Leeks, 254
  Green Macaroni and Cheese, 249
  Pasta Salad with Yellow Tomato Sauce, 240
  Penne with Mushrooms, Sun-Dried Tomatoes and Artichokes, 250
  Smoked Gouda Mac and Cheese, 248
  Spaghetti and Soyballs, 247
  Vegetarian Pad Thai, 255
pathobionts, 22
peanuts. *See also* nut butters
  Baked Plantain and Peanut Stew, 280
  Layered Rocky Road Bars, 321
pears
  Warm Pear and Snow Pea Salad with Miso Dressing, 230
  Winter Fruit Crisp, 317
peas (green)
  Couscous with Cilantro, Tomatoes and Peas, 259
  Green Pea and Asparagus Curry, 295
  Stir-Fried Mixed Vegetables, 300
  Sugar Snap Peas with Cherry Tomatoes, 296
  Vegetable Curry Rolls, 192
  Vegetable Fried Rice, 263
  Warm Pear and Snow Pea Salad with Miso Dressing, 230

pecans
  Layered Rocky Road Bars (variation), 321
  Orange-Flavored Breakfast Barley with Cranberries and Pecans, 149
penicillins, 47
Penne with Mushrooms, Sun-Dried Tomatoes and Artichokes, 250
peppers, bell. *See also* peppers, roasted red; vegetables
  Baked Springtime Risotto, 257
  Black Lentil Sloppy Joes, 271
  Grilled Vegetable Lasagna, 252
  Lentil Salad with Tomatoes and Tarragon, 241
  Pasta Salad with Yellow Tomato Sauce, 240
  Polenta with Fried Tomato, 260
  Roasted Red Peppers with Moroccan Couscous, 238
  Sautéed Eggplant Salad, 234
  Tofu and Chickpea Garlic Dip, 197
peppers, chile
  Baked Curried Tofu with Tomato Masala, 282
  Baked Plantain and Peanut Stew, 280
  Barbecue Barley and Sweet Potato Chili, 279
  Easy Black Beans, 274
  Eggplant with Green Chiles, 289
  Gazpacho Salsa, 205
  Refried Pumpkin, 210
  Spicy Tomato Curry with Poached Eggs, 152
  Turkish-Style Barley Soup, 220
  Vegetarian Pad Thai, 255
peppers, roasted red
  Chilled Yogurt Soup with Roasted Red Pepper and Pesto Swirls, 225
  Hummus with Roasted Red Pepper, 208
  Penne with Mushrooms, Sun-Dried Tomatoes and Artichokes, 250
  Quick Zucchini and Jerusalem Artichoke on Grilled Crostini, 198
pickles, 119
  Greek Bean Salad, 242
pine nuts
  Artichoke Salsa, 205
  Couscous Bake, 258
  Stuffed Mushroom Caps, 191

plantain. *See* bananas and plantains
pneumonia, 38
Polenta with Fried Tomato, 260
pollution, 21
polydextrose, 67
polyphenols, 91
polysaccharides, 24–25
portion size, 127
potassium, 80
potatoes. *See also* vegetables
    Crispy Coconut French Fries, 308
    Curried Spinach and Potatoes with Yogurt, 305
    Garlic Mashed Potatoes, 306
    Garlic Soup, 216
    Layered Artichokes and Potatoes, 307
    Malibu Tofu Scramble, 149
prebiotics, 40, 65–66, 68–69. *See also* fiber
    diet as source, 66, 109–13
    as disease treatment, 69–72
    food sources, 108–9, 130
    health claims, 73, 114–15
    and obesity, 65, 71
    recommended intake, 109
    safety of, 72
    supplements as source, 66–67, 114
Prevotella species, 27, 82, 83
probiotics, 41–42. *See also* bacteria
    food sources, 101, 117–20, 127, 128
    for GI conditions, 43–51
    increasing intake, 116–21
    for non-GI conditions, 51–55
    safety/risks of, 55–56
    supplements as source, 121, 122
    as therapy, 40, 42
    use with antibiotics, 50, 55
protein, 23, 26, 95–102
    fermentation of, 25, 26
    vegetarian sources, 96–99
psyllium, 61, 67, 131
    Banana Bread, 177
    Coconut Black Bean Brownies, 320
pumpkin purée
    Banana Flapjacks (variation), 157
    Refried Pumpkin, 210
pumpkin seeds (pepitas), 98, 99
    Arugula, Apricot and Crispy Chickpea Salad (tip), 229
    Pantry Muesli, 147
    Refried Pumpkin, 210
Purple Power Shake, 162

Q

Quick Zucchini and Jerusalem Artichoke on Grilled Crostini, 198
quinoa, 97. *See also* quinoa flour
    Coconut Quinoa Oat Granola, 146
    North African Carrot Quinoa Salad, 239
    Squash with Quinoa and Apricots, 303
quinoa flour
    Cocoa Banana Mini Muffins, 182
    Superpower Breakfast Cookies, 186

R

raisins. *See also* fruit, dried
    Curried Root Vegetables Masala, 302
    North African Carrot Quinoa Salad, 239
    Roasted Red Peppers with Moroccan Couscous, 238
    Super Health Bread, 174
Refried Pumpkin, 210
rice and wild rice
    Apple Rice Pudding, 313
    Baked Plantain and Peanut Stew, 280
    Baked Springtime Risotto, 257
    Cilantro Black Bean Burgers, 276
    Coconut Rice Pudding with Flambéed Bananas, 314
    Eggplant Pilaf, 264
    Lentil Tagine, 272
    Squash-Laced Wild Rice and Barley Casserole, 258
    Tomato and Onion Rice Pilau, 266
    Vegetable Fried Rice, 263
rice milk, 102
Root Coffee Blend, 171

S

Saccharomyces boulardii, 43, 44, 50, 51
salads, 228–42
    dressings, 232, 243–44
Salofalk, 76
salsas, 205–6
sauerkraut, 119
SCFAs (short-chain fatty acids), 17, 25, 26, 27, 58–59, 68. *See also* butyrate
seeds, 98–99. *See also* tahini; *specific types of seeds*

serving size, 127
sesame oil
    Mushroom, Tomato and Asparagus Toss, 294
    Stir-Fried Mixed Vegetables, 300
    Sugar Snap Peas with Cherry Tomatoes, 296
    Warm Pear and Snow Pea Salad with Miso Dressing, 230
sesame seeds. *See also* tahini
    Buckwheat Toast, 156
    "Roasted" Garlic, Hemp and Parsley Dressing (variation), 243
    Strawberry Sesame Banana Chews, 322
    Warm Pear and Snow Pea Salad with Miso Dressing, 230
    Whole-Grain Power Bars, 185
slow cooker recipes
    Apple Cranberry Bread, 175
    Artichoke and White Bean Spread, 209
    Barbecue Barley and Sweet Potato Chili, 279
    Caramelized Onion Dip, 202
    Cheesy Grits, 262
    Coconut Rice Pudding with Flambéed Bananas, 314
    French Onion Soup, Classic, 217
    Leek and Tomato Cobbler, 292
    Mushroom Barley Soup with Miso, 221
    Orange-Flavored Breakfast Barley with Cranberries and Pecans, 149
    Turkish-Style Barley Soup, 220
SMART goals, 133–34
Smoked Gouda Mac and Cheese, 248
Smoky Eggplant Dip with Yogurt, 203
smoothies and shakes, 162–65
snap/snow peas. *See* peas
sore throat, 38
soups, 211–26
sour cream
    Caramelized Onion Dip, 202
    Roasted Garlic Sour Cream Dip, 199
soybeans/edamame
    Green Pea and Asparagus Curry (variation), 295
    Soy Milk, 166
soy milk, 101
    Apple Rice Pudding, 313
    Crispy Buckwheat Tempehacon Waffles, 158

soy products, 96, 101. *See also* soybeans/edamame; soy milk
   Crunchy Tempehacon Bits, 159
   Penne with Mushrooms, Sun-Dried Tomatoes and Artichokes, 250
   Spaghetti and Soyballs, 247
Spiced Banana Walnut Pudding, 312
Spicy Kimchi, 288
Spicy Tofu with Vegetables, 281
Spicy Tomato Curry with Poached Eggs, 152
spinach, 99
   Artichoke Eight, 170
   Artichoke Quiche, 154
   Couscous Bake, 258
   Creamed Garlic Spinach, 297
   Curried Spinach and Potatoes with Yogurt, 305
   Dandelion Salad with Citrus Dressing, 232
   Green Macaroni and Cheese, 249
   Green Thai Curry with Spinach and Sweet Potatoes, 304
   Spinach Artichoke Bread, 179
spirulina, 96
spreads and dips, 158, 197–210
Spring Tonic, 169
sprouts
   Dandelion Salad with Citrus Dressing, 232
   Malibu Tofu Scramble, 150
   Vegetarian Pad Thai, 255
   Warm Pear and Snow Pea Salad with Miso Dressing, 230
squash. *See also* pumpkin purée; zucchini
   Baked Springtime Risotto (variation), 257
   Squash-Laced Wild Rice and Barley Casserole, 258
   Squash with Quinoa and Apricots, 303
Staphylococcus aureus, methicillin-resistant (MRSA), 32
stomach, 13, 49–51
strawberries
   Chilled Fruited Gazpacho, 226
   Coconut Milk (variation), 167
   Strawberry Freeze, 311
   Strawberry Sesame Banana Chews, 322
   Strawberry Yogurt Pie, 316
strep throat, 38
sugar, 12

Sugar Snap Peas with Cherry Tomatoes, 296
sulfonamides, 47
Summer Artichoke Salad, 231
Sun-Dried Tomato Barbecue Sauce, 257
sunflower seeds, 99
   Arugula, Apricot and Crispy Chickpea Salad (tip), 229
   Sunflower Seed Miso Butter, 160
Super Health Bread, 174
superbugs, 32
Superpower Breakfast Cookies, 186
supplements
   fiber, 61–62, 130–31
   iron, 94
   prebiotic, 66–67, 114
   probiotic, 121, 122
   vitamin B_{12}, 88, 131–32
sweet potatoes
   Barbecue Barley and Sweet Potato Chili, 279
   Crispy Coconut French Fries (variation), 308
   Curried Root Vegetables Masala, 302
   Green Thai Curry with Spinach and Sweet Potatoes, 304
Sweet Tart Smoothie, 163
Sweet Vanilla Buckwheat Almond Clusters, 188
Swiss Chard, Calabrese, 298
symbionts, 21

T

Tabbouleh, 236
tahini
   Hummus with Roasted Red Pepper, 208
   Sweet Vanilla Buckwheat Almond Clusters (variation), 188
   Tofu and Chickpea Garlic Dip, 197
Tasty Chickpea Cakes, 273
tempeh, 96, 120
   Crunchy Tempehacon Bits, 159
   Teriyaki Tempeh Satay with Peanut Sauce, 284
tetracyclines, 47
thyme. *See also* herbs
   Caramelized Onion Dip (variation), 202
   Citrus Dressing, 232
   Grilled Herb Crostini, 199
tofu, 96
   Baked Curried Tofu with Tomato Masala, 282

Barbecued Tofu Nuggets, 196
Grilled Vegetable Lasagna, 252
Malibu Tofu Scramble, 150
Spicy Tofu with Vegetables, 281
Toasted Tofu with Onion Miso Jam, 194
Tofu and Chickpea Garlic Dip, 197
Vegetarian Pad Thai, 255
tomatoes. *See also* vegetables
   Baked Curried Tofu with Tomato Masala, 282
   Baked Orzo and Beans, 277
   Baked Plantain and Peanut Stew, 280
   Barbecue Baked Beans, 275
   Barbecue Barley and Sweet Potato Chili, 279
   Basic Gravy, 153
   Black Bean Coconut Soup, 223
   Black Lentil Sloppy Joes, 271
   Cheesy Avocado Dip, 204
   Chilled Fruited Gazpacho, 226
   Couscous Bake, 258
   Couscous with Cilantro, Tomatoes and Peas, 259
   Fusilli with Leeks, 254
   Garden Vegetable Frittata, 151
   Gazpacho Salsa, 205
   Gazpacho Smoothie, 165
   Green Pea and Asparagus Curry, 295
   Grilled Vegetable Lasagna, 252
   Leek and Tomato Cobbler, 292
   Lentil Salad with Tomatoes and Tarragon, 241
   Lentil Soup Italian-Style, 222
   Lentils Bolognese, 270
   Mushroom, Tomato and Asparagus Toss, 294
   Pasta Salad with Yellow Tomato Sauce, 240
   Penne with Mushrooms, Sun-Dried Tomatoes and Artichokes, 250
   Polenta with Fried Tomato, 260
   Roasted Summer Vegetable Soup, 219
   Roasted Tomato and Pesto Soup, 218
   Sautéed Eggplant Salad, 234
   Spaghetti and Soyballs, 247
   Spicy Tomato Curry with Poached Eggs, 152
   Sugar Snap Peas with Cherry Tomatoes, 296
   Sun-Dried Tomato Barbecue Sauce, 257
   Tabbouleh, 236

tomatoes (*continued*)
Tomato and Onion Rice Pilau, 266
Tomato Basil Dressing, 244
Tomato Garlic Raita, 207
Tomato Mozzarella Salad, 233
Tomato Sauce, 246
traveler's diarrhea. *See* diarrhea, infectious
trimethoprim, 47
Triple B Health Muffins, 181
Tropical Smoothie, 164
tuberculosis, 32
Turkish-Style Barley Soup, 220
Tuzen (*Lactobacillus plantarum*), 49

U

ulcerative colitis, 21. *See also* inflammatory bowel disease (IBD)
ulcers, 49–51
urinary tract infections (UTIs), 51–53

V

vaginosis (bacterial), 53–55
vancomycin, 36, 47
vegan diet, 78, 79
health benefits, 81, 83, 84, 89
vitamin B$_{12}$ in, 86–88, 131–32
vegetables (mixed), 93, 99, 105. *See also* greens; juices; *specific vegetables*
Curried Root Vegetables Masala, 302
Spicy Tofu with Vegetables, 281
Stir-Fried Mixed Vegetables, 300
Vegetable Curry Rolls, 192
Vegetable Fried Rice, 263
Vegetable Stock, 212

Vegetarian Pad Thai, 255
Veggie Kabobs, 301
vegetarian diet, 77–79. *See also* vegan diet
adopting, 85, 142–43
health benefits, 78, 79–81
iron in, 89–94
and microbiome, 82–84
protein sources, 96–99
vitamin B$_{12}$ in, 86–88, 131–32
viruses, 34
vitamin B$_{12}$, 86–88, 131–32
vitamin C, 91
vitamin D, 102–3
vitamin K, 16

W

walnuts
Black Lentil Sloppy Joes, 271
Pasta Salad with Yellow Tomato Sauce, 240
Spiced Banana Walnut Pudding, 312
Whole-Grain Power Bars, 185
Warm Pear and Snow Pea Salad with Miso Dressing, 230
weight loss, 64, 79–80. *See also* obesity
wheat. *See* bran; bulgur
wheat dextrin, 67
Whole-Grain Power Bars, 185
Whole Wheat Buttermilk French Toast, 155
Wild Rice and Barley Casserole, Squash-Laced, 258
Winter Fruit Crisp, 317

Y

yeast, nutritional
Black Lentil Sloppy Joes, 271
Cheesy Shoestring Jicama Fries, 291
yeast infections, 117

yogurt, 117–18, 128
Apple Mint Smoothie, 163
Apple Rice Pudding, 313
Banana Berry Kefir, 162
Banana Orange Yogurt, 315
Chilled Curried Banana Coconut Soup, 224
Chilled Yogurt Soup with Roasted Red Pepper and Pesto Swirls, 225
Curried Spinach and Potatoes with Yogurt, 305
Homemade Yogurt, 159
Purple Power Shake, 162
Roasted Garlic Sour Cream Dip, 199
Smoky Eggplant Dip with Yogurt, 203
Strawberry Freeze, 311
Strawberry Yogurt Pie, 316
Superpower Breakfast Cookies, 186
Sweet Tart Smoothie, 163
Tomato Garlic Raita, 207
Tropical Smoothie, 164
Turkish-Style Barley Soup, 220
Whole Wheat Buttermilk French Toast, 155
Yogurt Cheese, 195
Yummy Asparagus, 287

Z

zinc, 104–6
zucchini
Garden Vegetable Frittata, 151
Grilled Vegetable Lasagna, 252
Malibu Tofu Scramble, 150
Quick Zucchini and Jerusalem Artichoke on Grilled Crostini, 198
Roasted Summer Vegetable Soup, 219
Stuffed Zucchini, 299
Veggie Kabobs, 301

Library and Archives Canada Cataloguing in Publication

Raman, Maitreyi, author
   The complete prebiotic & probiotic health guide : a vegetarian plan for balancing your gut flora : + 175 recipes / Dr. Maitreyi Raman, MD, MSc, FRCPC, Angela Sirounis, BSc, RD & Jennifer Shrubsole, BSc, RD.

ISBN 978-0-7788-0517-5 (paperback)

   1. Functional foods. 2. Prebiotics—Popular works. 3. Probiotics—Popular works. 4. Gastrointestinal system—Microbiology—Popular works. 5. Cookbooks. I. Sirounis, Angela, author II. Shrubsole, Jennifer, author III. Title. IV. Title: Complete prebiotic and probiotic health guide.

QP144.F85R35 2015   613.2   C2015-906863-0